Older Adults' Views on Death

Victor G. Cicirelli, PhD, is professor of Developmental and Aging Psychology in the Department of Psychological Sciences at Purdue University in West Lafayette, Indiana. He received a PhD in Developmental Psychology from Michigan State University. He has been a Postdoctoral Fellow at both the Institute for Cognitive Learning at the University of Wisconsin and the Andrus Gerontology Center of the University of Southern California and he held a Visiting Scientist Fellowship at the Max Planck Institute in Berlin. In addition to his teaching activities in gerontological psychology, Dr. Cicirelli's research interests include parent-child relationships in later life, sibling relationships, family support of the elderly, and dyadic decision-making by caregiving adult children and elderly parents. His most recent research work has been in the area of end-of-life decision-making and older adults' views on death. He is the author of *Helping Elderly Parents, Sibling Relationships Across the Life Span* and *Family Caregiving: Autonomous and Paternalistic Decision Making*, in addition to numerous journal articles and book chapters.

Older Adults' Views on Death

Victor G. Cicirelli, PhD

 Springer Publishing Company

Springer Publishing Company, Inc.
536 Broadway
New York, NY 10012-3955

Acquisitions Editor: Sheri W. Sussman
Production Editor: Sara Yoo
Cover design by Joanne Honigman

01 02 03 04 05 / 5 4 3 2 1

Library of Congress Cataloging-in-Publication Data

Cicirelli, Victor G.
    Older adults' views on death / Victor G. Cicirelli.
      p. cm.
    Includes bibliographical references and index.
    ISBN 0-8261-7012-9
    1. Aged—Psychology.   2. Death-psychological aspects.
  I. Title.
BF724.85.D43 C53 2002
155.9'37'0846—dc21   2002070597

Printed in the United States of America by Maple-Vail Book Manufacturing Group.

Contents

List of Tables

Preface

In my earlier work on end-of-life decision preferences of older adults, I could not help but be impressed by the great diversity of their views regarding the issues involved. Some of these views seemed difficult to explain, except in relation to the basic meanings and beliefs that they associated with questions of life and death. The desire to explore their views of death more fully inspired the work that led to the current volume.

Another stimulus for the present work was the realization that, with few exceptions, the existing research findings regarding death meanings and fear of death pertained to younger adults and the "young-old." This volume aims to fill this gap by looking at the views on death of those older adults aged 70 and up, that is, the age groups that are most vulnerable to death. I wanted to know whether their death meanings and fears of death contributed to their adjustment or maladjustment in the latter portion of life, or whether in fact their outlook on death might act as a constructive force to help them prepare for their eventual dying and death.

The study which formed the basis for much of this book was supported by the National Institutes of Health/National Institute on Aging Grant No. 1 R03 AG17279-01. I want to express my gratitude and appreciation to Dr. Sidney Stahl (Chief, Health Care Organization and Social Institutions, Behavioral and Social Research Program, National Institute on Aging) for his invaluable support and encouragement from the conceptualization of this project to its end.

In addition, I want to give particular thanks to all of the older adults who participated in the study, and their willingness and generosity in sharing at great length their thoughts, feelings, and beliefs about death. Some elders had experienced recent losses of loved ones and others suffered from a variety of ailments that made it exceedingly difficult for them to communicate their views; these individuals deserve particular appreciation for their contribution to the study. I am deeply grateful to all who took part in the study for their time and efforts.

1

Introduction and Study Method

WHY STUDY OLDER ADULTS VIEWS ON DEATH?

When we speak of older adults' views on death in this book, we are referring to their personal meanings of death, fear of death, and views of the dying process. Until recent times, most of the research knowledge pertinent to these topics has been gained from studies of younger adults. This is paradoxical, given the fact that older adults are the group with the greatest vulnerability to death.

Several factors have combined to spur interest in these topics in relation to older adults in recent years. Among these factors is the increased life expectancy of the population, with more elders living well past age 75 into their 80s, 90s, and 100s. At the same time, more older adults live with long-term chronic illness and face a lengthy period of decline before death. Advances in geriatric medicine, as well as increased use of high technology in medical care, make it possible to extend life for considerable periods of time without any likelihood of cure.

The grim prospect of living for indefinitely long periods of time under conditions involving a very low quality of life, characterized by pain, immobility, extreme dependency, and the like led to movements to establish the rights of older people to exert some control over the ways their lives end. The desire of many elders to avoid prolonging life through onerous and ultimately futile medical treatments resulted in the legalization of various advance directives for end-of-life care in all 50 states (Choice in Dying, 1993). Similar movements have aimed at the legalization of assistance with active means of ending life, such as assisted suicide and voluntary active euthanasia.

Numerous studies of older adults' attitudes and preferences regarding such end-of-life decision options have now been carried out, so that we have a better understanding of their feelings regarding such decisions. However, in order to more fully understand why elders make the kinds of end-of-life decisions that they do, we need to learn more about their basic views in regard to death. That is, we need to know about the personal meanings of death which older people have, about their various fears of death, and about the ways in which they look at the dying process. By understanding these areas more fully, we may eventually gain a fuller appreciation of these factors in the end-of-life decisions of older adults as they attempt to exert some control over their own deaths, that is, when, how, and where they will die.

DEMOGRAPHICS OF THE AGING POPULATION

Increased Number of Elders

Over the past century, both the number and proportion of adults aged 65 and over in the United States population has steadily increased, growing from only 3 million in 1900 to 35 million in 2000. While this tenfold increase in the population of the elderly was going on, the population as a whole sustained only a fourfold increase. The percentage of elders in the population, which was approximately 11% in 1980 is projected to increase to 20% by the year 2050, while the total number of older adults is expected to triple during the same period, going from 25 million to 79 million (U. S. Bureau of the Census, 1997). Looking at aging in another way, overall life expectancy has risen from 49 years in 1900 to 76 years at present.

In addition to the large overall increase in the aging population as a whole, the proportion of elders in three older age groups has been steadily changing to reflect elders' increasing longevity. In

1980, the percentage of the young-old (those 65 to 74 years of age) was 61%, the mid-old (those 75–84 years of age) was 30%, and the old-old (those 85 years of age and over) was 9%. By 2000, those percentages were 52%, 36%, and 12%, respectively, and by 2050, the percentages are projected to be 44%, 33%, and 23% (U. S. Bureau of the Census, 1997).

It is clear that the relative numbers of the mid-old and old-old are growing faster than the young-old, with the old-old the fastest growing group of older Americans (Perls, 1998). Their absolute size in numbers is projected to be very large by the middle of the 21st century. Most would agree that a prolonged life is good if it involves an active life expectancy, that is, living long and healthy rather than being full of diseases or disabilities (Rowe & Kahn, 1998). A large percentage of those beyond age 85 are relatively healthy, live in the community, and make decisions for themselves. Even among centenarians, about 30% are healthy and independent. For example, of the 160 centenarians participating in the Harvard study of centenarians, all lived until age 93 or 94 in extremely good health (Perls, 1998). However, at the present time, the majority of older people still decline in later life and die in their 70s, 80s, or 90s.

Incidence of Disease and Disability in Later Years

However, for many elders, disease and disability can begin well before the end of life and substantial numbers have chronic ailments. For example (U. S. Bureau of the Census, 1998), among the young-old, 32% of men and 25% of women suffer from various cardiovascular conditions, with the numbers rising to 43% of men and 36% of women among those aged 75 and over. Among the young-old, 30% of men and 38% of women have hypertension, with the numbers rising to 34% of men and 42% of women aged 75 and over. Among the young-old, 43% of men and 51% of women suffer from arthritis, with the percentage remaining relatively stable for men aged 75 and over but rising to 60% for the women. Smaller percentages suffer from such conditions as diabetes, chronic obstructive pulmonary disease, and kidney disease, not to mention vision and hearing problems, malignancies, muscular and skeletal problems, and various forms of dementia. Many older adults are afflicted with multiple conditions, and although many conditions can be controlled by medications for long periods of time, the ultimate course is a downward one.

Based on census information, 1% of people aged 65 to 74 and 7% of those aged 75 to 84 are in nursing homes. Among those aged 85 and older, the percentage increases to 22%, and for those aged 95 and over, the percentage rises to 47% (Manton, 1992; Rimer, 1998; Suzman, Manton, & Willis, 1992).

In sum, older adults are not only increasing in number but a substantial proportion are remaining in good health until quite late in life. Nevertheless, the majority still experience some degree of decline with increasing disabilities as they become older. There seem to be two subgroups of elders: one remaining relatively healthy and the other continuing to become less healthy as age increases. However, it is significant that both groups are near the end of their lives and must adapt to the special problems and tasks unique to that period of life, including facing death at some point.

According to statistics reported by Whitbourne (2001), the ten leading causes of death of older adults aged 65 and over were, in order, heart disease, malignancies, cerebrovascular, chronic obstructive pulmonary diseases, pneumonia and influenza, diabetes, unintentional injuries and adverse effects (e.g., falls), Alzheimer's disease, nephritis, and septicemia. It can be seen that the majority of these causes of death were from chronic conditions from which older adults may have suffered for a long time. Those living with chronic conditions have an increased vulnerability to death. Just how this vulnerability affects their personal meanings of death, death fears, and views of the dying process remains to be seen. It should in turn influence the desire to control when, how, and where they die.

RELATION OF ELDERS' VIEWS OF DEATH TO THEIR ADAPTATION (OR MALADAPTATION) IN LATER LIFE

It is important to consider whether the personal meanings of death and their death anxiety or fears of death contribute to older adult's adaptation or maladaptation in this last stage of life. A number of questions can be asked. Are the meanings of death generally positive or negative? Are death fears few or many? Is the view of the dying process realistic? How successfully older adults' adapt to the last stage of life will influence their decisions regarding the degree to which they desire to control their death.

If older adults see death in positive terms, for example, as the gateway to a blissful afterlife, as an opportunity for a reunion with loved ones who have passed on before, or as a release from the vicissitudes of aging, such views may help them to accept and adjust to their approaching death. This frame of mind could facilitate planning for one's death, orderly transfer of one's assets, as well as any desired adjustment or reconciliation in relationships with others. On the other hand, if older adults view death negatively as something to be dreaded and avoided at all costs, such views may lead them to increased efforts to safeguard health or to seek all possible medical treatments for any conditions they may have. They may avoid making timely plans for their eventual death, avoid any death-related topics or experiences, and attempt to suppress thinking about death.

For some, the recognition of their increasing vulnerability to death as they grow older can act as a spur to achieve certain goals in life in the remaining time left. These goals can be as varied as the individuals involved, for example, fulfilling a dream to travel to a particular destination, visiting friends and relatives to renew ties, erecting a building, contributing to efforts to bring about some objective for the community, planting trees and shrubs to beautify a neighborhood, learning something new, writing a book, setting down family history for the benefit of descendants, guiding a grandchild's education and launching in life, organizing one's possessions, and so on. The possibilities are endless. Setting goals to be achieved would seem to be adaptive in that it gives the aging individual purpose in life, thereby contributing to morale. It may be maladaptive if the individual overtaxes his or her resources, becomes frustrated over not achieving goals, or does not deal adequately with physical symptoms.

On the other hand, the recognition of increasing vulnerability to death can lead other elders to abandon any goals or plans for the future, regarding any such efforts as futile because they might not live to carry them out. They adopt a stance of living each day as it comes, and endeavoring just to get through each day. This may be adaptive if death truly is near because it avoids the frustration of not being able to achieve goals, but it comes at a price of having little purpose in life.

Which views are adaptive and which are maladaptive as the older adult draws nearer to death are yet to be determined. As yet, we know relatively little about the death meanings and death fears of older adults and their view of the dying process (or for that matter, their end-of-life decisions), and the relationship of these factors to their well-being. Since the population of advanced elderly adults is expected to increase greatly in size in the coming century, it is important to investigate these topics. By gaining such knowledge, we can suggest ways to help make the last stage of life more rewarding and fulfilling for older adults as well as to help them achieve the best possible death.

VIEWS OF DEATH IN RELATION TO END-OF-LIFE DECISIONS

Regardless of their degree of adaptation to the period of decline, older adults must eventually face death itself. Many want to participate in when, where, and how they will die. Because of technology and a change in societal values and norms, elders now have a number of options in end-of-life decisions. They can: (a) do nothing and simply live on a day-to-day basis until death comes naturally, (b) avail themselves of whatever treatments medical science has to offer in an attempt to extend life for as long as possible (such as organ transplants, replacement joints, artificial tissue replacements, dialysis, use of feeding tubes, and so on), (c) refuse or withdraw from medical treatments other than those needed to provide basic comfort (including refusal of treatments for ongoing chronic conditions as well as refusal of treatment for acute conditions, such as pneumonia, occurring above and beyond the chronic condition), living out their remaining days at home, in hospice care, or in a hospital or nursing home, (d) seek active means to end life, such as suicide, physician-assisted suicide, or voluntary active euthanasia by physician or family member, or (e) simply delegate any end-of-life decisions to a close family member or someone they trust rather than make decisions for themselves.

The end-of-life decisions they make have implications for their own quality of life and morale while they are still alive, as well as effects on their family and society. If they have death meanings, fears of death, and views of the dying process that decrease their morale, they may need counseling or special support services to help them not only rethink their end-of-life decisions but deal with their meanings, fears, and views. In regard to family and society, aging individuals may make an end-of-life decision to avail themselves of whatever modern medical treatments will keep them alive for as long as possible. Such a decision may increase family caregiving burdens as well as family and societal health care costs. At the other extreme, if these individuals wish to take active means to end their lives when they can no longer live independently, family caregiving burdens and health care costs might be less (assuming laws permitting assisted suicide or voluntary euthanasia were enacted throughout the country). Regardless of whatever kind of decision is made, it should be one which is in accord with the person's overall philosophy regarding life and death (including death meanings, fears of death, and views of the dying process).

To give the reader an appreciation of the various end-of-life decision options and their ramifications, each of five main options will be examined in turn.

Postponing Death for as Long as Possible

Most adults will try to live the latter portion of life in such a way as to extend life for as long as possible, adopting a moderate lifestyle including such measures as a healthful diet, exercise, and preventive health care. Such attempts at extending life are judged to be prudent means of attaining a successful old age. Despite such efforts, death becomes inevitable at some point. Nevertheless, some patients who are judged to be terminally ill do not wish to accept the fact that death is approaching. Instead, they seek every possible avenue to postpone death for as long as they can. In some cases, patients simply want more time to allow them to settle their affairs or to complete some personal goal. In other cases, patients hope to forestall death until a cure for their condition is found or they hope for some spontaneous cure. They are often willing to endure a drastically reduced quality of life in order to preserve their lives for as long as possible.

In other cases, regardless of the older person's views, family members often "want everything done" in order to extend their loved one's life, even if the patient is in a vegetative state. Some believe that life in any form is of value (Rubin, 1998), and others simply do not want to face the loss of a beloved family member.

Several recent studies have provided information on the extent to which older adults want aggressive interventions in order to sustain life. Eleazar et al. (1996), on the basis of case records for a national sample of frail elders, found that 10% of Whites, 19% of African Americans, 4% of Hispanics, and 10% of Asians wanted aggressive life-prolonging treatments. Other investigators (Cicirelli, 1998b; Danis, Garrett, Harris, & Patrick, 1994; Schonwetter, Walker, Kramer, & Robinson, 1994) also found that African Americans were more likely to want to have their lives preserved for as long as possible. Studies of patients who had previously undergone life-prolonging interventions (Danis, Patrick, Southerland, & Green, 1988; Mazur & Merz, 1996; Potter, Stewart, & Duncan, 1994) reported that these patients would be willing to undergo such treatments again in order to extend life for even a short period. Finally, in a study investigating the amount of time that seriously ill patients would be willing to trade for a shorter life in better health, Tsevat et al. (1994, 1998) found that most patients were unwilling to trade much of their remaining time in order to have better health. This was true even for patients in their 80s. Overall, it appears that there is a substantial group of elders for whom the will to survive is so strong that they are willing to undergo very aggressive treatments to extend life for even a short period.

Refusing or Withdrawing From Medical Treatment

End-of-life decisions to refuse or withdraw medical treatments needed to sustain life and to be allowed to die are preferred by many older adults who feel that further treatments are futile and serve only to prolong a diminished quality of life for an indefinite period of time (e.g., ventilators, tube feeding). Many elders fear being subjected to expensive medical treatments that do not restore health but are instead futile, and therefore seek to prevent such a state by refusing or withdrawing from treatment. Ethicists (e.g., Callahan, 1995) regard such a decision as morally acceptable, even though the patient's life may be shortened, because the course of the disease is regarded as the cause of death of the patient rather than the decision of the patient or the action of the physician.

Although opting to refuse or withdraw from life-sustaining medical treatments seems like a simple decision on the surface, it is much more complex than it appears. Although Cicirelli (1997) reported that 49% of a sample of older adults favored refusing or withdrawing from medical treatments in general if faced with a terminal condition and poor quality of life, other researchers have found that the percentage of older adults who would refuse or withdraw from treatment depends on the aggressiveness of the particular treatment. For example, in a study investigating preferences of advanced elderly regarding various treatment scenarios, Henderson (1990) discovered that 92% would refuse a respirator, 89% would refuse tube feeding, 78% would refuse CPR, 75% would refuse intravenous fluids, 41% would refuse antibiotics, and 21% would refuse oxygen. Other researchers had roughly similar findings (Cohen-Mansfield, Droge, & Billig, 1992; Diamond, Jernigan, Moseley, Messina, & McKeown, 1989; Schonwetter, Teasdale, Taffet, Robinson, & Luchi, 1991; Seckler, Meier, Mulvihill, & Paris, 1991; Tomlinson, Howe, Notman, & Rossmiller, 1990).

In addition to the type of treatment, the patient's state of health is an important factor in decisions to refuse or withdraw from treatment. Schonwetter and colleagues (1994) found that 34% would refuse CPR under current health conditions, 67% if acutely ill, but 92% if terminally ill, functionally impaired, or suffering from dementia. Demographic background factors also influence decisions. For example, Eleazar and colleagues (1996) found elderly Whites and Asian Americans most likely to refuse life-prolonging treatments and African-Americans least likely. Also, older adults of higher education, occupation, and income levels were more likely to refuse life-prolonging treatment interventions (Cicirelli, 1998b;

Danis et al., 1994; Mutran, Danis, Bratton, Sudha, & Hanson, 1997).
However, neither age nor gender appeared to affect decisions.
Other factors, such as the extent of knowledge about a particular
treatment, previous experience with the treatment, and the man-
ner of presenting decision scenarios all influenced decisions
(Malloy, Wigton, Meeske, & Tape, 1992; Schonwetter et al., 1994).

Among older adults' reasons for refusing medical treatment were
not wanting to be a burden to loved ones, not wanting to live with
physical or mental limitations, avoiding pain and suffering, not
wanting to be on life supports, wanting to limit costs, recognizing
the impossibility of a cure, and feeling that it was one's natural
time to die (Everhart & Pearlman, 1990; Moore & Sherman, 1999).

Only a few studies have considered the effect of personal and
social variables on older adults' decisions to refuse or withdraw
from treatment. These studies found no effect of locus of control,
self-esteem, loneliness, and social support and mixed effects of
depression on such decisions (Cicirelli, 1997; Cohen-Mansfield et
al., 1992; Sonnenblick, Friedlander, & Steinberg, 1993), although
they found that those who placed greater value on quality of life
and who had less religiosity were more likely to refuse treatment.
More relevant in the general context of this book are findings
(Cicirelli, 1997; Mutran et al., 1997) that fear of death was related
to less refusal of treatment.

Dying a Natural Death

Another end-of-life decision option is to simply allow disease and
aging to progress without medical treatment (other than comfort
care) until death comes "naturally." Some individuals just go on
with their lives on a day-to-day basis without making any plans as
to how they want to die until death overtakes them. Others plan
to enter hospice care for the last stage of life, renouncing any
thought of cure or life-sustaining treatment and receiving only
comfort care. It is difficult to estimate the numbers of elders seeking to die naturally, because such choices are not clearly distinguished from decisions to refuse or withdraw from treatment in
existing studies. Additionally, numbers of those elders who die nat-

urally at home without entering the health care system are unknown. One recent study of hospice care (Petrisek & Mor, 1999) found that about 450,000 deaths a year take place in hospice care, with the rate increasing by about 16% yearly.

Seeking Active Means to End Life

Even though the urge to survive is strong for most people, there are those who prefer to hasten their own deaths. If their state of health is very poor or they have been judged to be terminally ill, if there is no hope for a cure or remission, and/or if the quality of their everyday life is so poor as to become intolerable to them, they seek to end their lives rather than to go on. To do so, they have the option of suicide, assisted suicide (by physician or by someone close to them), or voluntary active euthanasia in which they ask another person to bring about their death.

Suicide

Given a dire state of health, Ditto and colleagues (1996) found that a majority of elders would prefer death over life. Whether they would take active means to end life is another question. Regarding suicide, Prado (1998) argued that it can be both rational and ethically justified when one is terminally ill and experiencing great suffering, although before doing so one should seek medical advice, put one's affairs in order, and leave an explanation to spare the feelings of loved ones. Suicide rates among older adults have been increasing in recent years, especially among the oldest-old ("Suicide rate," 1996). As compared to younger adults, those who commit suicide in old age are more likely to be stressed by illness, but are less likely to be stressed by other problems (Carney, Rich, Burke, & Fowler, 1994). Cicirelli (1998b) presented elders with various end-of-life decision situations depicting onerous symptoms and very low quality of life; only 7% indicated that they would favor suicide under such conditions.

Assisted Suicide

Because many elders who wish to take active means to end their lives when terminally ill lack the means, knowledge, or courage to carry out a suicide alone, they seek the assistance of someone else. In physician-assisted suicide, the physician provides the equipment, materials, and information on procedures but the patient must commit the final suicide act. Thus far, physician-assisted suicide is legal only in the state of Oregon. Although movements for legalization have arisen in other states, they have been unsuccessful thus far. Proponents and ethicists have debated the issues involved at great length and it has not been resolved.

However, substantial percentages of adults appear to favor physician-assisted suicide. In a recent Gallup poll (Moore, 1997), 61% of men and 56% of women favored legalization for a person who was terminally ill and in unremitting pain. An average of 40% responded that they would choose physician-assisted suicide for themselves under those conditions, although the percentage dropped somewhat when pain was not included in the question asked. In a similar survey of adults over age 60 (Seidlitz, Duberstein, Cox, & Conwell, 1995), 41% felt that physician-assisted suicide should be legalized, with views related to religiousness and ethnicity but not age.

In investigating whether older adults would choose physician-assisted suicide for themselves, Cicirelli (1997, 1998b) reported that from 12% to 21% of community-dwelling elders favored assisted suicide. Decisions were related to ethnicity, gender, age, education, religiosity, value for quality of life, and fear of death. Similar results were obtained in a national survey (Blendon, Szalay, & Knox, 1992), which found that 19% of respondents would ask a physician to prescribe a lethal drug if terminally ill.

Voluntary Active Euthanasia

An additional end-of-life decision option, although it is not legal anywhere in the United States, is voluntary active euthanasia. In this case, suffering and terminally ill patients request that the physician (or family member or someone else) end their lives and the physician acts to do so. There are lively ethical arguments both for and against this option (e.g., Callahan, 1995; Dixon, 1998), as well as considerable public support for its legalization. Leinbach (1993) reviewed poll results on this question from 1977 to 1991, finding that from 58% to 69% of adults favored legalization of euthanasia. In a quasi-longitudinal analysis, there was no discernible trend toward increased opposition to euthanasia as respondent cohorts aged; in general, attitudes for all age groups became more lenient over time.

Other studies investigated elder's views on whether they would desire voluntary active euthanasia for themselves if they were terminally ill and suffering an intolerably low quality of life. Cicirelli (1997, 1998b) found that 12% of senior-center participants and 20% of randomly sampled community-dwelling elders would prefer voluntary active euthanasia for themselves. The degree of acceptance of this option was related to ethnicity, gender, education, age, and religiosity, indicating that views vary depending on the characteristics of the respondent. Blendon and colleagues (1992) reported that 19% would favor voluntary active euthanasia for themselves. Although the percentages of older adults favoring physician-assisted suicide and voluntary active euthanasia for themselves are quite similar, MacDonald (1998) asked respondents to indicate their preference for one option or the other. They clearly preferred to have a lethal dose administered by a physician than assisted suicide with someone else's help. One reason for this preference appears to be that they want to share the responsibility for the act with someone in authority. (Physicians, in contrast, prefer assisted suicide because it allows the patient to assume a larger share of responsiblity.)

Delegating End-of-Life Decisions to Others

Although many older adults have made decisions about how and where they would like to die, and have formalized their wishes in some kind of advance directive document, others have not done so. High (1993a, 1993b) investigated older adults reasons for not completing an advance directive and found that about a third of the elders in his study favored allowing family members to make any needed end-of-life decisions for them. About two-thirds of these had spoken informally with family members about their views, and the rest assumed that there was some kind of tacit understanding with close family members regarding end-of-life care. Cicirelli's work (1997) supported High's findings, with 36% of older adults preferring to let family members (or someone else close to them) decide what kind of end-of-life treatment was best for them. Those adults who were older, of lower socioeconomic status, and/or African American were more likely to delegate end-of-life decisions to others. However, existing studies of the lack of agreement between older adults and their proxy decision-makers (see Cicirelli, 2001a for a review) indicate that family members may be unaware of elders' preferences or may base decisions on their own views rather than what they think the elder would want.

Implications of End-of-Life Decisions for Older Adults and Families

One can look at older adults' decisions regarding end-of-life care as simple preferences and no more. As such, they are important as they enable the older adult to face the end of life with some degree of control over the time, place, and manner of death, and with a sense of peace and dignity. However, in a larger sense, the older adult's end-of-life decisions are the culmination of that individual's entire set of views regarding death: the personal meanings of death, fears and apprehensions about death, and expectations about the dying process. Coming to a fuller understanding of these views and how they influence the last portion of life is the basis of the individual's philosophy about death.

METHODOLOGY OF THE EXPLORATORY STUDY

Threefold Means of Gaining Information on Elders' Views

In investigating elders' views on death, we used a three-pronged approach to gaining information. The first approach was to review available literature to discover what other researchers have found in the past. This was a challenging approach, because much of the existing research on death meanings and death fears has been carried out with younger adults. The number of studies specifically targeting older adults as subjects of research on death-related topics is relatively small. Another problem is that many of the existing studies have used only a broad "over 65" age category and did not attempt to determine age differences within that category. In looking at existing studies of younger adults, one can learn about approaches that have been taken to study views on death, generate hypotheses that might be of interest in studies with older adults, and reach conclusions about findings that might be generalized to older age groups. In looking at existing studies of older adults, one can reach some conclusions about what has been learned already and what needs to be investigated.

Using a single age range to refer to all older adults can be highly misleading, with the majority of individuals in their 60s and into their early 70s still relatively healthy, active, and independent, and increasing numbers of those in their 80s and 90s experiencing poor health, various disabilities, and lack of independence. In recent decades, gerontologists have employed various subdivisions of the age range (such as the young-old and the old-old, or the young-old, mid-old, and old-old, or the advanced-old, and so on), but these distinctions have rarely been made by those studying death-related topics. Consequently, in looking at existing research findings, we attempted to note the age range of the individuals studied in relation to the outcomes of these investigations.

Results of existing studies were examined to note how findings may vary by gender, ethnicity, socioeconomic status, and other background variables of interest. Some of these background variables have been investigated in relation to death-related topics, but others have not.

The second and third means of gaining information about older adults' death views both involved data from a small empirical study. A larger study was not carried out at this point in time because only certain variables relevant to the study of death views of older adults have been identified in previous studies. One objective of the empirical study was to identify those existing and new variables that would be important to investigate in larger studies. The first portion of the empirical study used existing instruments and quantitative analysis techniques to determine the relationship of elders' views on death to key demographic and contextual variables. The second portion of the study used a variety of qualitative techniques in open-end interviews to probe older adults' views. By doing so, we aimed to explore elders' views more fully, in order to identify important new variables for further study, and to determine whether the quantitative findings were borne out in participants' own words. Methods of qualitative analysis were used to identify themes in the qualitative protocols and to relate such themes to major background variables.

By using such a threefold approach, we were able to identify areas where the findings were convergent regardless of the approach as well as areas where the findings differed depending on the approach used. This supplementing of qualitative analyses of unstructured interview data (Addison, 1992; Strauss & Corbin, 1990) with quantitative analyses of data obtained using standardized assessment instruments, interpreted with reference to existing literature, is an example of methodological triangulation (Hendricks, 1996), used to obtain greater validity and depth for study conclusions. The outcome of this strategy is a richer understanding of elders' views than previously available as well as the identification of fruitful paths for future research.

Sample of Elders

Identification of the Sample

The sample of elders taking part in the study consisted of White and African American elders aged 70 and above, with the White sample located in Greater Lafayette, Indiana, and the African American sample located in the city of Indianapolis. It would have been desirable to use only a single site for the study. However, Greater Lafayette (the area surrounding Purdue University) had too few African American elders to yield a suitable sample, and considerations of time and travel costs precluded carrying out the entire study in Indianapolis where a plentiful population of older

African Americans lived. In both sites, potential participants were identified from such sources as voting records, lists of participants in our previous survey studies of older adults, senior citizen centers, retirement apartment complexes, church groups, and other organizations with memberships of older adults. In addition, those contacted early in the recruitment process were asked to nominate other potential participants for the study, a particularly useful technique for locating the oldest old.

It should be mentioned that each elder taking part in the study was first given full information about the general aims of the study and the types of information and views that they would be asked to provide, so that they could give full informed consent to the study. It is recognized that as a result the study sample involved those individuals who felt that they would be comfortable in sharing their views about death at some length in a personal interview.

Interviewing

Given the advanced age and the medical problems of many of the participants, interviews were paced so as not to tire them unduly. In some cases, there was a break in the interviewing to allow a brief period of rest; in other cases the interviewer returned to complete the interview on another day. In still other cases, the interview was rescheduled for another date if the elder was having a "bad day." Most, however, were able to carry out an extended interview without any apparent difficulty. In a few cases, the interviewer grew weary long before the elder showed the slightest sign of fatigue.

A few of the participants went to a great deal of trouble to share their views on death. One woman who had severe hearing problems was able to lip-read throughout the entire interview. Others managed to communicate despite the aftereffects of a stroke. All in all, it was a delight and privilege to interview the older men and women taking part in the study. Each of their life stories and viewpoints was unique and their willingness to share their thoughts with us was greatly appreciated.

Nature of the Sample

As previous researchers have indicated (e.g., Johnson & Barer, 1997), locating older adults aged 85 and above is particularly difficult. The population in this age group is still relatively small for any given area. Many are in nursing homes or other care institutions rather than living independently in the community. Many have problems of vision and hearing, memory loss, and other forms of cognitive disability. Also, lack of mobility, frailty, and specific medical problems may prevent them from participating in a study such as this.

The original plan was to include both men and women, Whites and African Americans, and those in their 70s, 80s, and 90s, with an approximately balanced representation from these groups. In addition, we hoped to include those who were healthy as well as those with health problems and various degrees of disability. However, smaller numbers of men and older African Americans in the population made this goal impossible to achieve.

The final sample of 109 elders included 93 women and 16 men; there were 68 Whites and 41 African Americans. Ages ranged from 70 to 97 years, with a mean age of 80.7 years (and a standard deviation of 6.9 years).

Subgroups of the Sample

For use in various analyses and for comparison purposes, the total sample was subdivided in different ways, depending on the type of analysis or comparison to be made. One subdivision was simply to group the sample into a younger group (age range 70–84) and an older group (age range 85 to 97 years). The younger group contained 76 elders and the older group contained 33. This subdivision into two groups was useful in only a few cases where comparisons with findings in the literature for young-old and old-old were made.

A second subdivision of the sample by age involved three age groups: 49 elders aged 70–79, 49 elders aged 80–89, and 11 elders aged 90–97. These groups were useful in several analyses, as well as for comparisons in the literature.

To obtain a more fine-grained subdivision of the sample by age, five age subgroups were defined: 70–74 (27 elders), 75–79 (22 elders), 80–84 (27 elders), 85–89 (22 elders), and 90–97 (11 elders). These groups were used in analyses testing for the possibility of age trends in variables of interest.

A different subgrouping of the total sample by ethnicity and socioeconomic status (SES) was used for many comparisons. Overall, the sample of Whites was higher in SES than the African American sample. In order to identify a group more similar in background characteristics to the African American sample for comparison purposes, the White sample was divided into two subgroups on the basis of their SES level. The Low SES White group was similar to the African American group in educational and occupational attainment, whereas the High SES White group was of higher educational and occupational attainment than either the Low SES White group or the African American group.

Cross-categorizations of the sample by gender, age group, and SES/ethnicity were used in making both quantitative and qualitative comparisons. Use of one type of categorization or another was dictated by the nature of the data being analyzed, as well as by particular questions of interest.

Quantitative Study: Approach, Measures, Analyses

The general objective of the quantitative study was to assess participants' views on death meanings, fear of death, and the dying process, and to relate these views to the participants' demographic background, religious behaviors and beliefs, health, morale, and family relationships. A structured interview-questionnaire was used to obtain this information, with individual interviews carried out by the investigator.

Demographic Variables

Six items were used to obtain basic background information. These were gender, age, marital status, employment (if any), educational level, and occupational level. Educational level and occupational level were each coded using the 7-point Hollingshead (1957) scales, with a high score indicating higher educational or occupational status. Hollingshead's socioeconomic status (SES) index was computed by summing four times the educational level and seven times the occupational level.

The basic demographic data are summarized in Table 1.1 for three groups: High SES Whites, Low SES Whites, and African Americans. Age was highest for the High SES Whites and lowest for the African Americans. The majority of all three groups were widowed. However, the greatest percentage of those currently married was in the High SES White group and the smallest percentage was in the African American group. Conversely, the greatest percentage of divorced and separated elders was in the African American group and the least was in the High SES White group. Nearly all members of all three ethnic/SES groups were retired. In terms of education, all of the High SES Whites had at least some college or vocational training beyond high school; 76% were college graduates or had postgraduate training. In contrast, only 12% of the Low SES Whites and 19% of the African Americans had some college or vocational training beyond high school. At the other end of the education scale, 12% of the Low SES White group and 37% of the African American group had nine or fewer years of education; none of the High SES Whites were at these education levels. Similarly, 88% of the High SES White group had occupations before retirement at the three highest levels on the Hollingshead scale, compared to 12% of the Low SES Whites and 22% of the African Americans. At the other end of the scale, only 7% of the High SES Whites were in unskilled or semiskilled manual occupations, compared to 46% of the Low SES Whites and 70% of the African Americans. These striking differences between the three groups were reflected in the mean SES index scores for the three groups: 63.8 for the High SES Whites, 35.7 for the Low SES Whites, and 32.3 for the African Americans, with a possible score range of 11 to 77 on the index.

The summary of the demographic characteristics of the three ethnic/SES groups indicates that the three groups represent a wide range of individual differences, particularly in terms of educational and occupational backgrounds. On the one hand, one might wish

TABLE 1.1 Demographic Characteristics of Three Sample Subgroups: High SES Whites (*n* = 42), Low SES Whites (*n* = 26), and African Americans (*n* = 41)

Characteristics	High SES Whites	Low SES Whites	African Americans
Age			
Range	70–97	70–93	70–88
Mean	83.90	80.54	77.54
Standard Deviation	7.20	6.72	5.07
Marital Status			
Currently married	28.6%	15.4%	2.4%
Widowed	59.5%	65.4%	65.9%
Divorced	4.8%	15.4%	26.8%
Separated	0.0%	3.8%	2.4%
Never married	7.1%	0.0%	2.4%
Employment			
Full or part-time	4.8%	0.0%	2.4%
Retired	95.2%	100.0%	92.7%
Never employed	0.0%	0.0%	4.9%
Education			
1–6 years	0.0%	7.7%	12.2%
7–9 years	0.0%	3.8%	24.4%
Some high school	0.0%	26.9%	29.3%
High school graduate	0.0%	50.0%	14.6%
Some college, vocational	23.8%	11.5%	12.2%
College graduate	23.8%	0.0%	2.4%
Postgraduate	52.4%	0.0%	4.9%
Occupation			
Unskilled manual	7.1%	11.5%	19.5%
Semiskilled manual	0.0%	34.6%	61.0%
Skilled manual	0.0%	0.0%	7.3%
Clerical, sales clerk	4.8%	42.3%	9.8%
Lesser admin., technician	26.2%	11.5%	17.1%
Manager, lesser prof.	38.1%	0.0%	4.9%
Major prof., owner	23.8%	0.0%	0.0%
SES Index			
Mean	63.81	35.69	32.15
Standard deviation	12.23	10.57	16.04

to achieve greater similarity of subgroups on the various background characteristics. On the other hand, the wide range of individual differences among study participants suggests that we would be more likely to sample a wide range of viewpoints on death-related topics. Because the study was exploratory in nature, with the aim of probing older adults' views on death in areas that have not been investigated thus far, the diversity in the sample is regarded as an advantage. However, the reader is cautioned to keep the diversity in background characteristics of the various subgroupings in mind when interpreting results. Results apply only to the particular subgroups indicated, but it is felt that findings of potential interest will stimulate further research in older adults views on death.

Personal Meanings of Death

Because previous studies of personal meanings of death carried out by other investigators involved qualitative analysis of respondents' written narratives, we were unable to find quantitative instruments to assess personal meanings in the literature. Therefore, the author's Personal Meanings of Death Scale (Cicirelli, 1998b), recently developed for a study of college students' meanings of death, was selected for use. This 17-item instrument measures four dimensions of personal meanings of death: Death as Legacy, Death as Afterlife, Death as Extinction, and Death as Motivator. Internal consistency reliabilities of the four subscales ranged from .66 to .73, levels considered adequate for group studies although not for individual diagnosis. Because the instrument had not been used with older adults, its use in the present study was considered exploratory.

Fear of Death

Unlike the area on personal meanings of death, several good measures of fear of death (i.e., death anxiety) were available for use. Because most investigators in the area now feel that fear of death is multidimensional in structure, four multidimensional instruments were considered for use: the Multidimensional Fear of Death Scale (MFODS) (Hoelter, 1979; Neimeyer & Moore, 1994), the

Revised Death Anxiety Scale (Tomer, Eliason, & Smith, 2000), the Collett-Lester Fear of Death Scale (Lester, 1994), and the Death Attitude Profile—Revised (Wong, Reker, & Gesser, 1994). The MFODS consisted of 42 items assessing 8 fear of death dimensions: fear of the dying process, fear of the dead, fear of being destroyed, fear for significant others, fear of the unknown, fear of conscious death, fear for the body after death, and fear of premature death. The Revised Death Anxiety Scale had 15 items assessing 4 dimensions of anxiety: nonbeing, pain, regret, and body concerns. The Collett-Lester scale had 32 items assessing 4 dimensions: death of self, death of others, dying of self, dying of others. Finally, the Death Attitude Profile consisted of 32 items measuring 5 dimensions of death attitudes: fear of death, death avoidance, neutral acceptance, approach acceptance, and escape acceptance.

The choice was a difficult one because all four measures have had considerable psychometric work, including factor analysis, and have good evidence for their reliability and validity. As might be expected, there is some overlap between the different scales. Ultimately, the MFODS was selected because there was a large body of research concerning its use, including older adults, because certain subscales of the instrument appeared to be particularly relevant to study aims, and because the author had used it successfully in previous studies with older adults (Cicirelli, 1997, 1998b). In retrospect, it might have been desirable to include the Death Attitude Profile as well, because the three subscales measuring neutral, approach, and escape acceptance of death would have been quite interesting in relation to older adults' views of death as they emerged in the study.

Dying Process

We were unaware of any existing instrument providing a quantitative assessment of views regarding the dying process, so an instrument was devised specifically for this study. To do so, 30 items were constructed to reflect the feelings, thoughts, and concerns that a person in the last stages of a terminal illness might have. The respondent was asked to imagine that he or she was dying of cancer and had at most a week to live, and indicate the frequency with which he or expected each thought or feeling to occur on a 5-point scale ranging from "never" to "most of the time." Factor analysis was then used to reduce the 30 items to a few subscales. Admittedly, such an instrument is purely exploratory until further research establishes its reliability and validity, but it is a first step in the absence of other available instrumentation.

Religious Behavior and Feelings

The literature on religiosity contains several instruments designed to measure various aspects of this concept. Religiosity is a somewhat elusive concept that encompasses several dimensions, and each of the existing instrument assesses certain dimensions and not others. Existing research has demonstrated a relationship between religiosity and well-being in later life (Koenig, Smiley, & Gonzales, 1988). It is not unreasonable to expect religiosity to be related to older adults' views of death as well.

For the present interview-questionnaire, several religiosity subscales were adapted from various sources to measure five aspects of religiosity. Organizational religiosity, the extent to which an individual participates in organized religious services and activities, was assessed by a five-item subscale of the religiosity measure used by Chatters, Levin, and Taylor (1992). A second four-item subscale of the Chatters and colleagues instrument was used to measure nonorganizational religiosity, namely, the extent to which an individual exhibits such behaviors as reading religious materials, watching or listening to TV or radio, and praying. Subjective (or intrinsic) religiosity, concerned with the level of religious commitment and the importance of religion in an individual's life, was assessed by three items adapted from Chatters and colleagues and from Krause (1993). Use of religion as an aid in coping with life was measured by four items devised for this study. Finally, a single item was used to assess change in religiosity, namely, whether older adults felt that they had become more or less religious since middle age. In addition to the measurement of various aspects of religiosity, elders were asked whether they were members (or otherwise affiliation) with an organized religion, and if so, what denomination.

Health

Because it was hypothesized that an older adults' state of health would be related to their views on death-related topics, several measures were used to assess the older person's health from three basic perspectives: global feelings of illness or wellness, presence or absence of illness and symptoms, and functional adequacy in terms of carrying out everyday activities.

Global feelings of health were assessed through a self-rating item. Self-rated health, although a single-item rating scale, has proven to be well correlated with a variety of other health indicators. Participants were asked first to rate their health in relation to others in their age group, and second to rate their health in relation to younger adults.

Two scales were used to indicate health in terms of the elders' illnesses and symptoms. First, a checklist of chronic illnesses was used, containing 20 of the most prevalent chronic conditions of older adults (U. S. Bureau of the Census, 1994; Villaverde & MacMillan, 1980). Elders were also given the opportunity to report other conditions not on the list. They responded first as to whether they had the given condition, and then rated its severity. Similarly, a checklist of symptoms was used, containing 42 common symptoms of older adults identified by Villaverde and MacMillan, with elders again given the opportunity to report other symptoms not on the list. They responded first whether or not they experienced the symptom, and then were asked to indicate how often it bothered them.

Functional health was assessed by two instruments: the Instrumental Activities of Daily Living Scale (IADL) and the Mobility scale (Lawton, 1972; Lawton, Moss, Fulcomer, & Kleban, 1982). The IADL measured the degree of help needed with instrumental activities of daily living, such things as telephoning, shopping, meal preparation, housekeeping, laundry, managing medications, managing finances, and grooming. (The companion Activities of Daily Living, which measured more basic activities such as bathing, dressing, eating, and toileting was not used because the population of older adults studied needed little help in these areas, if any.) The Mobility scale assessed the amount of help needed with such basic movement activities as walking, climbing stairs, rising from chairs, getting in and out of bed, and use of wheelchair.

One final perspective on health, life expectancy, was measured by asking elders first, how many more years they expected to live, and then how many more years they would like to live.

Morale

Although several indicators of emotional well-being have often been used in studies of older adults, including instruments measuring self-esteem, depression, loneliness, happiness, and morale, the Bradburn Affect Balance Scale (Bradburn, 1969) was selected for use in the present study. The scale has adequate reliability and validity, as well as a considerable literature supporting its use. Most important, it was used in the recent Johnson and Barer (1997) study of the old-old, in which they obtained interesting qualitative findings about older adults attitudes regarding death. We felt that it would be of value to compare results of the present study with Johnson and Barer's findings. The scale contains five items assessing positive feelings and five items assessing negative feelings, with the balance score the difference between the two sets of items.

Family Relationships

The final part of the quantitative interview-questionnaire was concerned with the older adult's family relationships. One hypothesis of the study was that losses of siblings and adult children through death would influence the way in which an elder looked at death. Therefore, data were gathered about each sibling in the family, including such information as birth order, gender, whether living or not, age (or age at death), proximity to elder, and feelings of closeness. Similar data were gathered for all adult children. From this basic information about the family, a number of quantitative variables could be defined for analysis.

(In the qualitative portion of the interview, further information about family relationships was gathered in regard to the wider kin network as well as siblings and adult children. Although most of this material was treated in the qualitative analyses, some summary rating variables were developed for the quantitative analysis. For example, a global rating of the older adult's family system, based on number of family members and the nature of family relationship in terms of closeness and functionality was made for use in analysis.)

Analysis

The analysis of data in the quantitative portion of the study used a wide variety of statistical methods, as considered appropriate to the data content and the aims of the study. It was considered to be complementary to the qualitative analysis, and was intended to provide support for hypotheses arising from the qualitative analysis, wherever possible.

In general, the analysis proceeded by first obtaining descriptive summaries of the data for the various measures of death meanings, fear of death, and the dying process, as well as the measures of demographic background, religiosity, health, well-being, and family relationships. For those scales newly devised for the study (e.g., the dying process), principle components factor analysis was used to reduce the overall number of items to a few salient dimensions. Correlational and regression analyses were used to probe relationships between measures of death meanings, fear of death, and the dying process and the other categories of variables (demographic background, religiosity, health, well-being, and family relationships). Analysis of variance techniques were used to compare the death views of the various age groups and to investigate possible age trends in the data. Analysis of variance was also used to compare the three ethnic/SES groups on the variables of interest. SPSS software was used throughout to carry out the quantitative analyses.

Overall, the findings of the quantitative analyses are interpreted within the larger qualitative frame of reference in order to gain the richest possible understanding of how the personal death meanings, death fears, and views of the dying process influence the lives of older adults. Of course, the findings must be regarded as provisional, given the facts that the older adults participating in the study constituted a convenience sample, the sample was relatively small and contained a limited number of men and of those over

90 years of age, and several of the instruments used were newly
devised for the study. Nevertheless, we feel that the insights and
information gained override the limitations of the study and offer
a basis for more sophisticated hypotheses for further study.

Qualitative Study

Whereas the quantitative approach to research offers careful and
reliable measures of phenomena and statistical tests of significance
in testing hypotheses about these phenomena, it tends to be limited because it deals with only those concepts for which adequate
measures are available. The qualitative approach to research, in
contrast, deals with the full richness of human experience, limited
only by the questions asked and the skill of the researcher in dis-
cerning relevant patterns in the narrative materials gathered for
analysis. The present study sought to bring together both approaches
to attempt to gain the fullest possible understanding of older adults'
views on death.

Unstructured interviews were used to elicit participants' personal meanings of death, fears of death, and conceptions of the
dying process, expressed in their own words. In addition, topics
concerned with religious beliefs and the influence of family relationships in relation to death-related topics were explored in the
interviews. This approach was designed to elicit views that respondents would not have a chance to express during the administration of formal quantitative instruments (Johnson & Barer, 1997;
Sankar & Gubrium, 1994).

A number of open-ended questions were prepared for use in
guiding the interviews, but the use of an informal conversational
tone was considered important to establish rapport and to give the
participants ample opportunity to express their full point of view.
In general, the interviewer allowed the conversation to flow in a
natural way, used questions to guide the interview as topics happened to come up. Probing questions were used when needed to
follow up on ideas and meanings that were introduced by the
respondent. Among the open-ended questions asked were the following: What is death? What does death mean to you? Do you ever

think about death getting closer: How has that changed the way you live? What do you think dying will be like? What kinds of feelings or emotions do you think you will experience? What do you think will happen to you after you die? What will your death mean to your family? When you think about death and dying, do you ever feel afraid or uneasy about it? What kinds of things bother you?

In relation to religious views, open-ended questions probed the relationship between views about the existence of God, the efficacy of prayer, and the meaning of death. Questions about family relationships explored the influence and support from various family members.

A multifaceted approach was taken in the qualitative study, supplementing the open-ended questions with other methods. One of these was the use of a sentence completion techniques in which study participants were asked to complete various sentence stems. For example: death is like _____; for old people death is _____; death is easier when _____; death is difficult when _____; when I think of being dead, I _____; death is always _____. In many cases, the sentence completion task elicited certain death meanings and views about death that did not spontaneously appear in the earlier portion of the qualitative interview.

A third approach was the use of three somewhat ambiguous drawings from the Gerontological Apperception Test (Wolk & Wolk, 1971). The rationale of this projective method was that, if thoughts and fears about death were suppressed from conscious awareness, they would appear as death themes when the respondent constructed a narrative about the subjects of the pictures. For example, one picture showed an older woman in bed and an older man entering the room carrying flowers. One possible narrative about what was going on in the picture and what was likely to happen might be that the woman had been ill but was recovering and would live a happy life with her husband (no death themes). Another possible narrative might be that the women had little time left before she died; her husband loved her so much that he soon died of a broken heart (two death themes). From these narratives, one can gain an idea of the extent to which thoughts of death influence the older adult's perceptions of otherwise neutral or ambiguous materials.

The entire interview was tape-recorded and transcribed for analysis. The basic analysis method of grounded theory (Addison, 1992; Strauss & Corbin, 1990) was applied to the qualitative interview protocols. Using open coding in line-by-line analysis of the first few protocols, categories of death-related concepts were identified. These were applied to new protocols, with new categories added as needed until no new categories appeared. After this initial step in the analysis procedure was completed, axial coding was carried out to identify conditions and contexts pertaining to the initial categories. Finally, selective coding was used to identify connections between categories. Hypotheses about connections between categories were verified by testing whether they applied to other protocols. By this means, a set of concepts used by older people in talking about death meanings, death fears, and the dying process gradually emerged. The QSR NUD*IST NVivo 1.0 computer software (Richards, 1999) was used in carrying out the qualitative analysis. It was a valuable tool in developing and applying coding categories, linking coding categories to attributes of the respondent and context, and verifying hypotheses about relationships between categories.

OVERVIEW OF THE BOOK

This volume can be regarded as an exploration of older adults' views on the broad topic of death. In carrying out such an exploration, each of the remaining chapters focuses on a particular topic and attempts to gain some understanding and appreciation of the ways that elders think and feel. The remaining portion of this chapter provides an overview of the remaining chapters.

Chapter 2 examines the sociocultural meanings of death and how individuals' views of death come about in relation to the social and cultural context in which they live. Existential philosophers have theorized that death loses its terror if one lives life in a meaningful and authentic way. Another perspective, derived from an evolutionary approach, is that although birth is necessary to perpetuate the species, the society and culture must also develop if the species is to survive. Both the individual and the culture are becoming increasingly complex, and have increasing capacity to deal with complex problems of life and death, including life span extension and even the possibility of life without death. The meanings of death held by the individual are developed in relation to the institutions in society that nourish the individual's capacity to function in that society. This chapter looks at the broad, general meanings of death characteristic of the society as a whole.

Chapter 3 goes on to look at the personal meanings of death held by the individual, developed in relation to that individual's niche in society and to the institutions of society, and shaped by a variety of idiosyncratic life experiences. These meanings are of subjective importance to the individual, whether or not they are shared by others. Various approaches to the study of personal meanings of death are reviewed, including personifications of death, death as metaphor, and death themes. The death themes revealed by elders in interviews are examined and related to age and other demographic variables.

In Chapter 4, fears of death (death anxiety) are examined. Although this is a much-researched topic, there has been little research dealing with the very old. In the qualitative interviews, most of the older adults studied appeared to have little fear of death; some indicated that they would welcome it. However, many actively avoided thinking about it. Quantitative analysis of elder's responses to a multidimensional fear of death instrument indicated that fear of death was in general low, with the strongest fear in relation to the possibility of bodily destruction. Fears did seem to vary with age, however, with the greatest fears expressed by those in their early eighties.

In Chapter 5, older adults' views and expectations about the dying process are explored. The right-to-die movement has asserted the rights of dying individuals to refuse or withdraw from futile and onerous medical treatments, under the assumption that the dying process would be one of pain, helplessness, and indignity. On the other hand, some research has found that the dying process is not one of protracted pain for most people. In the interviews, the older adults studied had somewhat vague views of what dying would be like. For the most part, however, they expected their own deaths to be relatively benign, simply passing away during sleep or a quiet fading away. Even if dying were to become a difficult process, they expected to be sedated and unaware. Most prominent in their expectations about the process were thoughts about their family, concerns about physical symptoms, and concerns about the duration and nature of the actual dying process.

Chapter 6 considers the many ways in which religious belief and spirituality influence older adults' death meanings, fears of death, and views about the dying process. The great majority of the older adults studied held traditional religious core beliefs involving the existence of a God, a conception of some kind of afterlife, and the importance of prayer to communicate with God. For most, their beliefs appeared to reflect a rote learning of religious teaching in childhood, without any mature examination. A minority of elders did not hold traditional religious beliefs, but had developed a personal philosophy of life that enabled them to view death with equanimity as a natural process. Most prayed regularly, seeking God's help and strength in dealing with their poor health and other problems, and gaining a sense of security and comfort thereby. They felt that their faith and prayers would help them through the dying process. Overall, the study findings support the hypothesis based on attachment theory that God is the ultimate attachment figure of humans, a hypothesis that is examined in detail in this chapter. Religion served many elders as a means of coping with the inevitability of death and the dying process, as well as helping to allay their fears.

Chapter 7 considers the proposition that declines in health in later years influence elders' views of death as the possibility of death becomes ever more likely. Study participants were assessed on a variety of measures of health, including medical conditions, functional adequacy, and subjective views. No matter what measure was used, a considerable range in participants' health was detected. Many elders in poor health viewed death as a relief or release from their physical problems and suffering. They did not want to live longer in their present state of health and some actively longed for death. Other participants who were in better health did not anticipate a difficult death when it finally came, expecting the dying process to be rapid and painless. Nevertheless, most accepted a period of poor health in old age as an inevitable part of life, with death as a natural culmination. The quantitative analyses, in contrast, found health to have only a modest influence on death-related views. In regard to personal meanings of death, those in better health were less likely to view death as extinction. They had less fear of the dying process, but more fear for significant others should they die. They also expected to experience fewer negative emotions and physical concerns during the dying process. Overall, the outcome of declining health appears to be a general realization of the finiteness of life, with only minor influence on specific views of death.

In Chapter 8, the influence of family relationships on older adults' views of death is considered. It is quite reasonable to suppose that those older adults who had close and supportive relationships with a circle of family and friends will view death in a different way than those who are relatively alone late in life. In the qualitative interviews, some elders who had considerable family support felt that family members would be greatly upset by their deaths, whereas others felt that family would take their passing in stride. Some who had weak or nonexistent family ties felt that family would not care about their deaths or care only about a potential inheritance. Some elders had family objectives that they wanted to achieve before their deaths, while others were concerned about conflicts, misunderstandings, or lack of communication with family members as they approached death. Those who had closer family relationships viewed death as a motivator for activities in their remaining life, and tended to see death as an extinction. Fear of death appeared to be related to sibling relationships and the proportion of deceased siblings in the family. In regard to expectations about the dying process, those with closer relationships with their adult children anticipated experiencing more negative emotions and more concerns about family. It would appear that the particular patterning of an older individual's family relationships influences not only their conceptions of death, but also the way they feel about leaving those loved ones behind.

In Chapter 9, an attempt is made to bring together the separate threads examined in the preceding chapters to gain a more integrated picture. The question addressed in the chapter is the extent to which older adults' death meanings, fears of death, and expectations of the dying process are interrelated and how they may depend on age, ethnicity, socioeconomic status, health, religious views, and family ties. Although other background variables influence elders' views of death to some extent, their religious orientation is the major influence for the majority, who seem to subscribe to the teachings of their particular church about death and the afterlife without much independent reflection. Elders' meanings of death are related to the kinds of fears of death and also to their expectations about the dying process. Also, fears of death are related to expectations about the dying process. Overall, meaningful patterns seem to exist, linking older adults' views about death to the larger context in which they live.

The final chapter, Chapter 10, considers conclusions drawn from the empirical study in relation to existing literature, identifies questions remaining to be answered in further study in this area, and draws implications for end-of-life decisions and care during the dying process. It is apparent that one cannot generalize research findings on views of death to all types of older adults and all types of situations. Some views varied with age, and it appeared that dealing with smaller age categories may better reflect important life changes for the older adult. Future research in the area needs to look for patterns in death views among subgroups of elders differing on demographic background, health, religious background, and family relationships. Future research also needs to include basic personality variables. Aspects of personality (both stable and changing) that are related to the way older adults live are also likely to be related to their views about death and may account for many findings. Earlier studies established some connections between older adults' fear of death and their end-of-life decision preferences. Knowledge of elders' personal meanings of death, their fears, and their expectations about the dying process should lead to a better understanding of their end-of-life decisions, and should also have important implications for care during the dying process.

2

Sociocultural Meanings of Death

The central theme of this chapter is that society and its institutions originate to satisfy the needs of its members and eventually perpetuate society itself. Cultural meanings develop as a way of regulating the group behavior of society members to carry out its functions. As part of this process, both certain societal institutions and concomitant cultural meanings develop to cope with the death of members of the society. Subsequently, both the general and specific cultural meanings of death provide the basic context for the development of personal meanings of death which the individual uses to help make sense out of his or her own eventual death, to prepare for it, and to guide him or her in carrying on daily living activities.

This book is primarily concerned with older adults' views of death, but it is important to consider the sociocultural meanings of death in order to provide a broader context within which to understand the significance of personal meanings of death, fears of death, and views of the dying process. For example, a cultural meaning of death might be that dead bodies in a society must be disposed of in some manner to help maintain a healthy and orderly society. As a member of society, the individual may participate in carrying out whatever cultural practices exist for such disposal, for example, burying the dead in the ground. Eventually, however, an individual may go beyond this to derive a personal meaning that one's body should be placed in an above-ground mausoleum so that one's bodily remains can be closer to God. Such a personal meaning of death is derived from the more general cultural meaning that dead bodies must be disposed of rather than simply left on the ground to decay.

Definition of Society

Society is more than a collection of individuals. It is a group of people who have existed for a long period of time, who are united by social relationships, who occupy a particular geographical territory, and who are relatively self-sufficient and self-sustaining (Gelles & Levine, 1999). Such groups of people share common or patterned behavior. Interaction and communication among individuals within the society lead to differentiation of roles and division of labor to maintain the functioning of society (Gelles & Levine, 1999; Marshall, 1980).

Society begins with the individuals who band together to satisfy basic needs in order to survive. Certain institutions develop not only to ensure survival but to help individuals adapt to changing circumstances and continue to grow during their lifetime. The death of individuals within the society initiates the development of certain institutions to help maintain society by protecting members of the society from premature death and dealing with the deaths of society's members when they occur.

Birth and death together make societies and their institutions necessary. From an evolutionary viewpoint, birth and death must continue to occur for the survival of the species. Society, institutions, and culture develop to ensure this process. Social interaction between individuals leads to common or patterned group behaviors that become institutionalized to ensure that the appropriate required tasks are carried out. For example, infants are helpless and must depend upon caregivers, usually their mothers, to be nurtured early in life. Secure attachment bonds between mother and infant ensure that infants will be fed, loved, and provided with the necessary care for at least the early stages of development. The interaction and organization of individuals into a society makes this more possible than mothers acting alone.

Innovations in society (e.g., developing new technology to pro-duce more food in a shorter amount of time) lead to a more efficient and advanced society which in turn allows societal members more freedom and time to further develop both society and themselves. The more the latter occurs, the more sophisticated and diverse institutions serving society's members become.

Definition of Culture

We have a basic need to create meaning to help interpret the world around us, including both the world of the living and the dead. But what is a meaning? A meaning is the interpretation that people attach to an experience. A meaning is established when a symbol is used to represent some other object or situation. For example, the symbol "chair" is used to represent the object that one sits on. When we now identify that object with the symbol "chair" the object has meaning. When we use symbols to interpret or represent our experiences we establish meanings that may be public or private. If others use the same symbols to interpret the same experiences then meanings become public (Baumeister, 1991).

Culture is a set of meanings created by society, manifested in values, beliefs, and norms to regulate the requirements of the societal institutions and the group behaviors necessary to fulfill these requirements.

Culture can be defined as all that in human society which is socially rather than biologically transmitted (DeSpelder & Strickland, 2002). This definition encompasses both material and nonmaterial components. Material culture consists of things (such manufactured objects as buildings and consumer goods) and physical manifestations of the life of a people. The nonmaterial aspects of a culture relate to the realm of ideas, beliefs, values, norms, and customs. Depending upon changing circumstances and subsequent reevaluation of the culture, individuals can and do change their culture over time.

Cultural values, norms, and beliefs regulate and advance development of institutions in society and the concomitant patterns of group behavior needed to carry out the functions of these institutions. This helps individuals gain a greater sense of certainty (or at least pre-dictability) and stability in the world they inhabit. And the more advanced the society, the better it can provide certainty and stability to its members from the unpredictability of both natural and social forces that could disrupt not only the functioning of existing society but its further growth as well.

Culture helps create a society that involves an orderly or stable world that allows individuals to satisfy needs, survive, and grow. As individuals assimilate cultural meanings, they have rules to guide their daily behavior in a predictable fashion. There is a sense of certainty that one is living in a stable and predictable world, thereby increasing one's sense of security and the opportunities for indi-vidual development. It also motivates one to learn and gain new knowledge about oneself and one's environment, and to learn the skills necessary to cope with a variety of problems. As individuals continue to experience greater occupational success and achieve-ments acknowledged by others, they also gain greater acceptance and status within society. They feel a sense of belonging and an increased sense of self-worth that makes it possible to deal more effectively with any threatening situations such as the uncertainty surrounding many circumstances of life.

Cultures can also change and develop over time by borrowing ideas and tools from other cultures, by inventions arising within the culture, by the advancement of technology, and by a crisis that forces change. In the end, individuals may become part of a more effective and efficient society and culture, which in turn enhances their confidence in themselves to cope with any unpre-dicted problems.

SOCIAL INSTITUTIONS CONCERNED WITH DEATH

Various institutions exist to maintain and promote the further development of society itself. Others may exist to satisfy the needs, development, pleasures, and leisure activities of individual mem-bers of the society. However, other institutions exist to deal directly with the death of societal members, and certain institutions func-tion indirectly to deal with certain problems associated with death (e.g., life insurance companies). Facing and dealing with death is the ultimate challenge of life and societal and cultural institutions help to prepare individuals for such a challenge.

According to Corr, Nabe, and Corr (2000), every society has some form of death system. They state that the death system may be "formal, explicit, and widely acknowledged in some of its aspects, even while it is largely hidden and often unspoken in other aspects . . . no society is without some system for coping with the fundamental realities that death presents to human existence" (pp. 78–79).

Direct Effect of Certain Institutions

Kastenbaum (1995) also maintains that every society has some form of death system, a system of institutions that formally or informally deals with the problems of death, dying, and bereavement in society. Each society's death system has its own basic components and typical functions. According to Kastenbaum, the components of a death system are: (a) people, those whose roles and institutions lead them to deal directly with death, such as medical examiners, coroners, funeral directors, and so on, (b) places, that is, specific locations that are identified with death, such as cemeteries, funeral homes, historic battlefields, hospital terminal wards, and so on, (c) times, that is, occasions that are associated with death, such as Memorial Day, the anniversary of a deceased family member, and so on, (d) objects, that is, things whose attributes link them to death, such as death certificates, hearses, obituaries, death notices in the newspapers, the gallows, electric chair, tombstones, shrouds, and so on, and (e) symbols, that is, objects and actions that indicate death, such as skull and crossbones, wearing of a black armband, use of euphemisms, and so on.

These components are put together in various ways to help carry out certain functions. It is these functions that are the core of the death system. These functions are carried out by societal members in various roles representing different institutions that deal directly with death.

Perhaps the most basic or general functions of society are to protect people from unnecessary or premature death, to assist the dying individual, and to deal with death when it occurs. Such functions can be accomplished in various ways by many specific institutions. According to Kastenbaum (1995), the following are among the important functions of the death system:

- *Development and use of warning systems to alert people to avoid life-threatening situations.* The weather bureau provides warnings for hurricanes, tornadoes, floods, blizzards, dust storms, and the like, whereas police departments and various civil preparedness agencies warn of forest or brush fires, avalanche conditions, tidal waves, earthquakes, fallen trees and electrical wires, and so on. Specific techniques can be used, such as periodic bulletins of changing weather conditions, sirens or flashing lights to indicate immediate danger in certain situations, or the erection of signs and barricades to limit access to dangerous areas. Such an approach can prevent unnecessary deaths by helping individuals to avoid or prepare for dangerous situations.
- *Development of more effective police agencies.* Establishment of police departments, development of emergency facilities (such as the 911 telephone system), and training of officers in lifesaving techniques all help to protect citizens from being killed by immoral or irrational individuals within the society.
- *Enactment and enforcement of laws and regulations to provide safe working and living conditions and to alert consumers to the dangers of products sold in the marketplace.* This includes such diverse activities as workplace regulations through Occupational Safety and Health Administration (OSHA), standards for housing and water supplies, warnings on products such as cigarettes, warnings regarding the side effects of certain products or medications, and so on.
- *Promotion of the improved diagnosis, treatment, and prognosis of life-threatening diseases.* This includes a variety of public health activities at both the national and local levels (e.g., vaccinations), as well as the provision of basic research funds to seek cures for other life threatening disease (e.g., cancer, AIDS).
- *Emergency treatment of dying individuals.* This includes the establishment and staffing of facilities to restore or save lives on an emergency basis, either in the field or in an emergency room or hospital.

- *Provision of care for the dying.* This includes establishment and use of various institutions such as home care, hospitals, hospices, nursing homes, and so on, to provide comfort and humane care to dying individuals.
- *Improvement of the quality of care for the dying.* Research, training of personnel, and establishing of standards for care of terminal patients are all directed to the objective of creating conditions so that a "good death" can occur. The well-known SUPPORT study (Steinhauser, Christakis, Clipp, McNeilly, McIntyre, & Tulsky, 2000) identified many of the desires of dying patients and their families members in regard to end-of-life care. These desires included such things as freedom from pain, being treated with dignity, being kept clean, knowing what to expect, being comfortable with one's nurse, trusting one's doctor, sharing time with loved ones and close friends, and so on. Societal institutions still need to implement many of these requests by patients so that terminally ill patients can die in comfort and dignity.
- *Determination of death and disposal of the body.* When a person dies, important societal functions are to examine the body and to pronounce the person legally dead (typically carried out by a physician or coroner), to establish the cause of death (which may entail an autopsy), to issue a death certificate, and to carry out disposal of the dead body (typically carried out by a mortician in compliance with legal requirements and the wishes of surviving family members). Today, disposal of the body involves many choices, such as cremation, burial underground, interment in tombs or mausoleums, burial at sea, or even propulsion of the cremated remains to outer space.
- *Carrying out of funeral rites and helping the bereaved survivors.* Religious institutions, funeral homes, government institutions, and so on provide forms for carrying out funeral rites, although these may vary depending on the religious beliefs of the deceased and family, or the former occupation of the deceased. Other social service institutions help the bereaved to deal with their grieving process (e.g., Widow-to-Widow, Compassionate Friends). Society may facilitate the grieving process by helping the individual to make sense of the loved person's death through the use of religious and philosophic beliefs.

- *Protection of society through socially sanctioned killing.* Laws and social institutions allow for the killing of either humans or animals under carefully defined conditions in order to help protect society when it is threatened, such as training citizens for war, capital punishment, justified killing of certain lawbreakers by police, slaughtering of animals for food, or exterminating them when they carry harmful diseases.

One might add another function to Kastenbaum's (1995) list:

- *Regulating the ending of life through rational suicide, passive euthanasia, and physician-assisted suicide.* Another societal function is to establish laws and regulations dealing with ending the lives of terminally ill individuals. This would include regulating the means by which rational suicide may be carried out (e.g., availability of barbiturates), establishing conditions under which medical treatment of the terminally ill may be refused, withheld, or withdrawn, and (in Oregon) establishing conditions under which physicians may act to hasten the death of a terminally ill individual. In addition, a developing function is to counsel those who desire to end their lives, and also help to prevent individuals from ending their lives if they are not ready for it (Cicirelli, 2001a).

All death systems have important functions in society, although just which functions are implemented and how these functions are accomplished varies from one society to another. Primitive societies may implement only a few of these functions, whereas modern industrialized societies may implement most or all of these functions, elaborated at highly complex levels.

Indirect Effects of Certain Institutions

Kastenbaum (1995) also indicates that various individuals carry out roles in other societal institutions that are indirectly related to the death system. They participate in death-related activities but they have other main functions in society, such as florists (floral tributes), insurance agents (life and accident insurance), and so on. The federal government provides Social Security and Medicare to provide for medical care and financial security of older adults, many of whom might die earlier without help. Pension plans through employers and various financial institutions provide additional financial security for later life and for the survivors of the deceased.

Lawyers and the court system provide for the establishment of such things as wills and trusts to assure that the wishes of the deceased are carried out regarding division of assets, the orderly payments of debts owed by the deceased, transfer of remaining property to rightful heirs, and so on. In addition, the legal profession can assist citizens to prepare legal advance directives (for example, living wills, durable power of attorney) to specify the wishes of individuals regarding care at the end of life should they become decisionally incapacitated, and to assist in securing the implementation of these wishes where necessary.

Educational establishments, public health agencies, spas, and health clubs attempt to alter individuals' lifestyles and instill healthy habits of living in hope of delaying the onset or reducing the rate of decline in chronic or life-threatening diseases.

Governments at various levels enact laws and enforcement procedures to promote public health and safety (such as making cars safer, requiring use of fuels with fewer pollutants, requiring use of safety belts, setting driving speed limits and other traffic laws, establishing strict standards regarding food additives and bacterial content, etc.) to protect people from ill health, injury, or death.

Many religious institutions within the society help to provide individuals with some sense of the meaning of life and death, give them solace when dying, and help them live their lives with greater well-being as they integrate religious beliefs into life.

The family influences the individual's death meanings, fears, and views of the dying process, as well as the way in which the individual interacts with the larger death system. Families may think, feel, and behave in ways that are assimilated by their individual members. Also, certain family members' attitudes regarding the grieving process for a dead loved one can shape the grieving responses of other individuals within the family.

The media (television, radio, newspapers, magazines, books, films, videos, cassettes, and compact discs) communicate ideas, values, and norms about death and also explore death-related issues. In this way, the ideas, values, norms, and beliefs of the culture are transmitted to large numbers of people, and changes in values and norms are promoted (e.g., the right-to-die movement). Sometimes individuals develop attitudes toward death or means of coping with death from the messages received. Additionally, the manner in which grief is expressed by families of famous people who died (e.g., the Kennedy family following the assassination of the president) may influence others to grieve in a certain manner.

Major events and forces acting on the society can bring about changes in the sociocultural meanings of death. For example, if an uncontrollable plague or catastrophic war were to cause the death of a large portion of the population, then the institutions of society may be forced to change which in turn may change the socialization processes influencing individuals in that society. In a further example, individuals may import new ideas from other cultures which change the sociocultural meanings of death, which in turn change various social institutions. The important point is that societal or publicly shared meanings of death existing within the present culture or new meanings arising from other influences are the basis for regulating the functioning of institutions that directly or indirectly deal with death. These sociocultural meanings, along with the unique characteristics and experiences of individuals, are the basis for the formation of the individual's personal meanings of death. The personal meanings of death are important at the individual level as they influence how a person will live, his or her reactions to death, and the preparation for his or her own death.

MULTILEVEL MEANINGS OF DEATH

As previously mentioned, the implementation of cultural values, norms, and beliefs by members of a society allow them to achieve, develop skills, and experience acceptance, support, and success in life which in turn increases their sense of security and self-worth. This allows them to cope with death, and the threat or fear of death in a more effective manner (Greenberg, Solomon, & Pyszczynski, 1997). This, of course, is not as true of primitive, preindustrial, and rural societies. In such societies, death is highly unpredictable and when it occurs, society is more interested in maintaining its survival as a collective unit than in emphasizing the individual (Marshall, 1980).

Death not only poses a fundamental threat to the certainty, order, and stability of society but also to the cultural meanings concerned with death. Broad cultural meanings of death may vary with different societies, e.g., some cultures may be fatalistic towards death, some may deny death, or some may defy or accept death. However, there seem to be multilevels of sociocultural meanings of death, and one may have to deal with them separately to understand their effect on society. With this in mind, four different levels of sociocultural meaning of death are identified.

Biological Meaning

The first level of death meanings is the biological level, where the occurrence of death is simply a fact of life. Even in primitive societies, others would know that death occurred when no further movement existed in the human body and when putrefaction took place. At this point, societies needed to develop ways of coping with disposal of the dead. However, to function more effectively, a second level of death meanings is involved.

Biosocial Meaning

At the biosocial level of death meanings, an attempt is made to determine the precise moment of death. Many functions of society depend upon this knowledge, which helps to determine whether or not a homicide occurred, who is the rightful heir to a particular inheritance, when organ transplants can be made, when the process of cryonics should begin, when people should be buried to avoid being buried alive (as can be the case in some cultures or underdeveloped countries where embalming is not allowed or practiced), when a person wishes to use the knowledge of the time left to live to control events that will occur following death, and so on.

However, the precise moment of death is not an objective fact, but is an interpretation of the process of death using a shared meaning by experts or of society as a whole. Unfortunately, society is still struggling to find a common shared meaning to define the precise moment of death. To do so, three issues must be resolved.

What Criteria Should Be Used to Establish Time of Death?

The first issue involves making a value judgment as to whether the precise moment of death should depend upon total cessation of all bodily functioning or upon the cessation of one or more key bodily functions (such as heartbeat or respiration). Additionally, judgments must be made regarding the existence of possible exceptions to a general rule for deciding whether a person is still alive or dead.

For example, when an individual's bodily functions are maintained by artificial means (e.g., use of a ventilator) is the individual still alive? For how long should society judge that person to be alive when life is maintained by artificial means?

A subissue is how to determine when total cessation of key bodily functions has actually occurred under natural conditions. Sometimes individuals are pronounced dead when there is no heartbeat or respiration, and yet they may be resuscitated if medical personnel are sufficiently persistent. Or spontaneous remission may occur, which suggests the existence of some kind of suspended animation. Even when all major bodily functions appear to have ceased, there still may be minute amounts of blood and oxygen still flowing that cannot be detected by our present instrumentation.

Some experts use lack of brain function as a criterion for death. But even when a person is considered brain-dead, one may still detect small local electrical currents occurring in certain parts of the brain. These are usually ignored because they seem to be random and do not seem relevant to regulating any function. But the fact of their existence would seem to violate the criterion of total brain death. (Of course, a less stringent definition of brain death is useful in avoiding delay in organ transplants.)

Irreversibility of Functioning

The second issue in determining time of death is to determine the time of irreversibility, that is, the time when reversibility of bodily functioning is no longer possible. One must be certain that, when a person is pronounced dead, there is no possibility that this state can be reversed. This is not always easy to accomplish. There have been cases when people were pronounced dead but later regained consciousness in a mortuary. In other cases, when there was an exhumation for some reason, it appeared that the individual had regained consciousness after burial because the body was turned or clothes were partially torn off.

One suggested criterion for brain death is that no electrical activity in the brain can be detected over a 24-hour period of observation. But is this a sufficient time period? How long should one wait? How many assessments of electrical activity should be made before one gives up? As medical personnel know, brain activity can be eliminated for a time by cold, alcohol, and barbiturates. Could other factors eliminate it for longer periods of time?

There is another possibility. With today's technology, skin, nail, or muscle cells can be detected to be alive and active well after a person is pronounced dead by other criteria (even if heart, lungs, and brain are not functioning). At some future time, reversibility of death may be possible working only with still living cells of an otherwise dead individual. Scientists might take any living cell from the body, and with sophisticated techniques generate other types of cells, reconstruct tissues and organs, and regulate the coordination of physiological systems to have a living human being again. In this futuristic case, the precise moment for pronouncing death would be changed dramatically from today's criteria. This indicates that the pronouncement of death doesn't necessarily correspond to what is considered final biological death. It is a biosocial judgment made at a given moment in time relative to the advancement of technology.

Philosophic Values

The third issue involved in deciding the precise moment of death involves philosophic values rather than technology. The question is: What are the criteria for deciding an entity is a living human being rather than just a living being? (This complicated issue is also related to questions surrounding abortion.) For example, suppose an individual's cerebrum is destroyed and he or she is in a permanent vegetative state. The brain stem is intact so there is spontaneous breathing, heart beat, and maintaining of homeostasis of chemicals in the blood but there will never be consciousness, awareness, or cognitive functioning again. Self-identity or personhood is gone forever. Some scholars would pronounce the person dead on the basis of cognitive death, i.e., no cerebral functioning. Other scholars would argue that the person is still alive because basic biological functions are still occurring. Who is correct? At the present time, the majority takes the second position. However, if positions were to shift, what would society do? If the person were pronounced dead, could one proceed to bury a biologically functioning body? Or should one keep such permanently cognitively dead people with a functioning body in a special institution until their bodily functioning finally stopped?

These issues make it difficult to determine not only when the precise moment of death occurs but whether a body is in fact dead. In turn, these issues have implications for society's decisions regarding disposal of a dead body. Determinations of death are not precise biological facts, but are relative to time and place based on biosocial meanings of death agreed upon by a given society. Thus, the pronouncement of death does not correspond to the fact of death; it can change relative to advances in technology and different conceptions of philosophy concerning the meaning of life and death.

Sociocultural Meaning

The third level of death meanings involves sociocultural meanings of death within a culture. It is concerned with the roles that societal members assume in carrying out the tasks of the societal death system. There are many issues here, depending upon the particular culture or subculture. For example, how does the culture of one's society determine disposal of the dead body? Is cremation allowed? Burial at sea? Disposal in outer space? Or simply a traditional underground burial? What are the funeral rites? What are the customs regarding the grieving process? What are the legal aspects of distributing the dead person's financial resources, and so on? In short, a society's cultural meanings regarding death would regulate these and other such death-related activities.

Common interactions and experiences with other members of society lead to the socialization of individuals to the common cultural meanings of death and their implications for practice in maintaining the function of society in dealing with the public concerns of death. This process is carried on from one generation to the next (Moller, 1996).

Death motivates society and culture to protect members against death or the threat of death and influences society and culture to develop institutions to provide individuals with knowledge, skills, values, and beliefs to help them cope with death. But the occurrence of death, especially the death of large numbers of people in some tragedy, or the death of a few prominent but loved people, or the death of key people needed to run the country, or the frightening death of victims of disturbed killers can be disruptive of the normal functioning of society. Such deaths may influence the sociocultural meanings of death to enable the society to deal with such situations.

Conversely, sociocultural meanings of death can have an influence on death itself or the threat of death. Social institutions erected to protect people from death may be modified in many ways to enable such institutions to educate, train, and support members to be better prepared for death, giving them greater confidence to deal with death when it occurs.

Sociocultural meanings of death are common or publicly shared meanings. Once formed, they continue to influence members of society as they are passed on from generation to another. Kastenbaum (2000a) has identified four sociocultural meanings of death that have persisted for at least a century and which will likely continue with perhaps some modifications into the future. They are: (a) death is a punishment for a life of sloth or sin, (b) death brings deliverance from misery, (c) death is a natural end to this life but is also the beginning to a better life that we can hardly imagine, and (d) death is a junkyard for the failed, worn, and obsolete.

As members of society are socialized to assimilate such sociocultural meanings of death, they are influenced to regulate group
behavior by implementing certain roles to deal with the dying and
dead in society. Sociocultural meanings of death are interpretations of how group members should view death, helping them learn
to alleviate death fears, and develop greater confidence in coping
with death more effectively.

Personal Meanings

The fourth level of death meanings involves the personal meanings of death (about which more will be said in the next chapter).
As individuals progress through the years of adulthood, their sense
of self-identity continues to develop and they begin to view themselves as a person independent of society as a whole. They go
beyond thinking about death according to roles and norms pre-
scribed by the culture to derive personal or unique meanings of
death, interpreting what death means for them relative to their
own identity, recognizing fears of their own death, and attempting to developing strategies to cope with death. Although personal
meanings of death may be loosely based on the sociocultural meanings of death, they are modified and shaped by the individual's
own experiences in life and by personality traits.

Personal meanings of death are unique or private to the person.
They may be extensions or modifications of shared cultural meanings or they may be entirely new innovations. Such personal meanings of death influence the way the individual lives his or her life
relative to the restrictions that death places on it, the individual's
reactions to the prospect of his or her own death as well as preparations for it.

This level of death meanings is not primarily concerned with
the deaths of others. It is concerned with the meanings of death
for a particular individual in relation to his or her own eventual
death, and the implications of these meanings for the individual's
own life on earth and any anticipated life after death.

In sum, the multilevel meanings of death indicate that death
can be experienced at various levels either separately or simultaneously. Also, the levels of death meanings can reciprocally inter-

act with one another. For example, if a terribly mutilated and decaying body is found near a highway, an apparent victim of a hit-and-run accident, at the level of biological meaning the body is clearly dead; at the level of biosocial meaning it may be difficult to decide on any criteria to determine the precise moment of death (which might be important to determine cause of death or settle questions of inheritance); at the sociocultural level of meaning, social customs may influence the disposal of the body (including such questions as use of cosmetic restoration, open- or closed-casket funeral ceremony, or immediate cremation); at the level of personal meaning, the death may influence survivors' personal meanings of death (perhaps leading them to conclude that the time of one's death is always uncertain, and that one must find better ways to deal with such uncertainty). Survivors whose death meanings have changed as a result of this death may seek certain laws to improve safety on the highways, which in turn may reduce the number of deaths where the precise moment of death cannot be determined, and also may allow formulation of better criteria to judge the occurrence of death without any qualification.

IMPACT OF DEATH ON SOCIETY

The death of society members can temporarily disrupt or permanently alter the way that society functions. The society will have to make a greater effort to restore and maintain its original functioning, or modify itself to reach a new level of functioning. In either case, societal changes may lead to cultural and personal changes in meanings of death, and the latter may in turn change how societal members and individuals deal with death. One needs to consider how changes in certain basic factors can alter the number of members in a society and hence disrupt societal functioning.

Demographic Changes

The impact of death on society can be felt through shifts in the birth and death rates of a country. If birth and death rates of a country or the world remain in balance, then a stable population is maintained. But if birth rates increase and death rates decline, then the population increases for all age groups, that is, there is a general increase in population.

In recent decades, the world population has increased from one billion to nearly six billion people (Ehrlich, 1968, 1990). Ehrlich warns that the population of the world could become so great that it might exceed the resources of the planet and eventually lead to one or more dysfunctional societies. Excessive numbers of people in a society relative to resources reduce the quality of life for most people in the society, and can lead to mass migration of people to other countries. Given such a situation, cultural meanings of death may change, that is, many types of death are considered more acceptable because the value of life itself is less important. (As a result, cultural meanings of death arising from population pressure may conflict with other religious or philosophic values of the same culture.)

On the other hand, birth rates may decline while death rates remain stable or increase. Singer (1999) discusses the views of experts who have begun to describe a trend which is called a demographic transition. Such a transition takes place when birth rates are changing from high to low or vice versa in modern society. The transition that is now occurring in modern society is that high birth rates are shifting to low birth rates. Experts had felt that birth and death rates would become relatively equal and the population of society would level off and remain stable. However, Singer goes on to conclude that this is wrong. Birth rates have declined in a number of countries but so have death rates (or at most the latter have remained stable). This means that certain countries are shrinking in total number of people but simultaneously increasing in the percentage of elderly people. This situation results in societies that cannot maintain their present total population or the balance between young and old. In order for the population of a society to replace itself, it takes 2.1 children per mother. Many countries in the world now have replacement rates below 2.1, achieving a population drain instead of zero population growth. This is a phenomenon occurring in many countries worldwide, e.g., United Kingdom, Italy, France, Germany, Singapore, and Japan. If this trend continues, world population will soon reach a peak based on earlier birth rates and then decline will be dramatic. Such a shrinking population involving fewer young people and proportionally more elderly will eventually be disruptive to society because qualified people will not be available to fill certain occupational roles needed to maintain the adequate functioning of society. Some societies may become dysfunctional to the point that the social order will have to change, which in turn may modify the cultural meanings of death.

The United States may escape this phenomenon to a certain degree because of the high level of immigration at the present time, but with continued immigration comes an increasing diversity of people that may go beyond an optimum level. (Individuals seem to prefer an ethnic/racially integrated society if equality between the groups exists, and intermarriage may accelerate integration. However, when inequality of resources and status exists between different ethnic/racial groups, they may voluntarily prefer separatism. If separatism were to increase in the United States, societal members may have difficulty interacting and communicating on the basis of similar values, beliefs, and norms, and balkanization of the country may begin to emerge.) In an extremely multicultural society, cultural meanings in general and cultural meanings of death in particular may change and become too diverse to reflect the common values, beliefs, and norms needed to maintain a cohesive society.

Sociocultural Meanings of Death for Different Age Segments of the Society

Another aspect of population change should also be considered. If the total number of people in the nation remains the same but there is a dramatic shift in the proportion of young, middle-aged, or elderly, then different age-related views of certain groups of people in society will determine the values, norms, and beliefs, possibly resulting in changes in sociocultural meanings of death.

However, this is an area (sociocultural and personal meanings of death for different age groups) where both existing knowledge and research programs are scarce. We do know from existing studies that the development of conceptions of death in childhood seems to follow a sequence beginning with personal conceptions of death in early childhood (e.g., death as sleep, or personification of death as a bogeyman) and ending with a relatively clear understanding of objective death by the preteen years. Gradual socialization of the child in matters related to death leads to the understanding of death's universality, irreversibility, nonfunctionality, and causality, and the beginnings of ideas about noncorporeal continuation after death (Brent & Speece, 1993; Nagy, 1948; Speece & Brent, 1996). Once such basic concepts have been established, whether as the result of a general maturing of thought processes or the result of specific experiences with death, other more enriched and elaborated sociocultural and personal meanings of death emerge and change over the rest of the life span.

However, our knowledge of both the sociocultural and personal meanings of death for adolescents, young adults, middle-aged adults and elders is limited for the society in general and for subgroups of society in particular. Even in terms of what we do know, it is difficult to determine the common or shared sociocultural meanings and independent personal meanings that might exist for each age group.

However, some general age profiles can be suggested. Aside from the subgroup of adolescents who have difficulty developing a sense of identity, who are overly sensitive, and who contemplate or carry out suicide, the majority of adolescents tend to be idealistic, romantic, and high risk-takers. Culturally, adolescents seem to perceive death as too remote to consider, despite frequent losses of their peers to drug overdose and auto accidents. It is not the length but quality of life that it is important for them. Feeling invulnerable, adolescents often risk death to prove their manhood or womanhood or to satisfy a need for excitement and adventure (Kastenbaum, 1995, 2000b).

Early adulthood is the time when most individuals break away from their parental home. The young adult is beginning a career, possibly getting married, setting up a home, having children, and so on. This is also the time when hopes, dreams, and ambitions in life all seem possible. Thus, for many young adults, death may mean the interruption of one's goals and the end of one's dreams in life. Such a shared cultural meaning of death would lead to the avoidance of activities or events (e.g., war) that might lead to the frustration of dying without attaining one's dreams. Thus, a society of predominantly young adults who are settling into careers and family life would tend to be a relatively more conservative society than one composed of predominantly late adolescents. Deaths forcing change in society would seem to be very disruptive.

By middle age, individuals begin to realize that changes in priorities may be necessary as they may not be able to fulfill all their goals and dreams. Death begins to mean a finitude of life; the middle-aged begin to experience their vulnerabilities due to declining physical and mental abilities. Also, there is a culmination of meaningful, ongoing relationships with spouse, children, siblings, other relatives, and friends. Death can mean the end of these important relationships. A society dominated by middle-aged people would also tend to be conservative, attempting to maintain all the material goods, wealth, and relationships accumulated over the years. Again, deaths that led to changes in society might be seen as quite disruptive.

In old age, people experience greater awareness of their closeness to death and many begin to prepare for life's ending. They may be motivated to try to find out whether life has meaning and purpose in spite of accumulated struggles and disappointments. It would seem that death-related forces changing society would not be as disrupting if society were predominantly composed of older people, as their vested interest in life would have begun to decline. Much more information is needed regarding the sociocultural meanings of death for all age groups but even more so for the elderly.

Different Types of Death

Different types of death may have impacts on society differing both in kind and degree. Mass deaths, as in wars or natural disasters, can be very destructive and disruptive to a society not only in terms of the mass killing of people but the need to rebuild society's infrastructure. Also, such mass deaths may threaten everyone's basic need for self-preservation. Alternatively, the death of a leader who is very important (e.g., the assassinations of President Kennedy and Dr. Martin Luther King) and the intense grief of members of the society may disrupt the functioning of that society for years to come. Thus, the number and status of individuals who die and the conditions under which death occurs are factors disrupting societal functioning. Other factors disrupting societal function may be the degree to which certain types of death are regarded as acceptable or nonacceptable by members of the society. Certain types of death may violate ethical standards or safety standards or they may involve conflict between different subgroups of society (e.g., abortion).

By reviewing some of the major types of death, one can get a better idea of how certain types of death can disrupt societal functioning and hence possibly shift sociocultural meanings of death.

Accidents

An accident can be defined as an unintentional act (Aiken, 2001). During 1997 (National Safety Council, 1999) 46.8% of accidental deaths were caused by motor vehicles, 18% by falls, and approximately 9% by solid or liquid poisoning. A smaller percentage was caused by drowning, fires and burns, suffocation, firearms, and gas or vapor poisoning. Motor vehicles have been the primary cause of accidental deaths for decades, with incompetence in driving, alcohol consumption, and vehicle defects important contributory causes.

From the perspective of location, falls are the top ranking cause of fatal accidents in the home, followed by poisoning by solids and liquids. Fires, burns, and deaths associated with fires are third, suffocation by ingested objects is fourth, followed by drowning, firearms, mechanical suffocation, and poisoning by gases and vapors.

From the standpoint of age, firearms are the leading cause of death in the 15 to 24 age range and the death rate for accidents due to motor vehicles is quite high. For those beyond age 74, accidents due to other factors, such as sensory defects and lack of motor coordination become more important.

According to Aiken (2001), fatal accidents that occur at home, in public, and at work are the result of the combination of unsafe conditions with unsafe acts by people in those conditions. A combination of unsafe acts and exposure to unsafe conditions increases the likelihood of accidents, including fatal accidents. Aiken also cited various studies relating personality factors to such accidents. For example, accident repeaters were less emotionally stable, were more hostile toward authority, were higher in anxiety, and had more problems getting along with other people (Shaw & Sichel, 1971). Another study indicated that people who were excessively ambitious with revengeful attitudes had a higher than average accident rate (McGuire, 1976).

If an accident happens purely by chance, little can be done and it is no one's fault. However, most accidents occur because of a combination of unsafe environments and unsafe behavior. For example, a young child who cannot swim impulsively jumps into the deep end of a pool with no lifeguard on duty. A teenager drives fast around a mountain curve and there is no outer rail on the road. An old man with slow reaction time drives up to a railroad crossing where there is no gate or red light. All these examples depict individual accidents. Each alone may not disrupt society but if the frequency of such individual accidents is high, then disruptions may occur.

Deaths from attacks by natural predators, although not considered to be accidental, are unexpected events that can cause great social upset and even panic if there are repeated attacks in a given area. Deaths off the New Jersey coast resulting from predations of a great white shark early in the 20th century are an example (Capuzzo, 2001).

Technological Accidents and Catastrophic Events

Certain types of accidents and natural events may kill many people simultaneously. They are termed catastrophic because they involve the deaths of large numbers of people. They occur in a brief period of time and bring sudden and great misfortune.

Such natural disasters include earthquakes, tornadoes, floods, tidal waves, cyclones, volcanic eruptions, mudslides, landslides, avalanches, forest fires or wildfires, crippling snowstorms, cold waves, heat waves, blizzards, lightening, and famines, with most of these events causing substantial loss of life (Brunner, 1999). For example, in 1925, tornadoes across six states killed 792 people. In 1935, the tidal surge accompanying a huge hurricane washed over the Florida Keys and swept 408 people to their deaths in the ocean. In 1981, a volcanic eruption of Mount St. Helen's, Washington, led to the death of 60 people. In 1985, a devastating earthquake hit Mexico City and surrounding states without warning, killing almost 25,000 people. In 1969, floods and mudslides in Southern California caused 100 deaths. The great blizzard of 1888 resulted in some 400 deaths. The list could go on and on.

Large-scale accidents include such things as train wrecks, multiple car wrecks, airline crashes, ships sinking, bridges collapsing, dams breaking, large building fires, and so on. For example (Brunner, 1999), the 1969 American Airlines crash in Chicago killed 275 persons, a 1990 night club fire in New York City killed 87, a 1993 ferry capsized off Haiti drowning over 1,000 passengers, and a 1993 train wreck on a bridge near Mobile, Alabama, killed 47.

Technological accidents may also cause loss of life at the level of catastrophic natural disasters and accidents. For example (Brunner, 1999), when a nuclear power plant exploded at Chernobyl in 1986, radioactivity was released over a large area with deaths estimated to be in the thousands. An explosion of a ship moored in Texas City, Texas, killed 516 in 1947. The worlds worst industrial accident occurred in 1984 when gaseous methyl isocyanate escaped from Union Carbide's pesticide plant in Bhopal, India, bringing death to 2,000 people living near the plant.

Natural disasters and accidents disrupt society not only in terms of the numbers of lives lost and the monetary damages. These catastrophic events affect the society in many other ways, such as the loss of certain people needed for societal functions in certain geographical areas, the degree of bereavement involved, and the agonizing appraisal that the accident could have been avoided, prevented, or its impact reduced if only certain precautions had been carried out (e.g., better warning systems could have been developed along with more efficient evacuation procedures of people from certain danger areas).

Killing

Intentionally or unintentionally causing the death of one or more members of one's own or other societies is regarded as killing.

However, different types of killing can be either encouraged, tolerated, or punished by the society.

War

War is sanctioned by society as a legitimate means of defending the national interest or protecting the homeland. However, there is often inconsistency or conflict between members of a society regarding the need and justification for a war. Different factions of society may be for and against war, for example, the Vietnam war, which was very unpopular among the younger generation and led to much social conflict. One might question war from the perspective of Judeo-Christian values or ethics, which hold that one should not kill. If so, what justifies the killing that takes place in a war? Why is killing viewed as murder in one situation but viewed as heroic in a war? Suppose one is facing an enemy soldier and is pulling the trigger to shoot when an officer yells, "The war is over! The enemy has surrendered!" But one's bullet leaves the gun just at that instant, killing the enemy soldier. Is it murder or heroism? Does a fraction of a second determine its meaning? Again, cultural conflict between those who participate in just wars, those who participate in unjust wars, and those conscientious objectors who refuse to participate in any wars may lead to disruptions in society and cultural conflicts, possibly modifying the cultural meaning of death.

Also, mega-deaths occurring in wars disrupt the functioning of society for many years (Aiken, 2001; Davies, 1996). In World War I, Germany had approximately 1,800,000 military deaths, Russia had 1,700,000, France had 1,400,000, Austria-Hungary had 1,200,000, Britain had 900,000, Italy had 600,000, Romania had 300,000, and Turkey had 300,000. In the World War II, the U.S.S.R. had 6,800,000 military deaths, Germany had 3,200,000, China had 1,300,000, Japan had 1,900,000, Poland had 700,000, the United States had 500,000, and Britain had 400,000. Such loss of life, along with the loss of money and property certainly caused great dislocations in these countries. These wars had political justifications. However, other wars throughout history were fought in the name of God to secure religious goals with great concomitant loss of life, such as the Crusaders vs. Moslems, Irish Catholics vs. Protestants,

Catholics vs. Puritans, Christians vs. heretics, Christians vs. Mormons, Jews vs. Arabs, Hindus vs. Moslems, and so on. From such examples, one can easily visualize the disruption of society when societies go to war over religious or cultural conflicts.

Genocide

Genocide is the attempt to kill or exterminate an entire ethnic, national, or religious group. One of most publicized examples was the Nazi attempt to exterminate the Jews. However, there are many examples throughout history (Kearl, 1989; Parkes, 1996; Rummel, 1995), for example, English-American settlers' attempt to exterminate the Native Americans, the Turks attempt to exterminate the Armenians in the early part of the 20th century, India's attempt to exterminate the Bangladeshi, the Chinese attempt to eliminate the Tibetans, the Serbs attempt to eliminate the Bosnians, the Hutu massacre of the Tutsi tribes in Africa, and so on.

Homicide

Homicide is the killing of one person by another. Justifiable homicide is killing in self-defense or to protect another person. In manslaughter, there is no intent to kill but the death of another occurs because of negligence, for example, reckless driving. Finally, murder is the intended killing of another. Second degree murder is deliberate but not premeditated, whereas first degree murder is both deliberate and premeditated.

Historically, about one third of murders in the United States are committed by family members, one third by coworkers or friends, and one third by strangers. The latter category has increased recently with an increase in brutal, motiveless, and random murders. One is more likely to die a violent death in the United States than in most other Western industrialized nations. The United States is a paradox; professing to be one of the most religious nations, but simultaneously being one of the most violent and with the highest crime rate. Over the decade of the 1990s, an average of about 20,000 people a year were murdered in the United States (Brunner, 1999).

Feticide

It is the killing of an unborn fetus, accomplished either by killing the mother (and indirectly killing the unborn fetus) or by killing an unborn fetus directly. Feticide has occurred through history in wars and for ideological reasons. Today, we have an ongoing controversy as to whether the killing of a fetus through abortion should be legal. This partially depends upon whether one considers the fetus (even in the early stages of growth) merely a living being or a living human being. Additionally, there is an issue surrounding the woman's autonomy to make a choice whether or not to bear a child. There is also an issue of justifiable feticide when abortion is carried out to protect the life of the mother. In any event, the issue is not settled and feticides continue to occur. Regardless of the numbers involved, the ongoing conflict disrupts society at an ideological level. The current debate over the use of unwanted embryos for stem cell research, in the hope of finding cures for various diseases, is an extension of the same fundamental argument.

In other countries (e.g., China and India), female fetuses are being aborted in great numbers as parents desire more boys (Dugger, 2001). The use of ultrasound technology has made such medical decisions easier. Disruptions to society continue a few decades later when young men cannot find sufficient numbers of suitable mates.

Infanticide

Infanticide is the killing of newborns, which has been practiced to some degree since ancient times. Some societies practiced infanticide as a means of ridding themselves of weak and deformed offspring or to eliminate births that violated cultural norms (such as infants resulting from rape or incest, or those conceived out of wedlock). China's policy of one child per family has led to the killing of newly born females because the family desired only a male, or second-born children in general (when abortion of fetuses was evaded in some way).

Filicide

Filicide is the killing of children. In the United States, filicide is most often the result of parental abuse or mental disease. In some poor countries, children have been sold into slavery to work as laborers under extremely unhealthy work conditions leading to their untimely deaths. However, the number involved is unknown.

Suicide, Physician-Assisted Suicide and Euthanasia

Suicide, physician-assisted suicide and euthanasia are other ways in which individuals may be killed, with considerable ongoing debate over whether such deaths are justified. Suicide involves the conscious intent of an individual to end his or her own life and the completion of such an act. In the United States, the suicide rate is highest for adolescents and the elderly. However, it is increasing for younger adolescents. Suicide by younger individuals, who have a lifetime yet to live, creates a crisis in cultural values. Suicide by the elderly, who choose to end their own lives rather than continue with an unbearably low quality of life, also creates a cultural conflict. Suicide goes against the beliefs of those who are religious. For others, rational suicide seems quite justified if terminal illness exists and/or if individuals themselves judge that there is no longer any quality to life.

Physician-assisted suicide takes place when the physician provides the information, material, and/or equipment for an individual to commit suicide. This is now legal in the state of Oregon but, again, is causing cultural conflict throughout the United States.

Euthanasia is the killing of an individual by another for humanitarian reasons, i.e., when terminal illness exist and/or no quality of life is judged to exist. Passive euthanasia (where a person is simply allowed to die by withdrawing or withholding life-extending medical treatment) is legal in the United States and is the basis for drafting living wills. Voluntary active euthanasia, where an individual requests the physician to kill him or her, is not legal in the United States, but it is legal in some other countries, e.g., the Netherlands (Williams, 2001). Because the world can now be regarded as a global village, what is allowed in other countries influences our own, facilitating greater societal and cultural conflict regarding such deaths.

Capital Punishment

Execution by the state, legally killing someone for committing a crime, is termed capital punishment. The death penalty is established by society for certain first-degree murders. At the present time, this is another area where cultural conflict exists as to whether or not to have a death penalty. Those who favor capital punishment feel that it deters crime and is less costly than imprisonment; they see no need for rehabilitation of a prisoner who has taken the life of another. Such proponents of capital punishment feel that "an eye for an eye" philosophy is justified; it is fair punishment for those who commit murders, and it is considered unlikely that an innocent man will be executed. Those who oppose capital punishment argue that it does not deter crime; it is not less costly, as sometimes prisoners stay on death row for years; an "eye for an eye" philosophy is not appropriate for a civilized society; some murderers may deserve a second chance and rehabilitation; capital punishment may result in the death of an innocent man (as recent DNA testing has indicated); and capital punishment is unfairly applied depending upon ethnic/racial background, gender, and socioeconomic status level. Existing data over the past 10 years ("Capital punishment," 2001) indicate that capital punishment does not act as a deterrent, inasmuch as homicide rates in those states with the death penalty range from 50 to 100% higher than homicide rates in those states without it. The very existence of such different views indicates that death by capital punishment disrupts society and is related to different social meanings of death.

Special Types of Killings (Mass Killer, Serial Killer, Terrorist, Political Assassination, Torturer)

These types of killings do not necessarily involve large numbers of deaths, but do threaten or frighten many people and hence can disrupt society. A terrorist kills others as a means of frightening the rest of society, calling attention to a political agenda, and undermining citizens' will to resist such an agenda. The most recent and the worst example of a terrorist attack in the United States involved the suicide airliner crashes into the World Trade Center in New York City and the Pentagon building in Washington, DC ("A nation challenged," 2002), which caused over 3,000 deaths and a great national disruption. Another example of a terrorist attack in the United States was that of Timothy McVeigh, who used a truckload of high explosives to bomb the Alfred P. Murrah Federal Building in Oklahoma City on April 19, 1995, killing 168 people and injuring more than 500 others (Kight, 1998).

A serial killer kills one person at a time, but may kill in a bizarre and fiendish way. Motives for such killings differ. For example, the serial killer Theodore Kaczynski (the Unabomber) sent bombs that killed 3 and injured 28 people as a way of protesting the organization of modern society. Other serial killers may have been motivated for sexual purposes or to satisfy a desire to kill. For example, Albert De Salvo, the Boston Strangler, killed 13 women in the Boston area after gaining entry to their homes and then sexually molesting them; John Wayne Gacy abducted and killed 33 boys in the Chicago area; Angelo Buono raped and murdered 10 girls and woman in the Los Angeles area, David Berkowitz, "Son of Sam," killed 6 people and wounded 9 others in the New York City area; and Jeffery Dahmer killed and sexually molested many boys in the Milwaukee area. These serial killers may not cause large numbers of deaths, but they can disrupt the functioning of society by the very nature of the killing. The killing is so brutal, random with no clear motive, and frightening that it is very unsettling to many members of society. People in the area feel that they could be the next victim.

A torturer induces prolonged suffering in his victims and may or may not kill them. This may be done to extract information, to force a recanting of stated beliefs, or for sadistic enjoyment. Examples of torture for political reasons were the Nazis in World War II and the Chilean government of Pinochet. In the late 1980s and early 1990s, two centers were started in the United States to help refugees who had been tortured in their own countries and were still suffering mental problems. They were the Marjorie Kovler

Center for the Treatment of Survivors of Torture in Chicago and the Center for Victims of Torture in Minneapolis. The victims served by these centers needed extensive clinical help to deal with the aftermath of torture.

In sum, the killing of people disrupts society in various ways. Killing may eliminate a large number of people, the killing itself may involve an initial cultural conflict between different societal members (e.g., the abortion issue), or it may involve the killing of a single person but one who is very important to the functioning of society. Whatever the type of killing, it may lead to serious disruptions in the functioning of society.

Disease

Death as a result of disease can come about as a result of communicable disease, chronic degenerative disease, or iatrogenic illness. Each of these has different implications for the sociocultural meanings of death.

Communicable Diseases

In the history of the world, communicable diseases have often resulted in plagues, epidemics, and endemics that have killed many people and caused serious disruptions to ongoing societies. The bubonic plague (or Black Death) is a classic example which wiped out a large portion of the European population in the 14th century. In the United States, the influenza epidemic of 1918 killed 500,000 people, the polio epidemic of 1952 killed 3,300 people, and the ongoing AIDS epidemic killed 391,000 people through 1997 (Brunner, 1999), all despite the efforts of public health agencies.

But now the increased international travel associated with a global economy has led to the exchange and transmission of communicable bacterial and viral diseases from one country to another. Movements of people, foods, animals, animal products, and various manufactured products make it easy to transmit diseases that otherwise would stay localized. The global interconnectedness includes the developing countries, which have large populations and where infectious diseases account for almost half the death each year. Half of these deaths can be attributed to three diseases: malaria, HIV/AIDS, and tuberculosis (Angier, 2001). Malaria kills more than one million people annually, the overwhelming majority of them children in sub-Saharan Africa. This portion of the world is also suffering great losses from HIV/AIDS. Of the 35 million people living with HIV or AIDS in the world, 25 million are in sub-Saharan Africa. Of the 5.4 million people who are newly infected with the virus each year, 4 million live in sub-Saharan Africa. Tuberculosis, once thought to be eradicated, is making a comeback as the bacteria spread through modern transportation systems. More recent problems with mad cow disease in Britain and Europe also was a concern in the United States.

The globalization of human and animal diseases now exists and is disruptive of various societies. Such diseases are a particular threat to the elderly, children, and others with weakened immune systems. They cause some social disruption in the United States as efforts are mounted to monitor the occurrence of these diseases, and to treat them when and if they occur.

Chronic Degenerative Disease

Some chronic conditions may be merely annoying or painful such as nearsightedness or osteoarthritis. But others can be fatal, such as diabetes, cancer, heart conditions, and so on (Kart & Kinney, 2001). As life expectancy has increased, chronic fatal diseases occur mostly among the elderly (Whitbourne, 2001). As the older population continues to increase, the medications and services needed to treat these diseases can cause serious problems for society.

Iatrogenic Illnesses

Iatrogenic illnesses are those that are contracted within a hospital or other medical establishment designed to serve the ill. Such an illness may be due to the carelessness or incompetence of the medical personnel, low standards of hygiene practiced in some medical institutions, or medical accidents (such as a mixup in medical prescriptions for two different patients). To the extent that such illnesses occur, suspicion and distrust of medical care providers becomes a problem in the society.

Effect of Type of Death on Sociocultural Meanings of Death

In summary, deaths of large number of people in catastrophic events, deaths of individuals who are admired and loved, deaths of people who have a key function to maintain the quality of an important institution, deaths of people at the hands of killers who commit bizarre, unexpected, brutal, and shocking acts that may threaten or frighten others, or deaths legalized by society but involving cultural conflict between societal members (abortion, capital punishment, war) can all be disruptive of societal functioning. Such deaths may necessitate changes in the organization of society and cultural values, and eventually the sociocultural meanings of death.

IMPLICATIONS OF SOCIOCULTURAL MEANINGS FOR PERSONAL MEANINGS OF DEATH

Death occurs in every society, and has many and far-reaching effects that people do not often realize immediately. For a society to deal effectively with the death of its members, it must develop a well-functioning death system along with sociocultural meanings of death that help to regulate the functioning of the system.

Although the extent of the effects of deaths may vary depending on the type of death and the individuals affected, some death-related events may disrupt society to the point where it can no longer function adequately or restore its previous state of functioning. This leads to societal changes, which in turn foster the emergence of new or modified cultural meanings of death to fit the new situation.

Individuals are socialized into cultural meanings of death by various paths, not surprising since the concept of death pervades almost every aspects of society and culture (DeSpelder & Strickland, 2002). Every culture has a coherent set of meanings or beliefs about death that societal members internalize through socialization and think about consciously or subconsciously in everyday life.

Such sociocultural meanings are part of the general culture and are learned by individuals formally or informally as they participate in societal activities. Sociocultural meanings of death pervade every aspect of society; they are part of religions, philosophies, political ideologies, the arts, television programs, and so on (Aiken, 2001). In addition to direct experiences with death, individuals in the United States have been exposed to thousands of deaths through television, films, theater, music, art, newspapers, and so on, all of which indirectly convey various sociocultural meanings of death (Kearl, 1989).

These sociocultural meanings of death are shared meanings of death by society but different cultural meanings of death can be more representative of certain individuals rather than the group as a whole. In other words, there are individual differences in the type and degree of socialization that people go through in assimilating certain cultural meanings of death; these individual differences may be the starting point in deriving personal meanings of death. The personal meanings arise from an amalgam of shared cultural meanings, the individual's personality, and the unique experiences in that individual's life.

Individuals may start with a group identity and tend to believe whatever the cultural norm about death has been, such that death is a transition to another life; that is, there is some form of eternal existence beyond death. Eventually, the individual separates himself or herself from the group or collective self and begins to think more independently. In this way, he or she continues to develop an individual sense of identity or sense of personhood. The individual may reflect more and come to new conclusions about the meaning of death that differ from the cultural meanings of death for the society as a whole. For example, he or she may now think that death is a personal threat to his or her existence; the individualized self which now has priority over identification with the group can be threatened by the uncertainty of duration of life on earth or the possibility of no life after death.

Although both sociocultural and personal meanings of death have their origins in society and culture, they may interact to stimulate further development of personal meanings of death. In short, the sociocultural and personal meanings are related and mutually influence each other but they serve different purposes. That is, individuals are socialized by society to assimilate sociocultural meanings of death, which influence group behavior as society attempts to solve societal problems concerned with death. In contrast, personal meanings are assimilated to help the individual deal with his or her own death and to lend meaning to his or her ongoing life before death occurs (Wong, 2000).

3

Personal Meanings of Death

WHAT ARE PERSONAL MEANINGS?

Beyond understanding the objective meaning of death as the irreversible cessation of all bodily and mental functions and the subjective meanings of death at the societal level, there are also personal meanings of death at the individual level. Personal meanings of death are unique to the individual even though others may coincidentally have the same unique meanings. Although personal meanings reported earlier in life can be a clue to later personal meanings, one must focus directly on the personal meanings of death of older adults if one is to understand their views because there are indications that personal meanings of death do change throughout the life span.

Personal meanings are primarily cognitive interpretations of objects and events in the environment, and occur prior to and serve as stimuli for emotional reactions. If personal meanings associated with death have negative consequences for the individual, they can generate various death fears and concerns about dying. Personal meanings may influence the way a given individual lives, the way in which he or she reacts to death, the fears of death that he or she might have, conceptions about the dying process, and the way that he or she prepares for death.

Although the primary task of this chapter is to identify the personal meanings of death for older adults, a further task is to relate the influence of certain sociodemographic variables to these personal meanings. All individuals are embedded in a particular society and their personal meanings of death are partially a product of the interaction of their characteristics and the culture they assimilate. This includes such important sociodemographic variables as age, gender, ethnicity, and socioeconomic status.

PREVIOUS STUDIES OF PERSONAL MEANINGS OF DEATH

Studies of older adults' personal meanings of death are quite limited. Therefore, a brief review of studies carried out at earlier life stages will not only give some perspective on changes in meanings over the life span but will provide some indication of the approaches to studying personal meanings taken by earlier researchers.

Although personal meanings of death have been found early in childhood (e.g., the perception of death as a bogey man), most developmental research has been concerned with how children come to grasp the objective notions of death (universality, irreversibility, nonfunctionality, and causality) as well as conceptions of noncorporeal continuation (e.g., Brent & Speece, 1993; Nagy, 1948, Speece & Brent, 1996). By late childhood, most children have an understanding of the fact that everyone dies sooner or later, that dead people do not come back to life, that dead people cannot carry on the functions of living beings, and that such things as severe illnesses, accidents, and homicides are causes of death. In a religious society, children also gain a notion that the soul but not the body can continue on after death.

A study by Noppe and Noppe (1997) found age differences in the meaning of death between children, adolescents, and young adults. Beliefs in the existence of an afterlife (heaven, hell, etc.) were greater among adolescents than among either children or young adults. Another study (Wenestam & Wass, 1987) identified such personal meanings of death as darkness, light, transition, afterlife, and annihilation. Some adolescents appear to see death as so remote that they associate few meanings with it, whereas others are very much preoccupied with death (Kastenbaum, 2000b).

Personal meanings of death are primarily cognitive interpretations of death based on personal experience. Some studies of death meanings of college students and young adults have carried out content analyses of free-response narratives concerning personal meanings of death, using responses to questions such as "What is death?" and "What does your death mean to you?" Researchers were then able to identify common themes found in the idiosyncratic narratives. Holcomb, Neimeyer, and Moore (1993) reported that two of the most frequent themes in personal death meanings were viewing death as involving continued existence in an afterlife and viewing death as nonexistence. Other researchers (Durlak, Horn, and Kass, 1990; Neimeyer, Fontana, & Gold, 1984) also identified death meanings involving an afterlife, death as extinction, and the impact of death on others. Although Durlak and colleagues studied a wider age range of individuals than the other researchers, they did not examine age difference in their findings. Regrettably, most studies did not involve older adults or, if they did (e.g., Durlak et al.), findings were not subdivided by age groups, providing little understanding of age differences in death meanings from a life span perspective.

In my own work (Cicirelli, 1998b), personal meanings of death were studied in college students ranging from 19 to 53 years of age. Based on earlier research, an instrument was constructed to assess the degree to which individuals viewed death as afterlife, death as extinction, death as a motivator for setting goals and achievements in life (thereby giving life meaning), and death as the opportunity to leave a legacy for one's heirs or future generations. The conception of death most strongly endorsed by these college students was death as motivator, followed by death as extinction, death as afterlife, and death as legacy. A younger subgroup (aged 19 to 25) tended to be more likely to view death as extinction than an older subgroup (aged 26 to 55), but less likely to view death as involving an afterlife.

Kastenbaum (1996, 2000b) used a variant on the above approaches to elicit death meanings, instructing young adults to consider a world without death. Among the themes identified in their responses were that a world without death would mean a loss of life's meaning and a loss of the possibility of an afterlife.

Still another research approach (Kalish, 1981; Kastenbaum & Herman, 1997; Ross & Pollio, 1991; Tamm, 1996) investigated adults' perceptions of death as a personification (such as a grim reaper, gay seducer, or gentle comforter) or as a metaphor (such as a falling curtain). These perceptions are interesting, but they are limited in that they do not indicate significant personal meanings that could potentially influence individuals' daily lives or future plans.

Finally, two recent studies of the oldest old (Johnson & Barer, 1997; Tobin, 1991, 1996), using naturalistic interview methods, offered some information about the way those aged 85 and above view death. Johnson and Barer carried out a six-year longitudinal study of 150 individuals in the San Francisco area who were at least 85 years old at the start of the study. Although some standardized personality instruments were used in the study, unstructured interviews were used to gather most of the information about this group. Death was among the topics considered. The oldest old realized that they were near the end of life and experienced a sense of the finitude of life, the need to consider death as part of living, and the need to make decisions in preparation for death. They spoke of death objectively and appeared to be philosophical about it. Most of their contemporaries were dead, and the great changes in society seemed to make it easier for them to leave this world. Tobin, who also studied the oldest old, noted that most of them saw death from a religious perspective as involving an afterlife.

In sum, previous studies have provided little information about the personal meanings of death held by the older adult. Although some changes with age are suggested by various studies, there has been little systematic investigation of differences in death meanings associated with age, gender, socioeconomic status, or ethnicity. Their value in helping to understand the views of older adults about death lies mainly in suggesting ways in which inquiry into the older adults' personal death meanings can proceed.

THE PRESENT STUDY

The primary focus of this chapter is the identification and understanding of the individual's personal death meanings. The general method of my exploratory study into older adults' views of death was described in Chapter 1. In regard to the exploration of death meanings, the approach was to use both quantitative and qualitative methods of data collection and analysis. It was hoped that a basic set of death meanings could be identified by both approaches, but that the qualitative method would reveal additional and perhaps novel death meanings held by older adults.

QUANTITATIVE APPROACH

The specific objective of the quantitative approach was to determine the extent to which older adults shared certain basic personal death meanings previously found in other studies with younger groups.

Description of the Scale

To assess the degree of preference for certain personal meanings of death, the Death Meanings Scale (Cicirelli, 1998b) was used. The scale assessed four major types of death meanings found among younger adults, and was originally developed for use with college students. In developing the scale, personal death meanings reported in existing studies were used as a basis for the construction of potential scale items. This collection of meanings, roughly categorized, is presented here because it gives the reader an appreciation of the variety of personal meanings of death previously reported:

1. Death means that one should live their life to fulfill certain goals, e.g., provide a legacy such as money, material goods, ideas; accomplish things to maximize the use of one's potential to make life worth living; accept responsibility to others and/or a higher being by living according to certain ethical rules values; continue to modify one's lifestyle as necessary to prepare for decline/dependency before death.
2. Death means reappraising relationships with others, e.g., it may mean separation from loved ones; it may mean that we become only a memory to others; it may involve anticipation of future reunion with loved ones; it may mean a concern for loved ones left behind; it may mean anticipated grief over loss of loved ones; it may mean an opportunity to outlive others to be a greater success in life; it may mean viewing people as eventually equal in the graveyard.

3. Death means potential experiences while living, e.g., it may mean pain and suffering while dying, it may mean the end of all one's yet unfulfilled dreams, it may mean that life is absurd with no value, significance or purpose; it may mean that life is worth living despite its finitude.

4. Death means loss or escape from unpleasant aspects of life, e.g., it may mean a relief from the struggles of life; it may mean suicide as an escape from failure to cope with life.

5. Death means subsequent outcomes, e.g., it may mean personal extinction; it may mean facing the unknown, it may mean an afterlife of eternal happiness with God; it may mean an afterlife of eternal damnation in hell as punishment for sins; it may mean an afterlife involving rebirth (reincarnation), it may mean an afterlife of being a wandering spirit counseling, guiding or threatening the living; it may mean the opportunity to die with honor and glory for a cause; it may mean a reunion with loved ones who previously died; it may mean an opportunity to recognize and praise another person's accomplishments in life, it may mean science will work to eliminate death.

A pool of items based on the above categories was field tested, and refined on the basis of item analysis and factor analysis (Cicirelli, 1998b). The final 17-item scale consisted of 4 subscales: Death as Legacy (5 items), Death as Afterlife (4 items), Death as Extinction (4 items), and Death as Motivator (4 items). These items are shown in Table 3.1. Individuals responded to each item on a 5-point Likert scale ranging from "1" (strongly disagree) to "5" (strongly agree), and subscores were formed by summing the appropriate items. Internal consistency reliabilities (coefficient alpha) for the subscales were: Death as Legacy, .72; Death as Afterlife, .73; Death as Extinction, .70; and Death as Motivator, .66.

For the older adults who participated in the present study, internal consistency reliabilities of the subscales were: Death as Legacy, .70; Death as Afterlife, .86; Death as Extinction, .65; and Death as Motivator, .71. In addition, factor analysis indicated that the four dimensions of the scale were consistent with those of the college student sample.

TABLE 3.1 Item Means on Personal Death Meanings Scale for Three SES/Ethnicity Subgroups

| Item | Group Means | | | F-test | Significance of Bonferroni tests | | |
	Group 1 Hi SES Whites ($n=42$)	Group 2 Low SES Whites ($n=26$)	Group 3 African Americans ($n=41$)		1 vs. 2	1 vs. 3	2 vs. 3
Death as Legacy							
5. Death provides the opportunity for others to recognize our accomplishments.	3.05	3.35	3.39	1.17	1.00	0.66	1.00
8. Death means the opportunity to leave a legacy (money, material goods, ideas) to others.	3.98	3.92	3.59	1.14	1.00	0.47	0.85
9. Death means the opportunity to die with honor and glory for a cause.	2.83	3.19	3.78	6.37***	0.72	0.02**	0.17
10. Death means the opportunity to outlive one's competitors.	1.74	2.31	2.32	3.64**	0.11	0.05**	1.00
16. Death is an opportunity to be praised for what we have accomplished.	2.36	2.96	3.15	3.90**	0.22	0.02**	1.00

(continued)

TABLE 3.1 *(continued)*

Item	Group Means			F-test	Significance of Bonferroni tests		
	Group 1 Hi SES Whites (n = 42)	Group 2 Low SES Whites (n =26)	Group 3 African Americans (n = 41)		1 vs. 2	1 vs. 3	2 vs. 3
Death as Afterlife							
2. Death means personal extinction. (Reverse scoring)	3.57	4.12	3.76	1.17	0.39	1.00	0.96
7. Death means reunion with our loved ones.	3.50	3.81	4.12	2.78*	0.92	0.06*	0.90
12. Death means the beginning of something beyond life on earth.	3.88	4.15	4.41	2.34*	1.00	0.10*	1.00
14. Death is the beginning of a new adventure in the afterlife.	3.69	3.92	4.24	2.34*	1.00	0.10*	0.83
Death as Extinction							
1. Death means pain and suffering.	2.33	2.54	2.32	0.30	1.00	0.66	1.00
3. Death means the end of one's dreams.	2.93	3.04	2.68	0.53	1.00	1.00	1.00
6. Death means separation from our loved ones.	3.76	3.85	4.10	0.89	1.00	0.59	1.00
11. Death means the loss of everything.	2.52	2.35	2.88	1.20	1.00	0.81	0.44

(continued)

TABLE 3.1 *(continued)*

| | Group Means | | | | Significance of Bonferroni tests | | |
| | Group 1 Hi SES Whites ($n = 42$) | Group 2 Low SES Whites ($n = 26$) | Group 3 African Americans ($n = 41$) | *F*-test | 1 vs. 2 | 1 vs. 3 | 2 vs. 3 |
Item							
Death as Motivator							
4. Having to die makes life seem more important.	3.19	3.88	3.17	2.67*	0.13	1.00	0.11
13. Death stimulates one to set goals.	3.26	3.38	3.61	0.79	1.00	0.65	1.00
15. Death motivates us to achieve.	3.00	3.19	3.83	4.92***	1.00	0.01***	0.13
17. Life gives death meaning.	3.57	3.62	3.85	0.74	1.00	0.75	1.00

*$P < .10$; **$p < .05$; ***$p < .01$

Death Meanings of Older Adults

Of the four death meanings assessed, two were concerned with the postdeath period (Death as Afterlife, Death as Extinction) and two with contemporary life (Death as Legacy, i.e., an opportunity to leave a legacy of goods or accomplishments for others, and Death as Motivator, an impetus to accomplish things in one's present life). Death as Afterlife was the most strongly affirmed meaning ($M =$ 14.4, $SD = 2.75$) and Death as Extinction the least ($M = 11.76$, $SD = 3.34$), with the two contemporary life meanings intermediate, Death as Motivator ($M = 13.82$, $SD = 3.71$), and Death as Legacy ($M = 12.19$, $SD = 3.38$, adjusted to a four-item scale for comparison purposes).

An important conclusion emerges from these findings. Although certain meanings were affirmed more strongly than others, elders held all four meanings simultaneously to some degree. It was not an either-or question. Death meant for them that eventually they would be with God or simply be nonexistent. Additionally, death meant being involved in their ongoing earthly life. Death meant making certain life choices so that they could leave behind a legacy of some kind to be remembered for. Also, death meant that their time on earth was limited and this fact apparently motivated them to accomplish things in the duration of time that they did have on earth. In short, personal meanings of death influenced both how older adults lived now and how they expected to exist beyond death.

Effects of Age, Gender, Ethnicity, and Socioeconomic Status (SES)

In the quantitative analyses of the Death Meaning scale, the four death meaning dimensions were assessed in relation to basic demographic background variables of age, ethnicity, gender, and socioeconomic status (as indexed by educational and occupational levels).

To examine age trends in the four death meanings, the total sample of older adults was divided into five subgroups: 70–74, 75–79, 80–84, 85–89, 90 and over. Death meanings varied with age only in the case of Extinction, which followed an inverted U-shaped curve. Viewing death as Extinction was greatest for those in the 80–84 age group, with Extinction scores for both the younger and older age groups falling off. That is, the 80–84 age group tended to see death as extinction to a greater degree than did other age groups. This was the first clue we had that those elders in their early 80s might be different in other ways. This time period seem to be a more sensitive period for concern with death meanings than other age groups.

Gender was related only to viewing Death as Afterlife, with a weak tendency ($p < .10$) for women to endorse Death as Afterlife more strongly than did men. Similarly, there was a weak tendency ($p < .10$) for African-Americans to view Death as Afterlife and Death as Legacy more strongly than did Whites. With regard to SES, those of higher SES regarded Death as Legacy ($p < .01$) and Death as Motivator ($p < .10$) less strongly than those of lower SES.

However, effects of ethnicity and SES were somewhat confounded, as the total group of White elders had a higher SES than the African Americans who took part in the study. To disentangle these effects, the sample of Whites was subdivided into two groups differing in SES, labeled High and Low. The Low SES White group was similar to the African Americans in educational and occupational attainment, whereas the High SES White group was of higher educational and occupational attainment than either of the other two groups. In comparisons of these three subgroups (using one-way analysis of variance), the death meanings of the Low Whites and the African Americans tended to be more similar to each other than to the High SES Whites. However, this difference was statistically significant only for Death as Legacy ($p < .05$), with the High SES Whites endorsing Death as Legacy less strongly than did the other two groups. These findings suggest that socioeconomic status level may be a more fundamental variable influencing the personal meanings of death than ethnicity per se.

(Older adults' responses to the 17 items of the Death Meanings scale are found in Table 3.1, with tests for differences between the High SES Whites, the Low SES Whites, and the African Americans on each of the items. The interested reader can gain a fuller appreciation of these older adults' thinking about death meanings.)

Summary

Of the four dimensions on the Death Meanings Scale, Death as Afterlife was the most strongly affirmed meaning and Death as Extinction the least, with the two contemporary life meanings (Death as Legacy and Death as Motivator) intermediate. However, the results indicated that the older adults' personal meanings of death are concerned with both contemporary life and an afterlife.

Age was the only sociodemographic variable associated with death meanings, and that was only in the case of Death as Extinction. The latter followed an inverted U-shaped curve indicating that those in the 80–84 age group perceived Death as Extinction most strongly compared to those in other age groups. Associations of other demographic variables with death meanings were weak at best.

QUALITATIVE APPROACH

The quantitative analysis was an attempt to begin to assess some core death meanings that we felt would exist for older people. However, we wanted to go beyond this, and felt the only way to do so was through a qualitative and exploratory approach.

The results of the quantitative analysis gave us some insights as how to proceed. The fact that death meanings were concerned with both contemporary life and afterlife indicated the importance of a continuum of time in relation to death meanings. Second, the possibility that older adults in their early 80s (a particular time period) were more sensitive to the meaning of death as personal extinction suggested to us that we develop a set of questions for interviewing that would follow a time dimension in the hope that it would reveal new death meanings held by older adults.

Interview Strategy

The specific strategy used in the qualitative method involved what we called a time-orientation technique. In this technique, we asked a set of questions designed to elicit death-related meanings associated with time. The questions were as follows:

1. How long do you expect to live? How long do you wish to live?

   We were interested in both parts of this question separately, if for no other reason than to determine how many elders might like to be centenarians. (Or, if not, why not?) Their reasons would reveal what death means to them. More importantly, we were concerned with the discrepancy between time expected to live and time desired to live. Theoretically, there were three possible discrepancy groups: those who expected to live longer than they desired; those whose expectations and desires were the same, and those who desired to live longer than they expected. We found older people in all three groups. The strategy then was to ask them why they felt the way they did, and presumably it would reveal directly or indirectly (allow us to infer) what death might mean to them.

   Following our time-orientation technique, we continued with the following question:

2. If you had 10 more years to live beyond what you expect, would you want this time and what would you do with it?

   Again, the strategy was to determine elders' reactions to the possibility of increased life, and to gain further clues as to their death meanings from their responses and reasoning. This was followed by a third time-related question.

3. If we could guarantee you perfect health and financial independence, would you want to live forever?

   This extension of the time dimension turned out to be very revealing. Finally, we asked a fourth question:

4. As you get older, do you experience or think about the nearness of death, i.e., death getting closer in time? If so, has it changed the way you think or live?

   This fourth question offered a somewhat different perspective, but also involved the time dimension in terms of perceived nearness to death.

5. Incomplete sentences task.

   A final portion of the qualitative interview did not fit nicely into the time dimension, although it could be construed in relation to time. It was a sentence completion task in which the elder was asked to complete several partial sentences dealing with death:

1. Death is like_____
2. For old people, death means _____
3. For young people, death means_____
4. For a man, death means _____
5. For a woman, death means_____
6. When I think of being dead, I_____
7. Death is always_____

In the remaining portion of the chapter, the study participants' responses to this of questions will be examined and compared. In so doing, we looked at subgroups of participants who were classified by age (70-, 80-, and 90-year-olds), gender (men and women) and by the ethnicity/SES grouping discussed in Chapter 1 (high SES Whites, low SES Whites, African Americans). We will begin by looking at the answers to question 1, and then continue with participants' responses to the remaining questions.

1. Death Meanings Expressed in Expected and Desired Durations of Life

Most people have some idea of about how long they are likely to live based on such things as their health, their lifestyle, how long others in their family have lived, and so on. Consequently, we asked the older adults participating in the exploratory study two questions about how they viewed the duration of their lives. First, "How many more years do you expect to live?" and then, "How many more years would you like to live?" From the responses to the first question, we were able to get some idea of whether an individual viewed death as meaning something remote in time or as meaning something close at hand. By looking at the difference between how long an individual desired to live and how long that individual expected to live we could get an indication of whether that individual viewed death as meaning a welcome relief from the struggles of life, an unwelcome fate to be postponed as long as possible, simply an accepted ending to life, or possibly something else.

As might be expected, the length of time that older adults expected to live was partially dependent on their age. On the average, those in the 70–74 age group expected to live another $13\frac{1}{2}$

years, those in the 75–79 age group another 9½ years, those in the 80–84 age group another 8 years, those in the 85–89 age group another 6½ years, and those age 90 and over expected to live another 3½ years. Clearly, death means a more remote event to those who are younger and a more imminent event to those who are older.

All saw death in terms of a limited life span. It was interesting that despite much recent media publicity about the increasing number of centenarians (e.g., Perls & Silver, 1999) none of our interviewees expected or desired to become a centenarian. Even those elders in their 90s who still manifested considerable health and vigor did not wish to live more than a few additional years. It may take awhile before culturally ingrained notions of the "fourscore and ten" as a good long life to yield to the emerging demographic realities.

The expected time left to live was no different for women than for men, for those who were married and those who were not, or for those of higher and lower socioeconomic status. However, African Americans in their 70s expected to live another 3 to 4 years longer than did Whites; this difference disappeared for the older age groups.

The difference between the desired and expected time left to live presented an interesting picture. On the average, these older adults desired to live about 2 years longer than they expected to live. However, such an average is somewhat misleading. For 50% of the older adults in the study, there was no difference between the two estimates; suggesting that death meant something to be accepted when one's time was up. However, 43% wanted to live longer than then they expected, anywhere from 3 to 15 additional years. This suggests a meaning of death as an unwelcome fate to be postponed at least for awhile. The final group, only 7% of the group, wanted to die anywhere from 1 to 9 years sooner than the time when they expected to die. All were women, but no other characteristics distinguished them from the larger group of their peers. For them, death appears to mean a welcome relief from the hardships of old age. One woman in her mid-70s explained,

I come from a family of long livers, but I wish I could go now.

The average difference between desired and expected years to live was no different for men and women, those who were married and those who were not, or for Whites of different socioeconomic status levels. However, the "desired minus expected" difference was about 3 years greater for African Americans than for Whites.

Finally, this "desired minus expected" difference was dependent on age, and was greater for those in the 75–79 and 80–84 age groups than for those either older or younger. This finding is of considerable interest, because the 80–84 age group was the one affirming the death meaning Death as Extinction most strongly, with the 77–79 group not far below. One can speculate that the younger group of elders in the study could view death as relatively remote for only so long, and that at about age 80 they experienced a strong sense of the finitude of life, but at the same time felt unready to leave life.

2. Death Meanings Associated With 10 More Years to Live

When presented with the opportunity to live an additional ten years beyond their expected time left to live, direct thoughts of death did not seem to enter the picture for our study participants. They certainly did not reject the thought of living ten more years (not even those individuals whose desired time left to live was less than their expected time left to live).

However, how they proposed to use the added years tended to reveal what they still wanted out of life, reflecting the meaning of life for them. And, because life and death are interdependent, their responses also reflect and allow us to infer their meanings of death. Looking at their responses for each gender by SES/ethnicity subgroup in turn will give us a change to see how views differ for the various subgroups and also examine how views change with age within subgroups. We begin with the group of White men of high socioeconomic status.

High SES White Men

Within this group, there was a very definite age trend in what they would want out of an additional ten years of life. The group of 70-year-olds was very future-oriented. Although they no longer have active careers, their theme was continued achievement; either intellectual or in public service of some kind. For example,

- I want to have a life of service; serve people.
- Achieve (read, get ideas, solve problems, partially build computer).
- I want to achieve, complete a book.

Some of these men also had concerns for maintaining improving family relationships, as well as references to personal goals such as travel. However, these seemed like minor themes for this younger group. For example,

- I want the love and affection of my family.
- Watch my children grow. Want to travel with wife.
- Improve relationships with my grandchildren.

Although there were only a few 80-year-old men, there was still some concern for continued achievement. However, there was a definite shift toward a greater concern for their own individual welfare. They want a more quiet life, to maintain health, and not to be a burden to society.

- I would like to continue what I am doing for the next ten years including some service to others, finish some meaningful projects, and keep my family happy. But I don't want to be a burden to society.
- I want good quiet living conditions, see people and make them happy. Only if I am in good health, would I want to travel.

In regard to death meanings, one could speculate that for the 80-year-olds, death also means decline in addition to death as a motivator for continued achievement.

Among the 90-year-olds, the dominant themes were concerns

about maintaining their health (i.e., physical and mental capacities) as well as a concern for being close to their families:

- I want to maintain my mental capacities. I want to continue reading and enjoy the news.
- I just want to be with family.
- I want to give more background (genealogy) to my nieces, nephews and grandchildren.

It seems that as age goes from the 70s to the 90s, these high SES men become less achievement and future oriented and become more concerned with the present in terms of maintaining their health and family ties. One might speculate that death meanings change from an emphasis on death as a motivator in earlier years to interpreting death as meaning bodily deterioration and loss of family in the later years.

High SES White Women

This group of White women seemed concerned with social goals rather than intellectual achievement, with family relationships a predominant concern at all ages. Yet, some age trends emerged. Those still in their 70s still had goals of helping others (volunteer work) and traveling in addition to family concerns. For example,

- I'm very concerned about my two children. I want to help them; I'm interested in their future and development rather than just enjoying them or depending upon them. I am concerned about their security and I want to help them get ahead. Also, I do love to travel.
- I like to travel, I have good friends, and I do volunteer work for the library. Unfortunately, I don't see my children often enough.
- I want to spend time with my loved ones. I want to see the future for my children and grandchildren, observe them growing up and see what they become.

For this age group, death seems to have meanings as a motivator for the achievement of certain goals and as leaving a legacy for family.

For the women in their 80s, helping others rather than satisfying personal needs seemed predominant. Included in their conception of helping others were volunteer work, making lonely people feel better, being useful or of value to people, and also helping their own family. For example,

- I want to be of value to people. I want to help them be happy.
- I want to help others; I want to make people who are lonely feel better.

Family was also very important to them. In addition to simply enjoying family relationships, they wanted to see their grandchildren grow up, and make sure their adult children were settled in life.

- I want health and happiness for my friends; enjoy seeing them and my family.
- I want to keep in touch with family and friends, and see how their lives develop.
- I want to enjoy my family and friends.

Finally, they wanted to remain mentally active but they were not necessarily motivated to attain some intellectual achievement goal; rather their interest in mental activity was more related to hobbies, games, and the like. One women said,

- I just want to keep using my mind. I have learned the computer and word processor, and send email to my children and grandchildren.

A few women were still interested in traveling but it was a lower priority than for those in their 70s, and a few mentioned maintaining health. However, the concerns for helping others and for family seemed to dominate the thinking of the 80-year-old group. One can infer from the emphasis on family in this context that death means loss of family.

The 90-year-old women differed from those who were younger in that maintaining their mental and physical health appeared to be a primary concern. For example,

- I want to maintain physical health.
- I want to have a normal mind and don't want to be dependent.
- I just want a comfortable existence.

At this stage of life, travel was not mentioned. Yet, the women in their 90s shared the concerns of the younger groups for relationships with family and friends and for helping others:

- I have a grandson who was in trouble but now seems to be on the right track. I want him to make it.
- I want to see my three granddaughters settled and happy.
- I want to do some good for somebody if I can.

It is interesting that for these older women, interest in family focuses not only on adult children but on their grandchildren's development. Curiously, only one person mentioned religion and concern for the afterlife. She stated,

- I want to be a good Christian and go to heaven.

As for death meanings for the high SES women, we can certainly infer that death could mean physical and mental deterioration, loss of family and friends, a motivator to achieve certain goals in life, and leaving a legacy through helping others.

If we are correct, it is most interesting that death meanings of these high SES women can be typified more as contemporary life meanings than as postdeath meanings (afterlife and extinction).

Low SES White Women

Several differences between the high and low SES women were apparent. In looking first at the low SES 70-year-olds, these women were much more self-absorbed and centered on their present life, which seemed to give them a reasonable degree of contentment. However, they didn't seem to give much thought as to what they would do if guaranteed another 10 years of life. They had no real commitment to future goals or achievements. For example,

- Just be at peace with everything.
- Not much. I'm satisfied with the way I am. I have a life that I can cope with.
- Peace, contentment, happiness.

They did show concern about their family members, but it was more a desire to be with them and enjoy their company rather than a concern for their welfare and development:

- See my kids more often.
- Maybe get my daughter and take a trip.

These 70-year-olds did express a little interest in helping others but to a much lesser degree than did the high SES White women.

In addition to goals of personal happiness, the 80-year-olds seemed more focused on dealing with their deteriorating health. For example,

- I don't want anything. I'm ready to die. Ten more years? I have no future.
- I want to be able to take care of myself.

Concerns for family relationships were second in importance:

- I'd like to spend more time with my family.
- I'd like everyone to be happy. I just want to get along.
- Just be happy, have my family come around.

One woman did say,

- I want to see my grandchildren and great grandchildren grow up and accomplish something.

But this expression of interest in their family member's development was an exception. These women were more interested in themselves and the present. They were preoccupied much more with survival than the White women at the higher socioeconomic levels, and thinking of future goals involving self-development or that of family members may have been too much of a luxury for them.

This concern for present needs also characterized the two women in their 90s whom we interviewed.

- I want to take care of myself and stay healthy, do things I like to do, and may see friends.
- I want more financial help and better health.

The goals of life for the low SES White women were more to survive, enjoy their children to some extent, and possibly give a little help to others. The possibility of having 10 more years of life didn't seem to change their outlook much. In general, there seemed to be shift from the 70s to the 90s resulting in less concern for others and more preoccupation with one's needs. There was no real concern for future goals dealing with growth at any age level. If death meanings reflect life meanings, then it would seem that the meaning of death for them would center on loss, that is, loss of bodily functioning and loss of family. It would seem that death means loss of everything, everything being synonymous with survival.

Low SES African-American Women

For the African-American women, goals for the next 10 years were focused primarily on relationships with God and family. In addition to just enjoying their family, they want to make sure that family members go to church and pay attention to God. For example,

- I want to continue to work for the Lord, pray for my family and get my son to go back to church.
- I want to be an example for my granddaughters and show them how to be better women.
- Our life comes from God; try to live as well as you can.
- I want my family delivered to God and to have good health.
- Practice my faith and get ready to meet the Lord.

Other goals for the future are simple and concrete and involve others. For example, a desire to have a nice home where a grandchild can play or staying healthy:

- I would like a new home and play with my grandchildren often.
- I want to be comfortable.

Others have interests and dreams to be fulfilled that they were unable to satisfy in the past, due to a heavy load of responsibility and lack of opportunity. These included both interests in learning new things and an interest in travel. For example,

- During the next 10 years, I would like to travel, take some tours.
- I would like to travel and meet new people. I want to do things that I haven't had a chance to do.
- I want to travel some, possibly California and Hawaii.
- I want to move into a nice apartment and travel a little.
- I would like to take up some crafts and go back to school.
- I would like to learn how to play the piano, learn crafts, and cro-chet and learn the computer.

Based on what they would do with their lives for the next 10 years, one might infer that their death meanings include death as a motivator (motivation to achieve, e.g. traveling, learning new things), death as legacy (insuring family members are on the right path), death as loss of family, and death as belief in God and an afterlife.

The 80-year-olds were similar to the 70-year-olds in their con-cern for God and family, but they were primarily concerned with maintaining health, being happy or contented, enjoying family and friends, and participating in their church. Their life seemed as if it involved a more relaxed pace than that of the 70-year-olds. However, unlike the younger group, they were not concerned with getting family members to go back to church, they were not con-cerned with traveling, they were not concerned with learning new things. They just wanted to enjoy a continuation of life in the pres-ent. For example,

- I would like to keep doing the same for the next 10 years: go to church, see friends, go shopping and take care of my house.
- I would like to keep doing what I do now: get up in the morn-ing, go to church, visit the senior center, call my boys, and visit friends.

- I just want to get along and have a good life.
- I want to be happy. I want the Lord to bless me and give me some money so I can get the things that I need.

This age group seems preoccupied with contentment in the present. For them, one might infer that death means loss of family, bodily deterioration, as well as an afterlife with God.

Low SES African American Men

Among the four African American men studied, the emphasis for the next ten years was more on financial security in old age for themselves and family members. They wanted money to fix up their home, money to help their daughters. There were secondary concerns for others and for religion. Some of the comments illustrate their views,

- I have love for people and great dedication to God.
- If I had the money, I would build homes and rent them to make money.
- I want to save money for my daughters. Also, I want to fix up my home before I die.
- I would like to help people as best as I can.

Again, one might infer that death meanings of this group of men included death as an afterlife with God, death as loss of family, and death as a motivator to achieve something.

3. Death Meanings Associated With Living Forever

Very few of the older adults we interviewed wanted to live forever, even if they were guaranteed good health and financial independence. The great majority did not want to live forever and their reasons were varied. Looking at the reasons by age, gender, and ethnicity/SES subgroups enabled us to find some reasons common to certain subgroups and from there to make some inferences regarding death meanings. We begin with the group of high SES White men, and proceed from there.

High SES White Men

Only two of the men in this category wanted to live forever, one in his 70s and one in his early 80s. These men looked at living forever as a great adventure. One commented,

- You know that life is laid out for you as a consequence of your activities. I would hope for broadening my activities, not lessening them no matter what age.

The rest of this group did not want to live forever. Among the 70-year-old men, some doubted that any guarantee of bodily and mental health would last, and they felt the need to reject eternal life if it included such declines. One man said,

- No, I cannot imagine that. I am a physician and I recognize that your systems do wear out.

Others were concerned with ecology and the quality of life on earth with so many people living forever. For example,

- To live forever would lead to all kinds of ecological questions, for example, where would we put all these people? If we continue to consume the earth's resources at the rate we do now, there would be no quality of life. Even now our quality of life is at the expense of other people. If we continue, disaster of some kind will occur.

Some felt that the generation gap would eventually become too great and it would be difficult to communicate and understand people.

- To keep up with each new generation would be too great.

Others took a religious viewpoint in that living forever would violate God's purpose.

- We were put here on this life with the purpose to serve God among his people, not to live forever.

- I think that God's purpose for man is to work and do good in a limited amount of time.

The men in their 80s echoed the theme that God's purpose would be violated by living that long. However, the 90-year-olds stressed difficulties in adapting to a changing society, the fact that there was no real purpose to living longer, and that they had already accomplished their goals in life. The age differences in views about eternal life reflect changing themes from either a sense of adventure about living long or a concern with the practical and moral problems that such a long life would bring (as expressed by the younger age groups) to a feeling among the oldest men that they had already fulfilled their mission in life and they saw no point in going on.

What death meanings can be inferred from the responses of these high SES men? Death means an afterlife, bodily deterioration, an ending to life's goals, an escape from a life of no purpose, death means opportunity for continuation of the species, and a legacy communicated to future generations.

High SES White Women

Only three women in this group wanted to live forever. They were in their early 80s and seemed to be an energetic and adventurous group. For example:

- I guess I'm not going to hurry death. As long as I'm productive to somebody and to society, I will appreciate life. Yes, I could live forever.
- If you can guarantee me health and independence, and I could learn to appreciate all the new technologies, yes, I'll take a chance.
- Yes, with friends, I could live forever.

The great majority of the high SES women, like the high SES men, didn't want to live forever. However, one can easily notice the differences in their reasons compared to those advanced by the men. They didn't want to live forever in a world without their children and grandchildren, or even without the rest of their family. Even their belief in an afterlife becomes intertwined with considerations of family. For example, one woman stated,

- No. I would not want to live in a world where my children and grandchildren are dead. They are a great source of satisfaction. Also, I believe in an afterlife, and if I want to see the rest of my family, I need to go to heaven.

Other women were concerned with becoming bored if they lived forever. A typical comment was,

- No, I think I'd get bored eventually. I think I'd run out of inspiration.
- No, I don't think so. I'd get tired of being around.

Some would not feel useful for such an indefinite time period. They already feel that their work here on earth is finished and they want to find out what follows this world. One woman said,

- No, I don't want to live forever. I would outlive my usefulness and wouldn't belong in this nasty world. My work on earth is accomplished and I'm curious about what happens next.

Other reasons were that they need to make room for the next generation and that cycles of life should be followed if one is to renew the life of the population. For example,

- No, I can't live forever. Old people must die so that there will be room enough for youngsters. I just feel that there is a time for everything, including a time to die.
- No, I think it is important that the cycles of life be followed, and the population of a country be renewed from time to time.

Another reason given was that they could not keep up with the times and would not fit in society; they would be out of touch with generations and technology. Some comments were,

- No, I would feel out of touch with the younger generation, and also technology. No thank you.

- No, because to other people, I would soon be an old fogy. I want to be part of other people. I'm not a hermit.

Among the 90-year-olds, there was a noticeable shift in the reasons for not wanting to live forever. This group was more concerned with their bodily health and loss of friends who couldn't be replaced. For example,

- Too many problems in life. Your body is bound to deteriorate. You couldn't guarantee that I'd never have any aches and pains. Unless everybody else was going to live forever too, I wouldn't know anybody.
- No, I would not want to live forever. The only way to live forever is if I could be real active again, maintain stable health, and stay that way. But then everybody else I knew would be gone. It goes against the grain of the way the world should go.

In summary, women in their 70s seemed to reject a long life if they were without family and reunion with God in the afterlife. In addition to concerns about family, women in their 80s emphasized more their need to be being useful, concern with boredom, following a natural life cycle, allowing room for a new generation to rejuvenate society, and concern for their own ability to fit in with a changing world. The 90-year-olds seemed more concerned about body deterioration and lost friends. However, the common thread in women's reasons for rejecting eternal life on earth is social: a concern for loss of family and friends and the impossibility of fitting in with new friends from continually new generations.

In general by rejecting living forever, death is accepted with a shorter life and the reasons expressed for this indicate the personal meaning of death for such people. For example, death means fulfilling God's plan, or being with God in the afterlife, or the loss of loved ones, or a natural outcome of bodily decline with age.

Low SES White Women

Among this group of women, five wanted to live forever. Four of the five felt a sense of adventure and excitement in the idea of living forever. For example,

- Yes, why not? I'd live life to the fullest.
- I'd like to see plays, movies, a lot of things, travel . . . seek new experiences.
- Yes, it would be fun to live forever. I'd work, help others, have fun.

The great majority of the low SES White women did not want to live forever for various reasons. Some felt that it would mean not seeing friends and family they cared about, either in this world or the afterlife:

- My children wouldn't live forever. I wouldn't be able to see the same people I love. It would be mighty lonely without them.
- I'd want to see my mom and dad again and my brother, and I'm convinced we'll be reunited. And I don't think this world is the greatest thing. I want to go to the next one.

Others cited religious beliefs *per se*. One stated,

- No, I do not want to live forever. My purpose in being on this earth to start with is to see God.
- No, I don't think we are meant to live forever.

A final reason not to live forever was a lack of purpose in doing so and hence a feeling that life would be boring. One woman stated,

- No, I wouldn't have any purpose, something that would last.

Age differences in views were also apparent among the low SES women as well as those of higher status. Compared to those still in their 70s, those in their 80s and 90s placed strong emphasis on loss of close relationships. For example,

- No, I would have outlived all my friends and relatives, and I would never wish for new friends. They would all be too much younger than me; they couldn't replace my old friends.
- No, because the rest of my family would be gone and I would be alone. I wouldn't be comfortable.

The older groups also raised the issue of a generation gap. For example,

- No, the world is changing too fast for me now, and I just don't think I want to face the computer age any more.

The death meaning of loss of friends and family was pervasive in the responses of these women, and to a much greater extent than in the responses of the higher SES women. Both groups of women also emphasized death meanings of fulfilling God's plans and uniting with God in the afterlife.

Low SES African American Women

Compared to White women, an even larger number of the African-American women expressed a desire to live forever, if that were possible. However, reasons for wanting to live forever were somewhat different and varied with age group. The 70-year-olds seemed to be attracted by a promise of having both money and health forever, enabling them to achieve freedom from lifelong concerns about finances and physical well-being. For example,

- If I had my health and plenty of money, sure, I'd like to go on.
- I would like to live forever and do the same things over and over again.
- I'd live from day to day like I'm doing now, and be contented.

In comparison to White women, this African American group didn't seem in search of adventure or excitement, but rather a simple and worry-free life.

Compared to the 70-year-olds, some of the 80-year-olds expressed altruistic and religious goals for extended life:

- Yes, I would like to live forever. If I had the money, then I could help somebody else . . . I could help build my church.
- Yes, I'd like to live forever, and be able to go to church and sing like a bird.

Others simply expressed a desire for more life. For example,

- I would want to live forever. Because life would be happy for me, it would be a better life.
- Yes, I would like to live forever because I like life.

Those who rejected any thought of living forever also cited reasons similar to those advanced by White women: concerns with bodily deterioration, the need to make room for newborns in the world, the generation gap, anticipation of boredom, a feeling that there is an appropriate time to die, and a desire to have an afterlife with God. A sample of the secular reasons follows:

- I don't think the body would hold up that long.
- No, I would be too old to take care of myself.
- No, because I want to get out of the way for the next generation.
- We must give somebody else a chance to go on.
- No, I would probably feel out of place. The people around me wouldn't have anything in common with me, and I don't think I would like that.
- There is a time to live and time to die. I want to live as long as I can, but you know you have to die.
- No, because I think after you get to a certain age you would be bored, and I don't intend to be bored.

Other reasons for rejecting eternal life on earth were related to religious beliefs:

- I don't think so. I'd rather live in heaven with God.
- I don't think the Lord would let me live that long. I wouldn't want to do anything to shorten my life, but I couldn't decide to live forever . . . it's in the Lord's hands and his judgment.
- You are not supposed to live forever. All the money and goodies you'd have wouldn't be so good as being with your creator or your maker. That would be the main thing.
- No, money isn't everything . . . God is love and that would endear me closer to him.

Although views of the different age groups were similar in most regards, the older group also expressed similar concerns about family relationships and friendships typical of the older White women:

- No, I don't want to live forever. It's not the world, it's the people and I would not want to live with them forever.
- I wouldn't want to live without my family and friends. New people wouldn't be the same.

Again, we attempted to infer death meanings from responses to a possibility of living forever. Following this procedure, death means bodily decline, death means loss of family and friends, death means symbolic afterlife through other generations, death means relief from a world that one cannot cope with, death means a natural life-death cycle, death means an escape from boredom, and death means being with God. For this group of African American women, being with God in the afterlife seems very predominant.

Low SES African American Men

Because there were only a few men in this group, findings are especially tentative. Two wanted to live forever for altruistic reasons,

- I would like to. I'd like to do things for others.
- Hell, yes. I'd build homes [for the homeless] and teach everybody to use their equipment.

The remaining two rejected living forever for religious reasons,

- No, I can't live forever when the Lord wants me to go.
- No, because that's not God's will that we live forever. I wouldn't want to do anything against his will.

In terms of death meanings, death as an afterlife with God was important for those who rejected living forever, whereas one might construe lack of death as a motivator toward altruistic acts for those who wanted to live forever.

Summary

Clearly, the great majority of older adults did not wish to live forever, although the proportion desiring to do so was greater for low
SES White women and African American men and women. The
desire to live forever declined with age among all groups. Those
who wanted to live forever were intrigued by the adventure of new
experiences and the possibility of altruistic acts and further achievement. Death meanings related to the perceived impossibility of living forever included death as fulfilling God's plan, death as being
with God in the afterlife, death as loss of loved ones, death as a
natural life-death cycle, death as a natural outcome of bodily decline
with age, death as an opportunity for legacy for future generations,
death as an escape from boredom and lack of purpose, and death
as an escape from inability to cope and adapt to changing times.

4. Death Meanings Associated With Approaching Death

Do You Ever Think About Death Getting Closer? If So,
How Has It Changed Your Life?

In their study of elders over 85 years of age, Johnson and Barer
(1997) found that as the very old perceived death to be getting
closer, they tended to simplify their physical environment and their
daily routines in order to make the activities of daily living more
manageable. In addition, they tended to reorder their priorities
and some created new roles that compensated for their losses.
Finally, they shifted their time orientation from the past or future
to the present, so that coping with day-to-day activities and finding happiness and contentment were the important things in life.
By changing their time orientation, these elders were able to enjoy
life while coming to terms with death.

As we found in an earlier portion of this chapter, the older adults
we studied had varying expectations of their time left to live,
depending on their age and other factors. The question asked here
explored the extent to which approaching death occupied their
thoughts and changed the way they lived. As before, we began by
looking at White men of high socioeconomic status.

High SES White Men

The majority of the men in the 70-year-old group had indeed thought about death getting closer, at least occasionally. And their activities had changed somewhat in response to their anticipated mortality. For example,

- Yes, I do think about death getting closer. It increases my appreciation for my wife and my family. I increase my reading and my listening to others.
- Yes, I do. I accept the diminution of my powers. I wonder about my financial resources, whether they will be sufficient. My associations with other people are less than they had been.
- Once in a while I think about it, but not often. I don't feel it influences me. I've slowed down quite a bit in what I used to do, but I still like to do a lot of things that I did and I do them.
- I would say, occasionally, yes. Two years ago I bought a new car, so I guess I plan to drive in it for awhile. I am not going to go down [*die*] very quickly. Although I have sort of peripheral thoughts about that.

Even those who claimed not to think about the nearness of death and denied its influence on their lives apparently did have a few thoughts about it:

- Nope, it doesn't. Because I'm operating the same at 76 as I did at 66 or 56. And I'm thinking that this can't go on forever but I accomplish the same things.
- You know, I think that every human being is kind of in denial, until he gets a message that he's terminally ill. He thinks that life is infinite. And that's one of the things that seem strange to me, that at 76, I know rationally that my life is only 6, 7 more years out, but today I feel like I am going to live forever. I feel like age 22.

The men in their 80s echoed the responses of the 70-year-olds, perceiving only minor influences of approaching death on their lives:

- I do occasionally. It influences me to some degree. I don't get carried away by that feeling. Since I'll be leaving a wife behind, I'd like to get the family business settled.
- I'd make no changes. I enjoy life as it is, and I'd like to continue as long as I can.

Even the 90-year-olds, except for one man, claimed not to be influenced by approaching death. That man had his affairs in order and was prepared for death. These contrasting views are as follows:

- I don't give death a thought. If I do think about it, it doesn't change my life at all. When I find myself at the age of 93, I wonder how I got here.
- I know it is inevitable. After all, I'm 90. I'm prepared for it. I've made all my funeral arrangements with my two sons. I've disposed of the property that I had as nearly as I can. I may have withdrawn more because, of the associates I had ten years ago, three fourths of them are gone.

Most of these high SES White men were still very much active in life and, although they thought of their own deaths occasionally, few had changed their lives greatly. What changes there were seemed to involve some reduction of activity, not major changes in their lives.

High SES White Women

Women of comparable socioeconomic status seemed to be somewhat more affected by thoughts of approaching death than the men. However, as many as half of the women at each of the three age groups (even the 90-year-olds) claimed to not think of death or to be affected by it:

- Not really. The attrition of friends has come. But I don't feel a sense of urgency. I just go along and take advantage of the opportunities that are presented to me.
- Not really. I don't think about it. No, I don't think I'd live any differently.

- No, I don't think about bad things . . . just the good things.
- I rarely think of that. I don't think it has changed me in any way.

Among the 70-year-olds who thought of approaching death, these thoughts did change their life to some extent. One had simplified her life somewhat, another kept her affairs in order, another was not forward-looking but lived from day to day.

- After all, when you are 79 years old, you know that you lived most of your life. I think I have simplified my life. I got rid of a lot of things I didn't need any more. You kind of do things the way you want to, live from day to day. I still see and talk to a lot of people, I think I am less brave about going out on my own now.
- Yes, I am getting older, so I think about it. I think about keeping our affairs in order.

A few of the women in their 80s who thought about death did not feel that such thoughts influenced their lives, but most had made some kind of changes: simplifying life, getting affairs in order, praying, getting prepared for death, reducing relationships with others, returning to their roots. We felt that they had a greater sense of urgency about the end of life than did those still in their 70s.

- Yes, I do. I know as I age I don't have the stamina to entertain my big family anymore and it does limit my physical activity.
- Of course. I've tried to simplify my life . . . giving things away . . . tried to arrange that everything will be as simple as possible to manage. I do pray more.
- Yes, I think about it but I don't do anything about it, except I try to live a good life and pray more.
- Yes I do. I see fewer people. I get out a whole lot less.
- Yes, I'd feel that way, especially if I'm ill. When I feel that death is nearing, I want to return to my roots and my family, so that I would be near those I love.

Those in their 90s were influenced by approaching death in similar ways to the 80-year-olds. One noticeable difference was that these oldest women did spend more time in prayer as a means of dealing with inevitable mortality. For example:

- Yes, I pray more, reduce my participation in things more.
- I think about it lots of times. I don't know if I am going to live the rest of this year. I've already called my son and written out the list of things I want to give to other people. It has changed me, as far as living here [*in senior housing*].
- Maybe I pray a little more.
- Yes, I think about death but I don't think about it as something I'm afraid of. I really want my granddaughters to know what the family stood for, what kind of life we had and hoped to pass on to them.

Low SES White Women

This group of women in their 70s was interesting. Although half indicated that they thought about approaching death whereas half did not, none felt that death had influenced them in any way.

- No. I live for today and look forward to tomorrow.
- No. I know I'm going to die, but I'm not going to do anything to hurry it.
- No. I don't think about it. If it happens, it happens.
- Yes, but I feel no need to change my life.
- Yes, But it doesn't bother me a bit.

A larger proportion of women in their 80s admitted thinking about their approaching death than was the case for women in their 70s, but most felt that thoughts of death had no influence on their lives. Of the few who suggested that their lives had changed, one woman attributed the change in lifestyle to aging, not thoughts of approaching death: For example:

- Yes, but I don't see death as being real close. I do take life a little easier and don't travel as much.
- No. I don't think that it will never come but I change because I'm getting older so I have to change my lifestyle . . . but not

because I think I'm going to die. The thought of death doesn't bother me.

- Yes, I think about it. It doesn't change my life but I treat my husband a little better.
- Yes, I think about death. I pray more, I try to simplify my life, and do all that I can do to help other people.

The two 90-year-olds in the group both said that, although they thought about death, they felt that approaching death in itself had not changed their activities:

- Yes, but I don't change the way I live.
- Yes. It hasn't changed the way I live but it makes me realize that things are harder. I don't have need for things now as I did when I was younger. You can't do the things you used to. I try to live as much as I can the way I had been living.

Considering the group of low SES White women as a whole, death seemed still too remote for the majority of these women to be concerned about it. This observation fits in with our earlier finding that they seemed to be oriented to the present and didn't look ahead. Whether they simply kept thoughts of their approaching death out of awareness or were not sufficiently introspective to think about death is not clear. One might infer that death as extinction was a predominant meaning for them, and they preferred not to think or talk about it.

Low SES African American Women

The African American women's responses to the question regarding approaching death were in sharp contrast to the low SES White women. The great majority in both age groups not only reported thinking about death, but also felt thoughts of death had led to changes in their life. Their own words say it best, for example:

- Yes, I do think about death. It leads to my working more. I appreciate people more, because I take time out to do it. There's one thing about death, you have no control over it. So I live each day preparing to die.

- Yes, I am getting older but now I live life in a way that I don't want to hurt anybody.
- Yes, it has changed me. Knowing that I'm eventually going to have to face death, I try to live in such a way that I have reasonable hope of the hereafter.
- Yes. It has made me simplify my life. I try not to spend time with unpleasant negative people, try to put my finances in order as much as I can.
- Yes, I think about death. I am trying to get things arranged to relieve some of the responsibility off of me in case something should happen so my daughter wouldn't be left with such a situation.
- Yes, sometimes I think about it. But then I look for new opportunities. Get up and get involved . . . new challenges, new experiences.

The views of the 80-year-olds were not too different from those of the 70-year-olds, feeling that their approaching death stimulated them to simplify their lives and increase religious activities.

- Yes, I think about death. Every time I get on my knees, I think about it, and that's day and night. Sometimes it gets too bad. I stop and close the door. I think about older people who go out to gamble, and they should live right in their last few years.
- Yes, I think about death. I try to read the Bible more and get to church more.
- Yes, I think about death everyday. I used to be a good time Charlie, now I begin to look after myself more, especially when you can't do as much.

The thoughts of approaching death motivated the African American women we interviewed to (a) want to help others more, try to do more things for others, (b) appreciate people more, (c) spend more time with family, (d) try harder not to hurt anybody, (e) try to live in such a way that they had a reasonable hope of the hereafter, (f) simplify or organize their life for themselves and their children, and (g) look for new opportunities and challenges rather than simply give up to death. The changes they attributed to the nearness of death were more concerned with improving social relationships with others and improving their relationship to God than with making their own lives simpler or more comfortable in a physical sense or with improving their own health status and dealing with disabilities. The concept of simplification of lifestyle advanced by Johnson and Barer (1997) was not observed in these African American women to any great degree, but possibly they were not sufficiently advanced in age.

Low SES African American Men

Only two men in the small sample of African American men responded to this question, and had thoughts of their approaching death. Only one felt motivated to try to improve the way he conducted his life:

- Yes, I think about death. I do try to be better and let my light shine to others.
- Yes, I think death will come.

Summary

After examining the views of both White and African American older men and women in three age groups, it is evident that many older people simply don't think about approaching death and therefore it doesn't influence or motivate them to change their behavior in any way. Others report that they did think about death either periodically or consistently, but again, such thoughts did not motivate them to change their behavior. One possible reason may be that the young-old felt that death was still too far away to worry about whereas the old-old may have felt too close to inevitable death to be concerned about changing their lives. Thus, we have no clear basis in their responses for inferring what death means to them.

Other elders, particularly the African American women, did think about getting closer to death and felt that nearness to death influences their behavior in various ways. Some felt that aging itself (rather than death per se) reduced their energy and mobility and motivated them to simplify their lives in the manner that Johnson and Barer (1997) described. The older adults we interviewed reported simplifying their physical environment by throwing away things, reducing their personal belongings, withdrawing from dubious social relationships, and carrying out procedures to put their legal, business, and personal affairs in order (e.g., making a will, instructing adult children as to their wishes).

However, simplifying life in preparation for death does not seem to be the whole story. The thought of death itself seemed to motivate some older adults to change their lifestyle or behavior in other ways, and this varied with the subgroups involved. For example, White men of higher socioeconomic status who were in their 70s sought to organize their lives to draw closer to their spouse, consolidate and maintain their financial status, and accomplish various intellectual goals. In contrast, those in their 80s and 90s did not appear to be motivated by approaching death in any particular manner. The situation among White women of higher socioeconomic status was somewhat different, in that those in their 70s and 80s were more likely to want to simplify their lives, while those in their 90s were motivated by approaching death to draw closer to their families and to pray more.

Among those of lower socioeconomic status who were in their 70s, there were some striking differences between White women and African American women as to the ways in which thoughts of approaching death stimulated them to change their lives. The White women placed emphasis on relationships with children, friends, or God. In contrast, the African Americans voiced a broader spectrum of changes in their lives. They wanted to help others more, to appreciate people more, to spend more time with family, to try harder not to hurt anyone, to try to live in a way offering hope of the afterlife, and to ask the Lord for strength and guidance. A few were similar to the high SES White men in that they wanted a certain degree of accomplishment and new opportunities and challenges rather than giving up in the face of death.

5. Meanings of Death From Sentence Completion

The sentence completion task did not ask the study participants to look at death at some future time, as in the questions using the time orientation technique, but asked them directly for meanings and associations with death at the present time. Responses to the seven incomplete sentences yielded a rich collection of death meanings overall. Many of these meanings were shared by the various age, gender, and ethnicity/SES groupings, and some were quite idiosyncratic. We will try to summarize these meanings for the group as a whole, pointing out group differences as appropriate. (Only two African American men responded to this task, so no comments will be made about this subgroup.)

Death Is Like . . .

Death meanings that were expressed across most ethnicity/SES, gender, and age groupings were death as a transition to the afterlife, death as an end of life or nonbeing, and death as unending sleep. The high SES White men and women did not go beyond these meanings in their responses. However, the low SES White women and the African American women expressed a wider range of meanings in addition to the more conventional meanings, including some death metaphors and some emotional responses. For them, death was a liberation from earthly problems, a new experience, just another facet of life, inevitable, being one with God, darkness and light, a dream, wonderful, and frightening, nightmare, a sting.

For Old People, Death Is . . .

Again, some meanings were found for all groups. They saw death for old people as meaning relief or a release from burdens and suffering, a hoped-for and welcome thing, a natural and expected reality, simple nonexistence, and as a transition to another life in heaven. Again, some more idiosyncratic meanings emerged from the low SES White women and the African American women. For them, death was also sleep, a dream, uncertainty, more acceptable, sorrow, and frightening.

For Young People, Death Is . . .

In sharp contrast to the meanings of death for old people, the meanings of death for young people tended to have quite negative connotation. Death for young people was seen by all groups as unimaginable, unthinkable, remote, unfortunate, unexpected, a surprise, premature, tragic, and unfulfilled goals. Additional meanings shared by the low SES White women and the African American women included death as unnatural, unreal, frightening, and sorrow. The responses of the African American women included such idiosyncratic meanings as death is God's plan, going to a better place, difficult, traumatic, a surprise, hard to accept, unknown, a closing, a punishment, unwanted, and a cutting-off of days.

For A Man, Death Is . . . ; For A Woman, Death Is . . .

Most of the older adults we interviewed did not feel that death was any different for a man or a woman and were unable to respond to these questions. However, some interesting differences were noted by those who did respond. For example, for a man, death means a loss of his contributions to society; for a woman, death means a loss of her nurturing the family. For a man, death is harder to accept; for a woman, it is easier to accept. For a man, death means regret over goals not achieved; for a woman, death means the end of things they want to do. For a man, death is inconceivable; for a woman, death is part of the natural cycle. For a man, death is devastating and degrading; for a woman, death is relief and peace. A man is more sensitive to death; a woman is just emotional. For a man, death means losing everything and a loss of control; for a woman, death means the end. For a man, death is frightening; for a woman it is unfair. The overall tenor of these difference is that to a man, death is a more momentous and negative occurrence, whereas for a woman death is a more natural and peaceful event.

When I Think of Being Dead, I . . .

A few responses to this sentence completion were typical across all groups: beginning an afterlife with God, reunion with loved ones in heaven, and a beginning of nonexistence. Some elders had no conception of what it would be like to be dead, and others simply wanted to avoid thinking or talking about it. The low SES White women and the African American women had a variety of additional thoughts about being dead. Some had to do with the possibility of an afterlife, such as a sense of peace, feeling like a shell with the soul gone, and worry about what will happen in the afterlife. Some thought that when dead they would feel concern about earthly details such as the funeral, what would happen to house and belongings. Some women felt that they would feel relieved when life was over, that they had completed their mission in life, and were glad to leave earthly cares and suffering. Another woman responded that the thought of being dead was a motivation to use the rest of her life to good advantage. Finally, some women felt that being dead would be a loss, that they would be sad and sorry to leave, and that they would miss loved ones and many things in life. As the reader can see, responses to this incomplete sentence involved many death meanings: death as afterlife, death as nonexistence, death as a motivator, death as a relief from suffering, and death as loss of loved ones.

Death Is Always . . .

Death is always inevitable, normal, universal, final, certain! These characteristics of the concept of death were mentioned by all groups of elders studied, as were meanings of death as a transition to the afterlife and death as extinction or nonexistence. Other responses were more idiosyncratic: Death is always an unknown, a mystery. Death is predestined and "on time" or it is unexpected, a shock. Death is separation from loved ones, and devastating to the family. Death is sad, frightening, terrible, or a welcome relief. Death is always trouble, a mess. Death is something for which one is never ready, or death is something to look forward to. Finally, death is always in awareness, always there in the back of your mind.

Summary

The wide spectrum of meanings elicited by the sentence completion task seemed to include a core centering around death as a
transition to the afterlife, death as nonexistence, death as loss of
family, and death as a relief from suffering. Important differences
in meanings emerged in that death for an old person was viewed
as expected and welcome, whereas death for a young person was
premature and tragic. Similarly, death for a man and death for a
woman evoked different shades of meaning. Above and beyond the
meanings shared by the majority of elders, the sentence completion task evoked a variety of meanings specific to an individual or
shared by only a few individuals. Many of these meanings appeared
to be the result of unique life experiences and circumstances.

DEATH MEANINGS IN OLD AGE: SOME CONCLUSIONS

Some people prefer the thought of living indefinitely but most
people do not. The older adults we studied regarded their life span
as a limited one, and most were contented with the length of life
they expected to have. Even though some (particularly African
Americans) desired a few more years of life beyond what they actually expected, none had aspirations to become a centenarian.

For various reasons, people value death as something desirable
compared to infinite life. It is not a question of accepting death as
an inevitable outcome, but of valuing and desiring it. However, it
is only through conscious awareness of the self as a living being
that man is led to interpret death or give it any meaning. We interpret or give death a meaning based upon life, the experiences of
living and assimilation of ideas from our culture.

Although there are many facets to the responses of the older
adults we studied, we were primarily concerned with their personal
death meanings. Other researchers and scholars have considered
personal meanings of death, but there has been little attention
paid to personal death meanings of older adults. Our approach to
identifying the personal death meanings of older adults was both
quantitative and qualitative, with a variety of qualitative techniques
being used.

First of all, the use of the Death Meaning Scale in the quantitative approach indicated that Death as Afterlife was the most strongly affirmed meaning, followed by Death as Motivator, Death as Legacy, and Death as Extinction. These four dimensions were validated by their repeated appearance among the variety of death meanings elicited by the qualitative approach, and were common to all groups to some degree. In the qualitative findings, men of high socioeconomic status were most likely to view death as a motivator for continued achievement in life. In contrast, women saw themselves as establishing a legacy for children and grandchildren through communication of their own standards and values as well as through active help.

Other death meanings derived from the time orientation techniques of the qualitative approach were death as meaning the loss of personal relationships, death as loss of functioning (bodily deterioration), and death as release from life's difficulties and suffering. New and more idiosyncratic meanings also emerged. Some seemed philosophical, such as death means a natural life-death cycle, death means life has no purpose, and death means rejuvenation of the species. Other new meanings were more personal, including death as a relief from coping with changes in society, and death as escape from boredom with life.

Curiously, the consideration of one's nearness to death seemed to evoke relatively few death meanings. Many elders asserted that they either never thought of themselves as approaching death or they didn't wish to think about it. Some felt that nearness to death motivated them to make preparations for it, such as settling their affairs.

The sentence completion task elicited the broadest spectrum of personal death meanings of all the methods used, centered around death as a transition to the afterlife, death as nonexistence, death as loss of family, and death as a relief from cares and suffering. An interesting point is that the personal death meanings of both men and women of high socioeconomic status seemed to be limited to these broader and widely shared conceptions, whereas the death meanings of both White and African American women of lower socioeconomic status included a wider variety of concepts as well as metaphors and emotional reactions.

Our study of personal death meanings in old age resulted in a better understanding of those meanings that appeared to be common to older adults, with little variation by age, gender, socioeconomic status, or ethnicity. It also resulted in an appreciation of all the unique death meanings and shadings of meanings that human beings associate with death.

4

Fear of Death

WHAT IS KNOWN ABOUT FEAR OF DEATH?

The Concept of Fear of Death

It has often been said that human beings are the only members of the animal kingdom who have a conscious awareness of the fact that they will die. Whether or not this is the case, such an awareness among humans is often accompanied by a sense of fear or anxiety related to the prospect of eventual death. Fear of death may not be a universal phenomenon, but it has certainly been an important influence in many cultures throughout the world. Dating from the earliest times, allusions to fear of death are found throughout literature.

The topic of fear of death (or death anxiety) has been a more general concern in Western cultures in recent times, manifested in the death awareness movement of the 1950s and in nearly a thousand articles on the subject up to the early 1990s (Neimeyer & Van Brunt, 1995). Fear of death continues to be an active area of inquiry for psychologists and other social scientists today. A computer search of the PsycINFO abstract database using the keywords "fear of death" and "death anxiety" turned up an additional 99 journal articles on the topic for the period 1998 to mid-2001 alone.

Fear of death can be defined as the anxiety experienced in daily life caused by the anticipation of the state in which one is dead (Tomer, 1994). It is regarded as an ongoing state in everyday life, in contrast to a more acute fear elicited by an immediate threat to one's life such as a gun at one's head or a natural disaster. Although some earlier authors made a distinction between death anxiety and fear of death, regarding fear as a reaction to an immediate threat of death and anxiety as a neurotic response unrelated to any immediate peril, Neimeyer and Van Brunt (1995) argued that such a distinction is "not compelling on conceptual or practical grounds (p. 52)." They concluded that the distinction was not maintained in operationalizing the concept in the construction of measuring instruments. In most cases the terms are used interchangeably in current literature and will be regarded as interchangeable here.

In a general way, the set of personal death meanings held by an individual is related to that individual's fear of death. As discussed in Chapter 3, personal death meanings are cognitive interpretations of death-related objects and events in the environment. In essence, they represent the totality of an individual's experiences with death either directly or vicariously in the general cultural milieu. If these personal death meanings have negative consequences for the individual, they can serve as a stimulus for fears of death.

Theoretical Explanations of Fear of Death

According to Tomer (1994), various theoretical approaches attempt to explain the causes of fear of death and its relationship to human behavior. Among these are existential philosophical approaches (e.g., Heidegger, 1962; Sartre, 1966) contrasting states of being and nonexistence, with fear arising from the contemplation of nonexistence. Self-realization theories (e.g., Maslow, 1968, 1970; Rogers, 1959) suggest that fear of death arises from awareness of approaching death and its threat to the fully functioning self. In search for meaning theories (e.g., Frankl, 1963; Maddi, 1970), the individual finds meaning through a purpose in life and a life scheme; to the extent that death is interpreted as part of the life scheme, fear of death is reduced. Personal construct theory (Kelly, 1955) holds that one develops a belief system of personal constructs that enable one to anticipate an orderly future; events outside the core system constitute a threat. Thus, when death is perceived as incompatible with one's construct system, death anxiety results. Stage theories (e.g., Erikson, 1963, 1982; Labouvie-Vief, 1982) view life as a series of developmental stages, each with a developmental crisis to be resolved before successfully continuing to the next stage. The penultimate stage (generativity vs. stagnation), arising when one becomes aware of the closeness of death, is successfully resolved when one is able to contribute to the development and well-being of future generations, with death anxiety resulting when one cannot transcend death in this way. The final stage of life (integrity vs. despair) is successfully resolved when one is able to view the self as an integrated whole and look back on a life well-lived. To do so results in a low fear of death, whereas to despair over past mistakes and lost opportunities in life results in greater fear. A more recent approach to understanding the fear of death is through path modeling (Tomer & Eliason, 1996, 2000a, 2000b). These authors envisage death anxiety as directly determined by three basic factors: past-related regret (the perception of not having fulfilled basic aspirations in life, future-related regret (perceived inability to fulfill basic goals in the future), and meaningfulness of death (perception of death as positive or negative, meaningful or senseless). All three are influenced by the salience of death for the individual (the extent to which one's own mortality is contemplated), beliefs about the self and the world, and the availability and activation of coping mechanisms. It is clear that certain elements are common to all the foregoing theories, involving a perception of approaching death and the resources of the self to deal with such a perception.

Terror Management Theory

At present, terror management theory (Becker, 1973; Greenberg, Solomon, & Pyszczynski, 1997; Solomon, Greenberg, & Pyszczynski, 1991a, 1991b) seems to be the most comprehensive and best supported of the existing approaches dealing with the cause and control of the fear of death. The basic assumption is that all humans are instinctively driven toward survival and continued existence, while at the same time they have knowledge of their inevitable mortality. As a result, there is a potential for them to consciously experience a terror of death. According to these theorists, the experience of such death terror would be paralyzing without some means of suppressing it from awareness. The basic task of the theory is to identify the factors helping to maintain this suppression. The theory holds that the core of death fear is fear of annihilation. Annihilation, or extinction of the self, is more than mere destruction of the body, but refers to the extinction of mind, spirit, and soul as well, that is, total nonexistence. Over time, individuals in various societies have developed cultural worldviews that characterize the universe or society as having rationality, predictability, and permanence. Socialization into any of these cultural worldviews provides protection against fear of annihilation, because it allows people to create standards of value for a meaningful life as well as ways of transcending death. If individuals become socialized and meet the standards valued by the culture, they attain a higher self-esteem and a promise of immortality. Self-esteem is regarded as the primary psychological mechanism whereby culture acts as a buffer to facilitate the individual's suppression of death fear. Self-esteem develops early in life as children interact with and meet the standards of their parents, who are representatives of the culture. The process is carried forward into adulthood, when individuals maintain or enhance their self-esteem by learning the teachings of the culture, participating in cultural rituals, attaining goals valued by the culture, fulfilling cultural roles, experiencing social validation in personal relationships, and using defensive responses when self-esteem is threatened.

Having faith in the truth of the worldview is also very important in facilitating and sustaining the suppression of fear of annihilation. The culture includes beliefs, values, and norms that allow the individual to create the illusion of being protected from death or eventually transcending it. By believing in the cultural systems individuals can achieve both literal and symbolic immortality (Lifton, 1983) and thus reduce the fear of death. Literal immortality refers to the belief that a noncorporeal aspect of the individual will live on indefinitely in some way. It is attained through religious beliefs concerned with a soul and afterlife. Symbolic immortality refers to the belief that individuals are represented by something or someone other than themselves that will continue to exist after they are dead. Individuals may continue to live symbolically by viewing children as extensions of themselves that continue through time, by feeling that they are valued parts of a culture that endures over time and beyond individual death, by making a permanent mark in the world through things that they produce or achieve, and so on.

Terror management theorists suggest two distinct modes of responding to conscious death concerns (Greenberg, Psyzczynski, Solomon, Simon, & Breus, 1994; Pyszczynski, Greenberg, & Solomon, 1999). First, individuals are motivated to use cognitive efforts to defend against death concerns, such as distraction, distancing themselves, and denying their vulnerability. Terror management theorists (Greenberg, Pyszczynski, Solomon, Simon, & Breus, 1994; Pyszczynski, Greenberg, & Solomon, 1999) suggest two distinct modes of responding to conscious death concerns, such as those evoked by external events. First, individuals use cognitive efforts (such as distraction, distancing themselves, denying their vulnerability, and so on) to defend against death concerns. As a result of such techniques, conscious death fears are reduced or eliminated and therefore are temporary. However, they may heighten the ongoing fear of annihilation at the subconscious level, intensifying the need to maintain suppression of this core fear of death. In the second mode of responding, individuals act to maintain this suppression by strengthening their self-esteem and defending their faith in the worldview. In other words, stimuli initially in awareness lead quickly to suppression of death concerns at that level, but the implicit knowledge of the threat of death and the subsequent fear of annihilation that are maintained within the individual outside of awareness may somehow signal the defenses of self-esteem and faith in the worldview (Greenberg et al., 1997). This signal effect implies that self-esteem and faith in the worldview may be related to fear of death assessed at the conscious level as well as acting outside of awareness.

Terror management theory argues that death concerns at the level of awareness are suppressed rather quickly. But terror management theory does not preclude the existence of knowledge and fears regarding death at the level of awareness; it suggests merely that the duration of such fears may be relatively brief.

In a recent chapter (McCoy, Pyszczynski, Solomon, & Greenberg,

2000), the theory was reexamined in relation to aging. A paradox of aging is that although one would expect aging adults to have increased fear of death accompanying their greater vulnerability in view of increasing age, illness, and general frailty, fear of death studies have consistently shown them to have a reduced fear of death in comparison to younger adults. At the same time, one would expect defenses against fear of annihilation to weaken because many sources of self-esteem are no longer available to aging individuals. They are no longer able to meet the standards of the culture due to declines in certain physical and cognitive abilities, obsolescence of previous roles in life that are no longer valued in a time of technological advances, loss of control over events, and the erosion of contemporary social supports making it more difficult to achieve social validation. Yet, existing research (Bengtson, Reedy, & Gordon, 1985; Dietz, 1996) indicates that self-esteem remains high for most older adults.

Another puzzling aspect of the relation of self-esteem to fear of death in the elderly is their apparent willingness to acknowledge the inevitability of death and deal with it at the level of immediate awareness. In this regard, Galt and Hayslip (1998) found that, compared to younger adults, older adults evidenced higher levels of overt death fear but lower levels of covert fear. If so, they may deal with fear by more direct means and gradually come to an acceptance of death. Feifel (1990) also views fear of death at different levels: a conscious level, a level of fantasy or imagery, and a nonconscious level. The way of thinking about terror management theory in relation to fear of death at different levels of awareness certainly fits in with Feifel's thinking.

McCoy and associates (2000) suggest that older adults use alternative routes for self-esteem maintenance other than through the consensual worldview favored by younger adults. These include socioemotional selectivity (Carstensen, 1992) to minimize contact with those threatening the self-concept, selective optimization with compensation (Baltes, 1997) to focus energies on those activities in which the aging individual can still achieve success, downward adjustment of standards to minimize discrepancy between real and ideal self (Ryff, 1991), cognitive reframing of events with optimistic reinterpretation, and reduced reliance on social consensus to avoid considering possible negative feedback. Additionally, elders are able to maintain self-esteem as well as gain a sense of death transcendence through generativity, a means of achieving symbolic immortality through transmissions of one's achievements in the culture to future generations (Solomon et al., 1991a). Terror management theory also holds that religious faith leads to the promise of literal immortality, the continuation of life in some form after bodily death. Expectations of both symbolic and literal immortality achieved through participation in the cultural worldview are hypothesized to reduce fear of death, and both are typically used by older adults.

Assessing Fear of Death

Assessing the extent of an individual's fear of death is not an easy matter, despite easy availability of a variety of measuring instruments at the present time. However, the diversity in such instruments reflects differences in their conceptualization, with some instruments probing anxieties at a more abstract level and others probing fear reactions associated with more concrete death stimuli. As a result, although most existing instruments consist of several subscales, there is only moderate overlap from instrument to instrument. More problematic are threats to validity raised by the tendency of some individuals to deny or suppress death fears from conscious awareness.

Various methods have been used to assess fear of death, including simple observations of behavior in response to death stimuli, psychophysiological responses to exposure to death stimuli (e.g., heart rate, galvanic skin response), content analysis of interview protocols, projective instruments, and psychometric scales. The psychometric scales, essentially self-report instruments, have been the most widely used in research as a result of their relative ease of administration and interpretation. Although some early studies (e.g., Bengtson, Cuellar, & Ragan, 1977) used only a single-item rating scale to assess fear of death, several more sophisticated instruments have been developed. A brief review of some of the most popular and well-supported of these instruments will give the reader a greater appreciation of the methodology involved and the variety of subscores being assessed. For a fuller review, see Neimeyer and Van Brunt (1995) or Neimeyer's (1994a) handbook. Because existing research articles report use of a wide variety of instruments, it is essential for the reader to be aware that there is no single and widely agreed-upon dimension of fear of death, but instead a rather large number of such dimensions that may or may not be measuring quite the same thing.

Templer's Death Anxiety Scale

The Death Anxiety Scale (Templer, 1972) consisted of 15 true-false statements, such as "I am very much afraid to die." The number of responses indicating agreement with a negative emotional item content was considered the measure of death anxiety. The scale had quite good test-retest reliability, but relatively low internal consistency reliability. Its brevity and ease of administration and scoring made it probably the most widely used instrument, especially in earlier research.

Subsequent factor analyses indicated that the scale was not unidimensional but contained anywhere from three to five separate dimensions (Neimeyer & Van Brunt, 1995), including a general death anxiety dimension, a dimension reflecting thoughts and talk about death, a dimension dealing with the subjective proximity of death, and a dimension reflecting fear of pain and suffering. Several revisions of the scale have been attempted by other investigators, the most recent of which was the Revised Death Anxiety Scale (RDAS) of Thorson and Powell (1994). The scale was expanded to 25 items, with 8 of these items given reverse scoring to eliminate response bias, and with a 5-point Likert response scale replacing the true-false format. Thorson and Powell indicated that a total death anxiety score could be obtained, as well as up to 7 factor scores including fear of uncertainty and missing out on things, fear of the pain associated with death, concern over disposition of one's body, fear of helplessness and loss of control, afterlife concerns, fear of decomposition, and concerns over leaving instructions as to how things should be done after one's death. The authors recommended caution in using the factor scores because they found different factor structures for those subgroups highest and lowest in death anxiety.

The Collett-Lester Fear of Death Scale

In its most recent form, the Collett-Lester Fear of Death Scale (Lester, 1994) assesses four aspects of fear of death: Fear of Death of Self, Fear of Death of Others, Fear of Dying of Self, and Fear of Dying of Others. The response to each of 32 items was made on a 5-point scale, ranging from "not disturbed" to "very disturbed." Although the test-retest reliability of the four subscales was satisfactory, subsequent studies found the factor structure of the instrument to be complex and only a partial match to the subscales.

The Threat Index

Of the various fear of death instruments discussed here, the Threat Index is the only one developed from a theoretical foundation. Kelly's (1955) psychology of personal constructs attempted to identify the core dimensions of meaning by which individuals organized and interpreted their lives.. In such a system, death was conceptualized as the ultimate threat to the individual's identity as a living being. The Threat Index (Neimeyer, 1994b) was devised to assess the degree of that threat. A recent form of the index contains 25 construct dimensions, each consisting of a pair of opposite adjectives (e.g., healthy-sick, strong-weak). The individual is asked to indicate for each dimension the extent to which he or she agrees with the left or right half of the construct, responding on a 7-point scale. The individual rates the 25 dimensions three times, first regarding "You or Your Present Life," then regarding "Your Ideal Self," and finally regarding "Your Own Death." To obtain a measure of death threat, one counts the number of times a dimension is scored on opposite ends of the response scale (1, 2, or 3 versus 5, 6, or 7) for "Your Own Death" as compared to "You or Your Present Life." The instrument yields a Global Threat measure as well as three factor subscores. (A brief form of the instrument consisting of only seven dimensions is also available.)

Death Attitude Profile—Revised

The Death Attitude Profile—Revised (Wong, Reker, & Gesser, 1994) is a 32-item instrument providing an assessment of five dimensions of overall death-related attitudes. The dimensions are Approach Acceptance (looking forward to death as the beginning of a new and glorious experience), Fear of Death (fear of the end of earthly existence and what may lie beyond), Death Avoidance (avoiding any thoughts of death or death-related subjects), Escape Acceptance (accepting death as an escape or relief from the burdens, pain, and suffering of life), and Neutral Acceptance (accepting death as a natural part of life). Wong and colleague view the Death Attitude Profile as providing a broader spectrum of death-related attitudes than fear alone, and consider an individual's profile of scores on the five dimensions to provide a more complete understanding of the way in which that person views his or her own death.

The Multidimensional Fear of Death Scale (MFODS)

The MFODS (Hoelter, 1979) consists of 42 5-point items yielding 8 subscales. The subscales include Fear of the Dying Process (including painful or violent deaths), Fear of the Dead (including avoidance of human or animal bodies), Fear of Being Destroyed (including cremation or dissection of the body for autopsy or organ transplants), Fear for Significant Others (including apprehension about the impact of the respondent's death on others), Fear of the Unknown (including fear of nonexistence and lack of knowledge about afterlife), Fear of Conscious Death (including concerns about falsely being declared dead), Fear for the Body after Death (including concern about decay and isolation of the body), and Fear of Premature Death (concerns about being unable to accomplish desired goals or experiences). Appropriate items are summed to yield the various subscores. Neimeyer and Moore (1994) reported extensive evidence for the factor structure of the instrument as well as the reliability and validity of the subscales. The MFODS is perhaps the scale with the best psychometric qualities of existing instruments.

Qualitative Interviews

In a study using a semi-structured interview to probe the fears and concerns about death and dying of nearly 200 homebound elders, Fry (1990) was able to identify 6 factors from factor analyses of 45 main fears and anxieties identified in content analysis of interview protocols. These included physical pain and suffering, fear of sensory loss, risk to safety of possessions, threats to self-esteem, fear of rejection by God, and fear of an unknown afterlife. It can be easily observed that several of these factors are highly similar to those found in a number of the fear of death instruments previously discussed, lending further validity to the self-report measures.

Previous Studies

Studies of fear of death in old age have focused mainly on the relationship of fear to age and other demographic variables. Personality variables, with the exception of depression, anxiety, and psychological problems, have not been explored in old age.

Taken as a whole, findings of existing studies of fear of death in old age tend to be somewhat inconsistent. The variety of measuring instruments used in different studies (ranging from single items to multidimensional scales and from self-report instruments to covert measures) means that it is difficult to compare findings of the studies when there may be limited overlap between the dimensions measured. Some instruments used are of doubtful reliability and validity. Studies have used varying methodologies and methods of analysis, again making them difficult to compare. Many studies have used small and nonrandom samples, making it difficult to generalize from study results to larger populations. Studies of older adults have often dealt with specialized samples (such as nursing home patients, volunteers at senior centers), and differences among the populations sampled have all contributed to the controversial nature of the findings. Despite this, there is surprising consensus among existing studies on certain points, and some general conclusions can be drawn regarding variables of interest to the present study.

Age Differences

Existing studies, although somewhat controversial, suggest that the
fear of death tends to be greater among younger age groups and
be relatively low for older people (e.g., Bengtson, Cuellar, & Ragan,
1977; Gesser, Wong, & Reker, 1987–88; Kastenbaum, 1992; Lonetto
& Templer, 1986; Neimeyer, 1988; Thorson & Powell, 2000). One
recent review (Neimeyer & Van Brunt, 1995) concluded that, in
general, fear of death had a negative linear correlation with age
from younger adulthood to old age. However, Neimeyer and Moore
(1994) reported that whereas most subscales of the Multidimensional Fear of Death Scale (Hoelter, 1979) declined with
age, Fear of the Unknown increased with age. The latter finding
is of interest, because even though multiple dimensions of fear of
death may exist, Fear of the Unknown represents a core concept
relevant to terror management theory, that is, the fear of annihilation or nonexistence after death.

The above studies reporting declines in fear of death with increasing age typically used "older adults" in late middle age or the young-
old as comparison groups. Although some studies included wider
age ranges, few individuals beyond age 70 were included in the
upper portion of the range.

Compared to the large number of studies of fear of death among
younger adults, relatively few studies of fear of death in old age
are found in the literature. Fortner, Neimeyer, and Rybarczyk (2000)
conducted a meta-analysis of 28 published studies and 21 disser-
tations and theses dealing with fear of death in adults ranging in
age from 61 to 87, and computed weighted average correlations
of age with fear of death. On average, the correlation of fear of
death did not differ significantly from zero, suggesting that fear
of death remains stable in old age. However, in the studies included
in the meta-analysis, most of the elders included in the various samples were in the 65 to 75 age range. What happens beyond age 75
is essentially unknown. Most studies have not included adults
beyond age 75, or if individuals up to age 85 and beyond were
included, they were not treated as a separate subgroup. In any
event, existing findings do not support the hypothesis that, among
older adults, increasing vulnerability to death with increasing age
leads to increased fear of death.

Johnson and Barer's (1997) recent unstructured interview study of the oldest-old provides information on fear of death among adults over age 85. According to these researchers, the oldest-old can accept death without fear. Death is no longer remote or abstract or something to avoid. They have no unfinished business in life and some are even bored with further living. What they fear is not death itself but the dying process, dreading a long illness in a nursing home and the thought of dying alone. Johnson and Barer felt that the oldest old have less to lose and can approach their death with equanimity. Death is also predictable, and hence, less disruptive to their lives and loved ones. They felt themselves prepared to die, and increasingly took death into account as they carried out their tasks, viewing death as part of living and facing it without fear. Overall, Johnson and Barer concluded that there is little or no fear of death in the oldest-old. Tobin (1991, 1996) observed a similar shift from a fear of nonbeing to a fear of the process of dying among the oldest old, as well as an increased acceptance of death. Such an increased acceptance does not necessarily mean that older adults are unconcerned about death. On the contrary, Kalish (1985) found death to be highly salient for older adults in that they both thought and talked about death more than did younger adults.

Gender Differences

A frequent conclusion of earlier studies is that, among college students and adults, women have greater fear of death than men (e.g., Davis, Bremer, Anderson, & Tramill, 1983; Young & Daniels, 1980). Using the multidimensional Leming Fear of Death Scale, Cicirelli (1998b) found that women reported greater fear on four of the eight subscales. In another study, women had less Fear of the Unknown than men on the Multidimensional Fear of Death Scale, although they had more fear than men on the other subscales (Neimeyer & Moore, 1994). Still other studies found no gender differences in death fear (Conte, Weiner, & Plutchik, 1982; Neimeyer & Dingemans, 1980; Neimeyer, Dingemans, & Epting, 1977) or differences using one measure and not on another. In general, although many studies found no gender differences, whenever differences were found, women reported greater fear than men.

One argument regarding any apparent gender differences was that they are artifactual results of women's greater expressiveness and depend on the type of death anxiety measure employed. In an attempt to resolve some of the controversy surrounding this research, Dattel and Neimeyer (1990) assessed fear of death in young and middle-aged men and women using two measures, one more affectively oriented (the Death Anxiety Scale) and the other more cognitively oriented (the Threat Index). Even when measures of self-disclosure and social desirability were used as controls in the analysis, women had significantly greater fear than men on the affectively oriented measure, although there was no gender difference on the cognitively oriented measure.

With regard to gender differences in fear of death in old age, the meta-analysis referred to earlier (Fortner et al., 2000), failed to find a significant gender effect. (Again, it should be noted that the bulk of the sample involved only the young-old.) It still needs to be determined whether gender differences in fear of death exist among the old-old and the very old.

Ethnicity

The few existing studies comparing Whites and African Americans on fear of death involved younger and middle-aged adults and had mixed findings. Some studies (e.g, Dodd & Mills, 1985; Young & Daniels, 1980) reported that African Americans had a greater fear of death than Whites, whereas other studies (e.g., Davis, Martin, Wilee, & Voorhees, 1980; Thorson & Powell, 1994) reported the opposite. Using a sample of nearly 400 elders attending senior centers, Cicirelli (2000) found no ethnic difference on six of the eight MFODS subscales, with Whites showing greater fear of the dying process and African Americans showing greater fear of conscious death. Overall, no clear conclusions are possible regarding ethnicity and fear of death.

QUANTITATIVE STUDY OF OLDER ADULTS'
FEAR OF DEATH

In the quantitative portion of the study, two instruments were used to assess older adults fear of death, (a) the Multivariate Fear of Death Scale (MFODS) which was discussed earlier in this chapter, and (b) an adaptation of a projective measure, the Geriatric Apperception Test (Wolk & Wolk, 1971). From these measures, one can not only get some idea of the relative strength of various dimensions of fear of death, but also how fear of death may vary for men and women, for those who are married and those who are single, for White and African American elders, for those who are of higher socioeconomic status levels and those who have lower status, and those who are very old and those who are less old. The latter is of particular interest because previous studies have included few elders in the old-old category, and this study will help to provide information about fear of death after age 75.

Multivariate Fear of Death Scale (MFODS)

Of the eight subscales of the Multidimensional Fear of Death Scale (MFODS) (Hoelter, 1979; Neimeyer & Moore, 1994), only four were used in our empirical study: Fear of the Dying Process (six items, pertaining to fear of painful or violent deaths), Fear of Being Destroyed (four items, pertaining to fear of bodily destruction, including dissection and cremation), Fear for Significant Others (six items, pertaining to the impact of the respondent's death on others and of others' deaths on the respondent), and Fear of the Unknown (five items, pertaining to fear of nonexistence and an uncertain afterlife). The major reason for using only four of the eight subscales was because the instrument was administered to the older adult sample as part of the larger interview-questionnaire and the time available to administer the battery was limited. The subscales selected for use were considered to be most relevant to the death concerns of older adults which centered around the dying process, physical decline, loss of family, and the afterlife. The remaining four subscales were Fear of the Dead (pertaining to avoidance of both human and animal remains), Fear of Conscious Death (including anxieties about falsely being declared dead), Fear for the Body after Death (pertaining to concerns about decay and isolation of the body), and Fear of Premature Death (pertaining to concerns that death will prevent one from accomplishing important life goals).

Neimeyer and Moore (1994) reported internal consistency reliabilities (Cronbach's alpha) ranging from .65 to .81 for the four subscales and test-retest reliabilities over a three-week period ranging from .61 to .77. For the participants in the present study, internal consistency reliabilities were .69, .69, .73, and .68 for Fear of the Dying Process, Fear of Being Destroyed, Fear for Significant Others, and Fear of the Unknown, respectively, values considered adequate for studies involving group comparisons.

Table 4.1 shows the means and standard deviations on the four MFODS subscales for the total group. On the average, the older adults in the study had a relatively low fear of death, although the size of the standard deviations indicates that a substantial proportion of the group has a greater degree of fear. Because the subscales contain different numbers of items, the mean per item (the mean divided by the number of items in the subscale) is also shown for each subscale in order to permit comparison between the different dimensions of fear. Fear for Significant Others was the strongest fear, closely followed by Fear of Being Destroyed, and Fear of the Dying Process. The weakest of the fears was Fear of the Unknown, which was not surprising in view of the extent of religious commitment among study participants.

Mean MFODS subscores for various groups, categorized by age, gender, ethnicity, and marital status are shown in Table 4.2. Analysis of variance was used in each case to determine whether differences in means were large enough to be significant.

Gender

Women scored higher than the men on all four fear of death subscales but this difference was large enough to be significant ($p <$ .05) only in the case of Fear of the Dying Process, where the mean score for women was 16.69 and for men was only 13.69.

TABLE 4.1 Mean and Standard Deviation of Study Participants on Each of Four MFODS Subscales, With Score Range, Number of Items, and Mean Per Item

Fear Subscale	Mean	SD	Range	No. of Items	Mean per Item
Dying process	16.25	5.17	6–28	6	2.71
Being destroyed	11.36	3.98	4–20	4	2.84
Significant others	17.51	4.99	8–30	6	2.92
The Unknown	10.39	3.23	5–20	5	2.08

Marital Status

The small differences in fear of death between those who were married and those who were widowed or divorced were insignificant from a statistical perspective, despite the fact that one might expect married women who have the support of a spouse to feel less vulnerable to death and hence have less fear.

Socioeconomic Status

To determine whether the index of socioeconomic status (SES), calculated from the educational and occupational levels attained by the individual, was related to fear of death, SES was correlated with each of the MFODS subscores. Correlations were negligible or very low for Fear of the Dying Process (.02), Fear for Significant Others (–.11), and Fear of the Unknown (–.15), but was statistically significant ($p < .01$) for Fear of Being Destroyed (–.37). Here those elders of higher socioeconomic status had less Fear of Being Destroyed than those elders of lower socioeconomic status. The areas touched upon in this MFODS subscale involved donation of organs and body parts, donation of body to science, and cremation. These were areas in which the integrity of the body after death was lost. It is not surprising that higher SES elders have a greater understanding and consequently less fear of these actions.

TABLE 4.2 Means and Standard Deviations of Four MFODS Subscales by Gender, Ethnicity, Age Group, and Marital Status

Group	N	Dying Process Mean	SD	Being Destroyed Mean	SD	Significant Others Mean	SD	The Unknown Mean	SD
Total Group	109	16.24	5.17	11.36	3.98	17.51	4.99	10.39	3.23
Age									
70–79	49	16.10	5.15	11.59	4.26	18.06	5.23	10.06	3.08
80–89	49	17.04	5.05	11.22	3.93	17.59	4.85	11.12	3.31
90–99	11	13.27	5.12	10.91	3.65	14.73	3.88	8.63	2.80
Gender									
Men	16	13.62	4.41	10.94	3.28	17.31	5.50	10.00	4.26
Women	93	16.69	5.18	11.43	4.10	17.55	4.93	10.46	3.05
Ethnicity									
White	68	16.81	5.06	10.40	3.77	17.01	4.67	10.26	3.31
African American	41	15.29	5.28	12.95	3.86	18.34	5.45	10.61	3.12
Marital Status									
Married	17	17.94	4.32	10.06	3.21	17.94	4.59	10.53	3.64
Single/Widowed	92	15.92	5.27	11.60	4.07	17.43	5.08	10.37	3.17

TABLE 4.3 Means on Fear of Death Subscales for Three SES/Ethnicity Subgroups, With *F*-test in the Analysis of Variance and Post Hoc Bonferroni Test for Differences Between Groups

	Group Means				Significance of Bonferroni tests		
Fear Subscale	Group 1 Hi SES Whites ($n = 42$)	Group 2 Low SES Whites ($n = 26$)	Group 3 African Americans ($n = 41$)	*F*-test	1 vs. 2	1 vs. 3	2 vs. 3
Dying Process	16.40	17.46	15.29	1.45	1.00	0.98	0.29
Being Destroyed	9.52	11.81	12.95	9.08**	0.05*	0.01**	0.67
Significant Others	16.26	18.23	18.34	2.12	0.34	0.17	1.00
The Unknown	9.95	10.77	10.61	0.66	0.94	1.00	1.00

* p < .05; ** p < .01

135

Ethnicity

Looking at the MFODS means for the White and African American elders (in Table 4.2), the scores for the African American group are higher than for Whites on Fear of Being Destroyed, Fear for Significant Others, and Fear of the Unknown, but the Whites scored higher on Fear of the Dying Process. However, in the analysis of variance, this difference was significant only for Fear of the Dying Process. In view of the fact that higher SES elders had less Fear of Being Destroyed than low SES elders, a further analysis was carried out comparing three groups: high SES Whites, low SES Whites, and low SES African Americans. (This analysis is summarized in Table 4.3.) The three-group analysis made it clear that the high SES White group had significantly less Fear of Being Destroyed than either the low SES White group or the low SES African American group, whereas the two low SES groups did not differ from each other. (The three groups did not differ on Fear of the Dying Process, Fear for Significant Others, or Fear of the Unknown.) One can conclude from this analysis that differences in socioeconomic status, rather than ethnic differences, were responsible for the observed differences in Fear of Being Destroyed.

Age

In looking at the means for the three age groups (70–79, 80–89, 90 and over) in Table 4.2, one can observe a slight decline with increasing age for Fear of Being Destroyed and Fear for Significant Others. However, these apparent age effects were not large enough to be statistically significant. In the case of the two remaining fear subscores, Fear of the Dying Process and Fear of the Unknown, the 80–90 group appeared to have greater fear than either the 70–79 age group or the age 90 and over group. This inverted U-shaped relationship was significant at the .10 level for Fear of the Dying Process and at the .05 level for Fear of the Unknown.

To examine these age differences in fear of death in greater detail, we used five age categories (70–74, 75–79, 80–84, 85–89, and 90–97) instead of three and employed trend analysis in the analysis of variance to test for the presence of both linear and quad-

TABLE 4.4 Age Subgroup Means and *F*-tests for Trend for Fear of Death Subscores

	Age Group							Tests for Age Trend	
Fear of Death Subscale	70–74	75–79	80–84	85–89	90–97	*F*		*t*(lin)	*t*(quad)
Dying Process	15.67	16.64	18.07	15.77	13.27	2.83*		–1.73	–2.88*
Being Destroyed	11.22	12.05	11.33	11.09	10.90	1.57		0.71	–1.02
Significant Others	18.33	17.73	17.78	17.36	14.73	0.90		–2.31	–1.61
The Unknown	10.07	10.04	11.63	10.50	8.36	2.01		–0.77	–1.71*

* $p < .05$; ** $p < .01$

ratic trends (see Table 4.4). In regard to both Fear of the Dying Process and Fear of the Unknown, there was a significant quadratic age trend, that is, an invert U-shaped age curve. Fear was greatest in the 80–84 age group, and was less in the 70–74 and 75–79 age groups and progressively less in the 85–89 and 90–97 age groups. (As in the three-group analyses, there was no effect of age on Fear of Being Destroyed and Fear for Significant Others.) When the analyses were repeated while controlling statistically for effects of SES, gender, ethnicity, and health, the results were unchanged.

The U-shaped age curve showing the relationship of Fear of the Dying Process and Fear of the Unknown to age is interesting. Of course, such a finding would need to be repeated with a larger and more representative sample of elders and perhaps with a longitudinal study. At this point, one can only speculate as to what might explain such a result. However, the finding is particularly intriguing because the high point among the age subgroups comes in the late 70s or early 80s, a period when there is some kind of transition from a young-old category where large numbers of older adults are still active and vital to an old-old category characterized by increasing physical decline. One can hypothesize that as individuals age, there comes a point where the likelihood of death (extinction of all earthly life) becomes more salient in terms of the expected life span, and there is a concomitant increase in fear of death. According to Wong (2000, p. 29), "the psychological defenses of denial and avoidance eventually fall in the face of mounting evidence of aging and dying. That is why, sooner or later, people need to come to some form of death acceptance in order to overcome the fear of death." In our data, such an acceptance of inevitable death may be indicated by the reduced fear of death in the older adults who had reached their late 80s or 90s.

The Gerontological Apperception Test

The second approach to assessing death fears involved the use of a projective measure, the Gerontological Apperception Test (GAT) (Wolk & Wolk, 1971), an adaptation of the more general Thematic

Apperception Test. In using the GAT, a series of ambiguous drawings depicting an older person in a particular setting is presented to the subject of the study one by one, and the individual is instructed to "make up your own story about what you see" and later asked "What do you think will happen next?" Responses are scored for the number of themes depicting some kind of loss.

For purposes of the present study, only three of the pictures from the GAT set were used, with responses scored for the number of themes referring to death. The first picture depicted an older woman in bed (possibly a hospital room) and an older man entering the room smiling and carrying a container of flowers. The second picture contained three standing figures, an older woman (with gender possibly ambiguous) and a younger man and woman. The older woman is looking downward with a serious expression (and possibly a scowl) on her face; the younger people also look serious and possibly concerned. The third picture depicts a younger man seated behind a desk, with some kind of certificate on the wall, and an older man with a concerned expression standing near the desk. Responses to each picture were transcribed and the number of death themes counted. A death theme consisted of a mention of the death or impending death of one of the figures in the drawing, with each separate mention of death counted. A total score was obtained for all three pictures.

An example of a response to the first picture in which the respondent mentioned no death themes is as follows:

- She is a convalescent. She needs attention, and he is bringing her flowers. It pleases her and pleases him to do it. Maybe it's his wife. She will soon get better and go home and they will be happy.

In contrast, a response in which death themes are evident is the following:

- A gentleman (maybe husband or son, minister, or brother) has a true concern for a sick female, and he brings a token of blossoms. I believe he has had some relationship to her and his flowers say what he thinks of her. I think she is on her way out, she is so skinny. He will leave, thinking that he has left a gift of himself, and she will accept it as a gift of praise or love. I think that she will die and so will the flowers. He will bear up and go about living.

In the above segment, three death themes can be identified: "she is on her way out," "she will die," and "so will the flowers."

Examples of responses to the second picture follow. The first contains no death themes:

- This woman feels that her son and his wife have not been supportive. She tells them she is lonely and they feel guilty, But their lives are filled with jobs, etc., and things will go on in the same cycle. Eventually they will find a way to spend more time with their lonely mother and they will all be happier.

The second response contains one death theme, "going to end her life."

- I imagine they are family. The older woman has given them bad news. Something she has learned about her health. She's got something that is going to end her life, and it's hard for them to take.

Examples of responses to the third picture follow. The first contains no death themes:

- A man receives news about his health that is not good. However, the doctor is very supportive and gives him hope for the future.

However, the second contains one death theme, "he is going to die soon."

- The young fellow is the man's attorney. The old man knows he is going to die soon. He is trying to get his affairs in order. He's giving the attorney instructions on how to distribute his money.

The total number of death themes in the older adults' responses to the GAT ranged from 0 to 4; 22% of the group had no death themes, 30% had one, 34% had two, 10% had three, and 4% had four. For the total group of elders, there was a mean of 1.43 death themes (*SD* = 1.06). There were no significant gender differences, but there was a weak trend at the .10 level of significance for the number of death themes to decline with age. The 70–79 age group had an average of 1.51 themes, the 80–89 age group had 1.37 themes, and the group aged 90 and over had 1.30 death themes. When the three ethnic/SES groups were compared, there was a weak effect of the ethnicity/SES dimension. In probing this effect, the low SES Whites had more death themes (1.62) than either the high SES Whites (1.34) or the African Americans (1.39). Finally, there was no significant correlation between the GAT and the four subscales of the MFODS.

Admittedly, the GAT is a weak instrument of unproven validity for the measurement of fear of death beyond its face validity. It was used as part of our frankly exploratory approach to areas where few other instruments exist. The few findings described in the preceding paragraph are of borderline significance. Nevertheless, there are a couple of points of interest. First, as a projective tool, the GAT aims to assess covert fears, that is, those fears not acknowledged by the conscious mind. The lower GAT scores obtained by the older age subgroups in the study as compared to the younger subgroups supports the conclusions of Galt and Hayslip (1998) that older adults have less covert death anxiety than younger adults. This finding also seems reasonable in light of the observation of Johnson and Barer (1997) that there is greater acceptance of death and less fear at older ages. The second point is that the greater number of death themes identified by the low SES Whites is not surprising given the greater variety of idiosyncratic emotional and figurative death meanings reported by this group. With a richer set of meanings associated with death stimuli available to them, they may more readily respond to the ambiguous pictures of the projective instrument in terms of death themes.

QUALITATIVE STUDY OF OLDER ADULTS' FEAR OF DEATH

Qualitative information relating to older adults' fear of death was obtained most directly from responses to the interview questions:

Do you have any fears about death? What kind of fears? Does dying itself bother you? Does it frighten you? Secondary information was also gained from the question: What kinds of feelings or emotions do you think you will feel when dying? Additionally, some study participants made pertinent spontaneous comments in other portions of the interview.

In carrying out the qualitative analysis, themes were identified that were considered relevant to fears of death and dying. Elders' views were examined for three age groups (70–79, 80–89, and 90 and above), three ethnicity/SES groups, and the both genders. Although limited by availability of the sample in certain categories, results are discussed for the following major categories: high SES White men, high SES White women, low SES White women, low SES African American women, and low SES African American men. Within each of these larger categories, responses of 70-year-olds, 80-year-olds and 90-year-olds were examined in turn, again depending on the availability of the sample.

High SES White Men

This group of men was highly articulate, but many simply evaded any talk about fears associated with death and dying. Whether they have suppressed all such fears, whether they do have fears but find it unmanly to talk about them, or whether they have intellectualized their fears in order to exert control over them is unclear. However, the 70-year-old men who did respond displayed a range of views:

- That's one of the things you don't talk about.
- I have my affairs in pretty good order. Death is just another bump in the road.
- I have some peripheral thoughts about it. I see death as a process. I doubt that I would feel emotions. [*He goes on to discuss his achievements, including some projects he has undertaken to benefit the community.*] It diminishes my apprehension or anxiety about the phenomenon of death.
- Like most people, I still have thoughts and fears about death, because what happens after death is still unknown. But I also

know it's inevitable, and I have a tendency not to keep worrying about something I have no control over.

- I think every human being is kind of in denial until he gets the message that he's terminally ill. I think I'm not afraid of death. I do have some anxiety about the process of dying—not with death itself. I don't have any fear at all of the unknown. [*He goes on to describe an incident in World War II, when his unit was given orders that appeared suicidal.*] I knew that shortly I would be dead. Fortunately, the order was canceled, but at that time I thought, well, when I'm dead I won't be feeling anything, and I've been pretty cold and miserable for the last month . . . I think when I die, I know what the result is. I will be dead. . . . Certainly there is anxiety about the process of dying and how painful that may be, but not about being dead. I don't worry about being dead. Ha, ha!

One 80-year-old man voiced some "emotional concerns," although he avoided referring explicitly to fear.

- I have never been real worked up about death. It's something that's going to come. I have to feel understanding about it. When death is near, there may be some emotional concerns.

The 90-year-olds seemed a bit more adjusted to the prospect of death.

- Death is inevitable and I'm prepared for it. I don't fear it. There is no point in fearing it. I might fear an auto accident, because that's not inevitable. I'm adjusted to it. The thought of dying doesn't bother me.
- I have never given death a thought. It doesn't frighten me or whatever. I know it's going to happen. When my time is up, it's up.

High SES White Women

The High SES women were somewhat more willing to express their views than the men, but many refused to dwell on thoughts about fears of death. However, a few of the 70-year-olds voiced some concerns.

- I don't think about death. When I'm dead, I'm dead, so why worry about it. I can't have any anxiety over something that has absolutely no solution.
- I guess I have a little anxiety. You just kind of reluctantly go through it [*death*].
- I have fears of dying. But death is just another stop on the journey. It doesn't arouse any fears in me.

Among the 80-year olds, some indicated that they did not dwell on thoughts and fears about death.

- I rarely think of death.
- No, I don't dwell on anything like that. I was awfully close to dying, but I truly gave it no thought whatsoever.

Others thought about death, but denied feeling any fear.

- No, I don't worry about death. I don't think dying is a terrible, terrible thing to experience.
- I don't think I'll be frightened.
- Someone was always dying in our family, and I appreciated growing up not afraid of a corpse. Those things have no fear for me.

Although one woman admitted some fear, others felt they were prepared to die without fear.

- I'm sure I'll feel afraid, because it is the unknown. But I don't dwell on it or think about it that much.
- No fears, I'm just prepared to take whatever comes.
- No, I won't be frightened because I've lived my life. Pain doesn't frighten me, because they have ways to deal with that.

The 90-year-olds also expressed a range of views, some admitting fear and others denying it. But some appeared to have developed a true acceptance of death.

- I think death will be frightening, at least at first—the idea of pain. But it will be a relief.

- I don't worry about death. I don't think about it, period! No, I wouldn't be frightened. It would be my time to go, clearly.
- Why should I fear it? I have no control over it.
- No, I won't be frightened. I have a feeling that it's time. I'm ready to die.
- I don't think of death as something to be afraid of, because I'm not. The one thing I'm afraid of is suffering an awful lot. One of the things that has made me so unafraid of dying is that we're all growing older and we all know we're going to die. It's just which one of us is next.

Low SES White Women

Like older adults of higher socioeconomic status, many of the women in the low socioeconomic status group also claimed to have little or no fear of death. For example, some women in the 70-year-old group stated,

- I don't think about dying that much. It doesn't bother me. I don't think I'll be afraid to die.
- You have to die sometime. I don't think about it. If it happens, it happens.
- I won't be frightened, I'll feel relief.

Some other felt some degree of fear of death:

- I feel apprehensive, but I don't think I am frightened.
- I think I'll have a lot of fear. Everyone does.

The 80-year old women also displayed a range of responses when asked about their death fears. However, a number of women seemed to be more actively concerned with keeping any thoughts about death and dying out of their awareness. For example,

- I don't think it is productive to spend a lot of time thinking about this sort of thing.
- I wouldn't be frightened. I don't think about it. You shouldn't think about it.

- The thought of death doesn't bother me. I just don't dwell on that.

As with the 70-year-olds, some did admit to feelings of fear and apprehensions about dying and death:

- I might be frightened. I don't know.
- I'm not afraid of dying, but I am afraid of choking to death.
- I worry that I'll be in a lot of pain.
- I think we're all just a little bit afraid of dying.

Although there were only a few 90-year-olds in the low SES group, these women seemed to have developed a somewhat more philosophical approach to death.

- I don't think that much about dying. I don't think I'll feel afraid. I never did fear death. You were to die and go to heaven and there would be life hereafter.
- Truthfully, I don't think that much about dying and death. I live one day at a time. [*She talks about her parents who both died of heart attacks.*] If I had a heart attack, I'd probably be a little frightened.

Low SES African American Men

There was only a small number of African American men participating in the study, and only one man in his 70s chose to comment regarding fears of death and dying,

- The closer I get to death, the less it worries me. I have no fears now.

Low SES African American Women

This group of women expressed a wide variety of views regarding any fears of death and dying. Some of the 70-year-olds denied thinking about death or having any fears:

- I just don't think about being dead.

- I don't think about being afraid, not even when I was young.
- Death is the last thing I think about. I never think about dying.
- Dying is not frightening.
- I don't think I'll be afraid. I've had some close calls and I could have died.

Others see death as a natural and expected event:

- There's a time to live and a time to die.
- Death is a natural thing.

Some have developed an attitude of acceptance of death:

- I live each day preparing to die. I have complete trust and acceptance, because everything dies.
- I don't think about dying. There is a state of mind you get in when you approach death. I don't think I'd be afraid.
- You can't get around it, you just have to accept it.
- It's easier when you accept that you are going to die.
- Sometimes I think about death in my bed. If I die, I die. I have no fears, period!

Some of these 70-year-olds viewed death not as frightening, but as a positive thing, a source of relief from illness and burdens:

- If I'm in pain, I'll feel relief.
- I look on death as wonderful, no more pain.
- I don't have that much fear of death. I think there will be a better life ahead.

Still others admitted that they had certain other fears:

- I don't think I'd be scared of dying, but I'll probably be scared, thinking of leaving my family.
- If you haven't lived right, you're scared. That's what is frightening about death.
- I have some feelings of fright, because it is unknown. My greatest fear is having something like cancer and being in a lot of pain for a long time. I fear that more than actual dying itself.

Like many of the 70-year-olds, some of the 80-year-old women asserted that they felt no fear of death:

- No, I'm not afraid of dying.
- I never had any fears. If I had, I wouldn't have been doing the things I was doing when I was younger.

One woman saw death more positively,

- I believe I'll feel relief.

Other women appeared to have various degrees of fear of death and dying. In some cases, statements were complex and revealed some ambivalence. A few revealed a great deal of fear:

- I just don't think about whether I'm going to die tomorrow. But when I die, I'll probably feel some fear.
- I think about death every day. I'm going to be frightened to die.
- I think about death all the time, that someone may break in and murder me. I'll feel relieved, I'm sure, when I'm dying.
- Every time I get on my knees I think about it, and that's day and night. Sometimes it gets too bad, I stop and close the door. The idea of what I will go through in dying bothers me.
- I think dying will be nice, just nice. And I am not afraid of it at all. The idea of what I might go through while dying doesn't bother me at all. I think I'll feel relief. I have no fears, other than of suffering for long time. I didn't even think about it earlier in life.

OLDER ADULTS' FEAR OF DEATH: SOME CONCLUSIONS

After considering the findings of both the quantitative and qualitative studies, one cannot help but be struck by the great variability in older adults' attitudes regarding death. At a time of life when they are becoming more and more vulnerable to death with each passing year, it seems paradoxical that many elders have little fear of death itself and little fear of dying. At the other end of the scale, some report having considerable fear of death, particularly of the dying process. This fear of the dying process at first glance seems to support Johnson and Barer's (1997) conclusion that the very old do not fear death but do fear the dying process. However, many of the older adults we interviewed seemed to have little or no fear of the dying process.

Some elders reported that they never think about death and others asserted that they have no fear of death. In particular, a few of the older men seemed to manifest a rather strong denial of any fears of death. One is led to question whether such denial implies, as terror management theorists (Greenberg et al., 1997; Solomon et al., 1991a, 1991b) suggest, that these individuals have effectively suppressed fear of death from immediate awareness, or whether there is a conscious attempt to control disturbing thoughts about death by refusing to dwell on them. McCoy and colleagues (2000) have argued that older adults use a variety of techniques to maintain high self-esteem despite the losses of aging, and this enables them to deal with fear of annihilation. Some of the older adults mentioned activities to benefit the community or activities to promote the welfare of their descendants. On the one hand, such activities can be interpreted from the perspective of terror management theory as gaining a kind of symbolic immortality and thereby lessening fear of death. On the other hand, interpreted from the perspective of Erikson's (1963, 1982) stage theory, fear of death can be transcended through contributions to the development and well-being of future generations.

Although fear of death had some relationship to demographic background characteristics, these relationships were neither strong nor extensive. For example, women had greater fear of the dying process than men, but this gender difference did not extend to other dimensions of fear of death. Apparent effects of ethnicity on fear of death appeared to be primarily due to social class differences, but again these differences did not extend to all dimensions of fear of death.

In regard to age differences in fear of death, an inverted U-shaped curve was found for fear of the dying process and fear of the unknown but not for other dimensions. The quantitative study suggested that these fears may reach a peak in the early 80s, tapering off at later ages. The qualitative findings seem to support such a view for two reasons. First, the greatest mention of fear of death was found in the low SES groups in their 80s. Second, those elders in their 90s seem to show an increasing acceptance of death, with some actively looking forward to death as a relief from problems of aging. Qualitative findings of this sort indicate that future quantitative studies might take advantage of a more broad-spectrum measure of attitudes toward death, such as the Death Attitude Profile—Revised of Wong and colleagues (1994), to tease out feelings of approach acceptance (looking forward to death as a new and glorious experience), escape acceptance (accepting death as a relief from suffering), neutral acceptance (accepting death as a natural part of life), and death avoidance (avoiding any thoughts of death or death-related subjects) from a core fear of death. All of these nuances of views relative to death were observed in the interview protocols of our older adults. The very diversity of views that we noted may be better tapped by a profile of death attitudes of this sort.

The qualitative interviews also lead us to speculate that the life experiences with death and loss may have something to do with the degree of fear of death experienced by older adults. Some elders were present at the death of a parent, spouse, or other relative and observed these deaths to be quiet and peaceful; in turn, they expected similarly benign deaths for themselves and appeared to have little fear of death. Others were present at the protracted deaths of loved ones who experienced a great deal of pain and other onerous symptoms. It is not surprising that such a critical life event would be followed by greater fear of death. A few adults had themselves come close to death on a previous occasion, and now felt that death was nothing to fear. Such life experiences have not been found to be related to fear of death in younger adults (Neimeyer & Van Brunt, 1995), but this hypothesis has not been examined with older adults. Investigations into the influence of such experiences might make use of the path modeling theoretical approach of Tomer and Eliason (1996, 2000a, 2000b).

In sum, there is considerable evidence that many older adults do fear death, whereas others seem to have managed to cope successfully with such fears as they approach the end of life. Yet, the factors explaining such fears are still not well understood.

5

Views and Expectations About the Dying Process

WHAT DO WE ALREADY KNOW?

The Dying Process as a Stage in Life

The dying process represents the last stage in life when people proceed through changes leading to death. For some, this process is rapid and relatively benign, whereas other experience a protracted and difficult death. According to Cloud (2000), a third of dying people spend at least 10 days in intensive care units where they have to deal with pain, suffering, and futile attempts to cure them or at least extend life. The right-to-die movement has asserted the rights of dying individuals to refuse or withdraw from futile attempts at cure when cure is either impossible or highly unlikely. Many people feel that it is more meaningful to use this last period of life to continue self-growth at the psychosocial level rather than to become preoccupied with attempts at cure.

When considering the dying process, one must realize that individuals who are going through the process are still living while dying. Thus, care for the dying involves not only attempts to reduce the negative aspects of dying but also attempts to improve the quality of living at the same time.

Dying consists primarily of a progressive decline in biological functioning of the individual. There is a decline in health status and an increase in physical symptoms as one moves closer to death.

Negative cognitive and emotional changes directly related to physical decline may occur. At the same time, these changes may be accompanied by other more positive cognitive and emotional changes related to the meaning of dying and the significance of the outcome of dying for the individual. But one must first understand the process of dying before one can hope to improve the quality of living while dying. However, this may be difficult until the beginning and end points of the dying process in our culture are established. These are necessary if one is to begin to study and gain a complete understanding of the dying process.

On a theoretical level, dying can be defined as the beginning of an irreversible decline in physical functioning that inevitably leads to final death. It is theoretical because no one can be absolutely certain when irreversibility begins. And it is not absolutely certain that decline inevitably leads to final death.

However, on a practical level, dying can be said to begin when physicians or medical personnel make the judgment that decline is irreversible. For example, a person may be judged to have 6 months or less to live, which qualifies that person to receive funds for hospice services, given the possibility of a wide margin of error in judgment. Another possible point at which dying may be said to begin is the moment when the physician communicates the diagnosis to the patient and the latter accepts it. Complicating the latter definition of the onset of dying is the fact that in today's multicultural society, communicating the fact that he or she is dying to a patient may violate the cultural norms of certain ethnic groups (e.g., some Mexicans and Koreans). These groups may feel that it is permissible to tell the family that a patient is dying but cruel to tell the patient directly. Above and beyond cultural norms, some doctors have inadequate social skills and do not know how to communicate such sensitive information to a patient or they are embarrassed to do so. Thus, what is acceptable to communicate may not be so easy from a psychological viewpoint.

Similarly, it can be difficult to determine when dying ends. As discussed in Chapter 2, the criteria of death may be the cessation of blood and oxygen circulation, or cessation of activity in the entire brain, or both, but death or "deathing" is a process, and it can be difficult to determine the precise moment of death during this process. The judgment of death is not the same as final death itself. To give an extreme example, suppose that one is pronounced dead in the year 2001, based on the criterion of cessation of entire brain functioning. But even when this criterion is used as a basis for the pronouncement of death and the body is lying in the morgue, there may still be some localized brain activity and continued growth of certain body cells (e.g., nail cells). To carry the example further, suppose that in the 22nd century, medical science and technology can reverse the process of decline so that, beginning at the cellular level, one can reconstruct organs, systems, and the body functioning as whole. Then, based on more advanced technology, pronouncement of the precise moment of death would have shifted.

Even today, as science and technology progress, it becomes more difficult to give a final answer as to when the precise moment of death has occurred. That is, it is difficult to determine irreversibility with absolute certainty. This problem is further complicated by the difficulty in reaching a consensus on what constitutes a living human being. For example, if legal and cultural standards were to change so that complete cessation of cerebral cortex functioning is the sole criterion for pronouncing a person dead, one could legally have a corpse in which there is spontaneous circulation of oxygen and blood due to continuing brain stem activity in the absence of cortex functioning. On the other hand, one might legally decide that the precise moment of death occurs at the psychological level when a conscious demented patient no longer reveals any personhood or self-identify. Of course, these examples of criteria for death are not legal at the present time, but they illustrate how the criteria for the precise moment of death may evolve as society and culture themselves continue to evolve. Therefore, the measure of the duration of the dying process may always be evolving and somewhat approximate. Such approximations may leave out short time periods at the beginning and the ending of the dying period, when certain interventions could make a difference in the outcome.

In the present study, we asked our participants to anticipate what their dying would entail even though they were not yet dying. We wanted to compare their ideas with the existing knowledge of the dying process to determine how realistic they were in understanding what to expect in this last part of their lives. It may be that since they themselves are old, they have witnessed the dying process of family and friends or have gone through their own life-threatening experiences. Such experiences might give them a more accurate understanding of the dying process. On the other hand, if they have no understanding of what to expect at the end of-life, then perhaps some educational intervention would help them to prepare and cope more effectively when their own dying process begins.

Physical and Health Changes in the Dying Process

During the dying process, there are general declines in health status and various physical symptoms emerge. Regardless of individual differences in dying, when the patient has only a few weeks or days to live, a common core of symptoms seems to be present. These physical symptoms may be attributable to various sources: the disease itself, the side effects of medical treatments (e.g., certain medications, chemotherapy, radiation), and deficiencies in eating, sleeping, or activity.

Although many authors have described the variety of physical symptoms that occur near death, (e.g., Emanuel & Emanuel, 1998; Fago, 2001; Field & Cassel, 1997; Gavrin & Chapman, 1995; Lawton, Moss, & Glicksman, 1990; Lynn et al., 1997; Morris, Suissa, Sherwood, Wright, & Greer, 1986; Rees, Hardy, Ling, Broadley, & A'Hern, 1998; Turner et al., 1996), these symptoms are described below following the categorization presented by Hurley, Volicer, and Mahoney (2001):

1. Pain includes both intensity and duration; it may be periodic or constant. Studies show that nearly half of Americans die in pain, surrounded and treated by strangers (Cloud, 2000). Pain may have different origins and be categorized as somatic, visceral, or neuropathic, and hence be treated differently. It may be due to the disease, toxic effects of the treatment, a severe preexisting condition, or all three of these factors. Uncontrolled pain interferes with all aspects of a patient's functioning, and can be very demoralizing.

2. Anorexia-cachexia syndrome is a condition involving reduced appetite (anorexia) and wasting of muscle mass (cachexia). Decreased food intake means that the energy a patient gains from eating does not cover the energy that he or she expends. Cachexia is common to terminal cancer patients and also to those with AIDS and dementia.

3. Weakness, tiredness, and fatigue (asthenia) may be caused by both disease and treatment. It may also be the result of malnutrition and disrupted sleep patterns. Extreme fatigue can interfere with a patient's ability to move, bathe, go to the toilet, and so on. Even dizziness and falls may occur under these conditions.

4. Dyspnea (shortness of breath) and cough are caused by an inability of the lungs to work in proportion to the demands of the activity. It may result from a number of conditions. Difficulty in breathing requires either an increase in ventilation or a decrease in activity.

5. Nausea (the feeling that one might vomit) and vomiting are common symptoms among patients with terminal cancer and AIDS. They are also frequent side effects of certain medications and therapies such as chemotherapy.

6. Dysphagia is the difficulty some dying patients have in swallowing food and liquids. Neuromuscular diseases and cancer are common causes of this problem. Inability to swallow will affect hydration, nutrition, and administration of medications.

7. Bowel problems may involve constipation, which can be caused by certain medications, emotional stress, reduced intake of food and liquids, or decreased activity. Diarrhea is less common than constipation in cancer patients but is considerably more common in HIV-infected patients. Bowel incontinence is a major disability for dementia and stroke patients, causing serious burdens to patients, their families, and other caregivers.

8. Mouth problems of dying patients include dry mouth, sores, dental and gum problems, and infections. These symptoms, which are uncomfortable or painful in themselves, tend to make eating, drinking, and taking medications unpleasant, and thus may lead to dehydration and malnutrition.

9. Skin problems also may cause distress, arising from an underlying disease, treatments, or both. Problems include itching,

dryness, chapping, acne, sweating, extreme sensitivity to touch, dark spots, and pressure sores. The patient also may experience cool limbs with a warm body, and mottled skin. In additions to causing physical discomfort, patients may perceive skin problems as embarrassing.

10. Lymphedema is tissue swelling due to the failure of lymph drainage. It may be caused by infection or therapies such as surgery and radiation. It may limit mobility, cause discomfort, and be unsightly.

11. Ascites is the accumulation of liquid in the abdomen, which occurs in 14% to 50% of terminal cancer patients and in most patients who die of liver failure. It causes feelings of bloating and discomfort from stretching.

12. Other symptoms that may occur are insomnia or sleeping too much, urinary problems (such as diminished production of urine), excessive secretion of bodily fluids, neurological problems (such as disorientation, dizziness, and decreased ability to see), and general agitation and restlessness.

According to Fago (2001), the signs of approaching death in the last few days of life are: reduced level of consciousness, anorexia and decreased thirst, disorientation with or without visual and auditory hallucinations, restlessness, irregular breathing patterns, excessive pulmonary secretions, decreased urine production and incontinence, and progressively cool, purple, mottled extremities. Fago points out that people should know what to expect to help them cope with these last days of their life.

Psychosocial Changes in the Dying Process

Psychosocial symptoms can occur as a direct result of physical decline, or as a result of an individual's reflections on the meaning of dying and its outcomes. Johnson and Barer (1997) stressed that very old people do not fear death but they do fear the dying process. Similar fears of dying have been reported in other studies. Anxiety, depression, confusion (e.g., having difficulty in recognizing family members), and dementia are common psychological symptoms experienced by those who are dying (Field & Cassel, 1997; Gavrin & Chapman, 1995; Hendin, 1973).

Although Kubler-Ross (1969) has been widely criticized for her pioneering work in describing stages of the dying process, some of her ideas are still valuable. The Kubler-Ross stage theory of dying hypothesized that terminally ill patients go through five stages involving shifts in emotional reactions during the dying process. When one becomes aware of being terminally ill, one experiences shock and denial, followed by anger, then bargaining, depression, and finally acceptance. There is no need to describe these emotional reactions as the Kubler-Ross theory is well-known and is a classic in the field. Despite criticisms, there are elements of truth in her position. For example, whether or not the emotional reactions follow a fixed sequence, occur simultaneously, or do not occur at all (for some emotional reactions), the theory does describe what some patients experience during the dying process. Kubler-Ross's work does make one appreciate the importance of emotional reactions during the dying process, as well as the necessity for the patient to deal with them. Finally, the emphasis placed by Kubler-Ross on acceptance of death with dignity and courage certainly does not apply to all patients, but it is part of the original impetus of the self-growth movement, that is, attempting to promote self-growth during the dying process. Acceptance of death was a humanistic approach, a stage where self-reflection and growth could still take place at the end of life. This was a positive aspect of dying, rather than merely viewing the body as an object to be subjected to the tubes, machines, and medications of modern technology (Moller, 1996).

Pattison (1977) divided the dying process into three phases (that roughly correspond to Kubler-Ross's (1969) stages of emotional reactions). Pattison's phases also concentrate on the many diverse emotional experiences associated with dying. In the first phase, anxiety reaches its peak as one first faces the awareness of dying. One is bewildered, confused, and threatened, leading to a peak level of anxiety. As one begins to adjust to the initial crisis, one may then have to cope with many other emotions or fears in the second phase. This phase may be short in duration, occurring near death, or it may involve a long duration possibly extending over years where one is in the hospital intermittently and must adjust to different fears. In fact, Pattison calls this a "dying while living" period, which takes on a very relevant meaning here. Some of the fears that Pattison discusses are fear of physical deterioration of one's body, loss of self-control (i.e., becoming increasingly dependent on others), pain, loneliness, having to deal with remissions and relapses, dealing with sexual desires, dealing with medical personnel in trying to obtain a complete diagnosis and adequate treatment, and so on. As in Kubler-Ross's (1969) approach, one finally reaches a third phase in which the reality of death is accepted as being imminent.

Glaser and Strauss (1968) identified trajectories for dying patients that indicated the duration and rate of their physical decline prior to death. All dying has duration (or takes time). However, when duration is combined with the shape or direction of the course of decline, then one obtains a trajectory of dying. The direction of dying may vacillate from decline to improvement, attaining a plateau, then a slow decline followed by rapid improvement and further rapid decline, and so on. All this vacillation will occur within a certain duration or period of time. One can have trajectories representing the individuality of dying, that is, unique trajectories for particular individuals.

However, some overlapping of individual trajectories exists, leading to the possibility of classifying some common core trajectories that fit various subgroups of patients. According to Glaser and Strauss (1968), one core trajectory occurs when the duration of dying is known and the direction or shape of the dying process is known, as when the dying patient is expected to last only a few hours and decline will be steep. Such a swift, abrupt decline may be due to a heart attack, a serious accident, or complications in surgery.

Another core trajectory occurs when the duration of dying is unknown and the direction or shape of dying is unknown. This is typical of many fatal chronic illnesses, for example, certain kinds of cancer and heart conditions. It may also involve a slow trajectory in which much custodial care is needed, such as in multiple sclerosis.

A third trajectory is found when both the duration and course of the illness are unknown, but both can be determined within a short time period (e.g., after exploratory surgery, awaiting a pathology report after surgery, waiting to see if illness responds to treatment, and so on).

One other core trajectory occurs when the duration of dying is known but the direction of dying is unknown, for example, when a patient has a bad heart but there is no chance for a transplant. The medical staff may be on constant alert for emergency treatment involving intensive care that may or may not result in death.

One final core trajectory is found when the duration of dying is unknown but the direction of dying is known. This trajectory might involve a case of leukemia where the patient vacillates many times from slow improvement to rapid decline, then remains at a plateau, then experiences further decline, and so on.

Medical personnel can formulate a trajectory from a diagnosis, followed by a prognosis to use as a guide to change treatment or care at different points in the trajectory. Such trajectories or expectations of dying can also be formulated by family, friends, and the patient. These trajectories may or may not match those of the medical personnel, but both kinds of trajectories may influence the behavior of others toward the patient as well as the patient's own behaviors.

Accompanying the trajectories of physical changes during the dying process, one can formulate cognitive/emotional trajectories, that is, ideational and emotional changes directly associated with the physical changes or ideational/emotional changes associated with the meaning and significance of dying and motivated by the patient's personality. Such trajectories can represent the unique expectations of a sequence of physical and cognitive-emotional changes that will occur during the patient's dying process.

Many trajectories can be identified that lead to useful classification schemes. An important and well-known scheme is that formulated by the Institute of Medicine (1997). The first trajectory is sudden death from an unexpected cause, such as an accident. The second trajectory is that of steady decline, such as cancer. The third trajectory is a long period of chronic illness with gradual decline and periodic crises that may result in sudden death, for example, congestive heart failure.

An interesting study that illustrates the vacillation of a psychological trajectory (Chochinov, Tataryn, Clinch, & Dudgeon, 1999) was carried out to assess dying patients' continued will to live. The researchers worked with 168 mostly elderly cancer patients admitted to a palliative care facility in Manitoba between November 1993 and March 1995. The subjects of the study were screened to make sure that they had the mental competence and physical strength to participate. Patients completed a questionnaire twice a day and continued in most cases until shortly before death. They rated themselves on a 100-point scale measuring pain, nausea, shortness of breath, appetite, drowsiness, depression, sense of well-being, anxiety, and activity. They also rated the strength of their will to live on a scale with "complete will to live" and "no will to live" at the extremes.

Chochinov and colleagues (1999) found that patients' will to live fluctuated greatly from time to time; within a 12-hour period, the patient's will to live could fluctuate by 30% or more. Over a 30-day period, the fluctuations were as great as 70% leading to the conclusion that the will to live is highly unstable among cancer patients. Most of the patients were enrolled in the study 24 hours after being admitted to the center, and initially anxiety was the single most important factor weakening their will to live. Later, depression became the most significant factor determining their will to live, and as death grew closer, physical distress replaced mental anxiety as the main factor weakening the will to live.

Although the results probably would be different for different types of subjects, diseases, and contexts, the work of Chochinov and colleagues (1999) is important in that it demonstrates a unique sequence or trajectory during the dying process. It is a sequential process concerned with changing needs, symptoms, and feelings that appears to be needed to fully understand the dying process when considered along with concomitant causal changes in the person and the context.

Based on observational studies in hospitals, Glaser and Strauss (1968) developed a context awareness approach to dying. Acting as participant observers, they monitored the interaction between terminal patients and medical personnel. Their observations were coded into four types of awareness contexts, that is, degrees of awareness by patients as to whether they were judged to be dying. The first is called "closed awareness," a state in which patients do not know that they are dying, and the medical personnel does not tell them. The second context is "suspected awareness," a state in which the patients suspect they are dying and attempt to find out the truth in various ways, but the medical personnel avoids telling them. The third context is "mutual pretense," where patients and medical personnel both know that patients are dying but both continue to pretend otherwise. They avoid the issue and usually discuss mundane topics. The fourth context is "open awareness," where patients and medical personnel know the patient is dying and there is opportunity for truthful dialogue.

Seale, Addington-Hall, and McCarthy (1997) analyzed a subset of data from a survey carried out in the United Kingdom of 3,698 relatives, friends, and others who knew a sample of people dying in 1990. Using the typology of awareness context developed by Glaser and Strauss (1968), the prevalence of different awareness contexts was determined. Open awareness of dying, where both the dying person and the respondent knew that the person dying, was the most prevalent awareness context. This was particularly the case regarding cancer patients, and represents a change since 1968 when closed awareness (where the respondent knows, but the dying person does not) was more common. Compared with people in closed awareness, people dying in full awareness are more able to plan their own dying process. They can avoid to a greater extent the possibility of dying alone, they have greater influence on where they will die (e.g., at home), and they express more openly their wishes as to how they want to die (e.g., through euthanasia). In short, study respondents felt that patients tended to feel a greater sense of satisfaction when they had more control over when, where, and how they die. It is this context that allows for further self-growth during the period of living while dying.

According to Schroepfer (1999), each awareness context provides different opportunities and costs for reducing discomfort, fear, and isolation, and increasing growth, sharing, and acceptance. Furthermore, both Kubler-Ross's (1969) and Glaser and Strauss's (1968) positions sought to reduce stress by helping the patient to finally gain acceptance of death. But Schroepfer also felt that acceptance of death is related to perceived control over death, which in turn helps to reduce the degree of stress. Many people today die in a hospital or nursing home, with a much smaller number dying at home. In such institutions, they experience a depersonalized environment, follow rigid schedules, are perceived as helpless by medical personnel, and know that death is inevitable. Such factors lead dying people to experience a loss of control in their lives, which in turn influences the stress of the dying process itself.

Singer, Martin, and Kelner (1999) gained insight into the dying process by determining some of the needs of dying patients. They carried out a qualitative study involving interviews and working with three groups of patients who were either on dialysis, had HIV, or were residents of a long-term care facility. They attempted to determine the kind of end-of-life care that these dying patients desired. Five domains of quality of end-of-life care were identified. First, patients did not want prolongation of dying if it meant the possibility of living on machines, living like a vegetable, or being in a coma with no hope of enjoying any further quality of life. Second, patients felt strongly about controlling their dying process, making whatever decisions were involved so long as they could do so, and having a proxy of their own choosing to be in control when they could no longer make decisions. However, control did not mean making every minute decision on a day-to-day a basis, but rather an overall sense of control over the course or events with their views in general respected and followed. Third, they wanted their loved ones spared any unnecessary burden during their dying process. For example, they did not want loved ones to be burdened with providing physical care or making decisions about life-sustaining treatment without their input. Fourth, they wanted their loved ones to maintain communication with them, talking with them about their dying. Maintaining communication while dying was a very important part of end-of-life care. Finally, dying patients wanted to have adequate treatment for pain and other symptoms (such as vomiting, diarrhea, breathlessness, and so on). In short, dying patients wanted to have loved ones with them, wanted to maintain communication, wanted to exercise some control over the dying process, and wanted to eliminate pain and other distressing symptoms.

Steinhauser and colleagues (2000) evaluated the agreement among family members, physicians, care providers, and patients regarding end-of-life care, and found that all agreed that patients wanted to have freedom from pain, anxiety, and shortness of breath, to be kept clean, and to maintain contact or physical touch with others. This study is interesting because it brings out the dying patients' need to remain in contact with others.

Although the concept of trajectory is used to track paths of health decline and disease during the dying process, some (Bradley, Fried, Kasl, & Idler, 2001) make the point that one can also conceptualize and use trajectories to track multiple qualities of living near the end of life, i.e., a quality of life trajectory above and beyond a dying trajectory. Quality of life is dynamic and changing during the dying period but, if trajectories can be used to track quality of life, knowledge of such trajectories would help clinical practice in the future to benefit terminally ill patients and their families.

Bradley and colleagues (2001) identified various domains in which quality of life could be enhanced for dying patients if intervention takes place at the right time during the trajectory of dying. Such domains involve enhancing religiosity, spiritualism, social support, perceived control, elimination of pain (especially severe and uncontrollable pain), and maintaining communication and physical presence with family and friends. It is hoped that improving care in these domains would not only help the patient deal with dying but simultaneously maintain or improve quality of life close to death. However, to attain this goal, researchers need to further identify the characteristics of quality of life while living near the end of life.

The foregoing review of existing knowledge of the dying process identifies various declines and changes occurring during the dying process. Those who advocate the satisfaction of certain emotional needs or attainment of goals for self-growth during the dying process also imply that certain physical needs exist and should be satisfied.

In summary, one can state that as health declines during the dying process, the patient is likely to experience many physical symptoms (including various levels of pain), lack of support from others, inadequate control of the dying process, various specific fears of dying as well as general death anxiety, concerns about dying alone, depression, and so on. Overall, it is anything but a pleasant process.

THE PRESENT STUDY

The foregoing review of present knowledge of the dying process served as background for our present study of older adults, and led to several questions to guide this portion of the study:

To what extent do older adults, who are only anticipating their eventual dying, think in the same manner or reveal any of the same needs of patients who are actually dying?

Do older adults identify any particular emotions or feelings that they expect to have to deal with when dying?

Do they think sequentially in terms of any trajectories or expectancies that they will have to face?

Do they think in terms of any awareness context surrounding their dying, or any larger environmental context involving family, friends, or medical personnel that might have an influence on their dying?

Do they think in terms of any continued self-growth that can occur while they are dying?

QUANTITATIVE DATA AND ANALYSES

As in other areas, we collected both quantitative and qualitative data in the hopes that the various approaches and data sources would complement each other and provide greater insight into the way in which older adults view the dying process. The quantitative data regarding the dying process centered around the Dying Process Scale, a measure devised for this study.

Description of the Dying Process Scale

Because study respondents were not dying, we asked them to imagine themselves in a hospital with terminal cancer and only five days to live. To find out how our subjects viewed dying under these conditions, we developed an instrument involving 30 items presenting topics that a dying person might focus on during the last few days of life. In responding to each item, study participants were asked to indicate how often they anticipated the topic to occupy their thoughts, using a 5-point scale (never or rarely, occasionally, often, very often, and most of the time or always) with "5" indicating the most frequent response.

Table 5.1 presents the items and study participants' responses, with means (*M*) and standard deviations (*SD*) for the group as a whole, arranged according to rank order of the means. Looking at the mean scores for each of the 30 items, one can identify the topics that study participants anticipated thinking about most and less often. Things they would think about *very often* (item means in the range of 3.5 to 4.5) were their relationships with God and their family, and missing their family members. Things that they anticipated thinking about *often* (item means in the range of 2.5 to 3.5) were physical pain, physical symptoms, feeling depressed, thinking about their past life, thinking about dying quickly, feeling a sense of hopelessness, and feeling totally helpless, wanting to spend time talking to doctors, nurses, and other patients, experiencing sorrow, thinking about life with their mate, thinking about siblings, thinking about how they are being treated in the hospital, and focusing on getting through each day. Things that they would anticipate thinking about *occasionally* (item means in the range of 1.5 to 2.5) were a miracle to save their life, what will happen when they die, feeling lonely, feeling a need to control their life, being preoccupied with side effects of medication, experiencing changes in moods, spending time thinking about ideas, thinking about bodily appearance, feeling frightened, not wanting to see people now, feeling uncertain about when they will die, and feeling a great sense of emptiness. Things they anticipated thinking about *never or rarely* (item means less than 1.5) were feeling angry and feeling bitter.

In general, one can observe from Table 5.1 that these elders' relationship with God and relationships with family would be their most frequent thoughts or concerns. And the least frequent would be feelings of anger or bitterness. Most interesting is that feeling depressed, feeling frightened of dying, and feeling a need to control one's dying were not high on the list, although the current literature on patients actually in the dying process suggests that they would be.

TABLE 5.1 Means and Standard Deviations for 30 Dying Process Items for the Group as a Whole

Rank	Item No.	Item	Mean	SD
1	12	I think about my relationship with God.	4.04	1.17
2	3	I think about my family and how I miss them.	3.61	1.33
3	30	I focus on getting through each day.	3.33	1.38
4	11	I think about my past life.	3.23	1.30
5	18	I spend time talking to doctors and nurses.	3.20	1.14
6	17	I spend time talking to other patients.	3.13	1.22
7	14	I think about dying quickly.	2.94	1.41
8	16	I feel totally helpless.	2.88	1.43
9	1	I focus on the physical pain that I have.	2.83	1.42
10	25	I think about how I'm being treated.	2.77	1.34
11	24	I want to spend more time with siblings.	2.74	1.38
12	6	I feel depressed.	2.62	1.43
13	23	I think about the life I could have with my mate.	2.58	1.37
14	15	I feel a sense of hopelessness.	2.57	1.40
15	22	I experience sorrow.	2.57	1.34
16	2	I concentrate on my physical symptoms.	2.52	1.28
17	4	I think about a miracle saving my life.	2.49	1.48
18	20	I spend time thinking about ideas.	2.44	1.29
19	29	I feel sense of emptiness.	2.39	1.36
20	21	I think about my bodily appearance.	2.38	1.44
21	5	I wonder what will happen to me when I die.	2.36	1.37
22	19	I experience changes in mood.	2.36	1.31
23	27	I don't want to see people now.	2.35	1.29
24	13	I am preoccupied with the side effects of medication.	2.32	1.21
25	7	I feel lonely.	2.30	1.25
26	26	I feel frightened.	2.21	1.20
27	10	I feel a need to control my life.	2.10	1.30
28	28	I feel upset by the uncertainty of when I will die.	2.00	1.24
29	8	I feel angry.	1.45	0.83
30	9	I feel bitter.	1.38	0.85

Descriptors corresponding to item means: most of the time = above 4.5; very often = 3.5–4.5; often = 2.5–3.5; occasionally = 1.5–2.5; never or rarely = below 0.5.

On the other hand, thoughts related to the hospital context seem important, e.g., getting through each day, spending time talking to doctors, nurses and other patients, and thinking about how one is being treated in the hospital. Thinking about one's past life fits in with a life review concept, which various authors (e.g., Butler, 1963; Erikson, 1959) suggest is important for older people near death. In general, emotional reactions of various kinds seem to have less priority than dealing with the dying situation. For example, by talking to doctors, nurses, and patients, a patient might learn of new ideas for dealing with the cancer condition.

Factor Analysis of the Item Scores

A principal components factor analysis with varimax rotation was carried out to explore the presence of underlying factors in the instrument. Although nine factors with eigenvalues greater than 1 were identified, an examination of the scree plot in combination with a consideration of the content of items with loadings of .4 or greater on the factor led to retention of only the first five factors. These factors represented 23 of the 30 items and explained 51% of the variance in the data set. They were labeled as follows:

Emotional reactions. This factor included eight items describing emotions associated with dying such as feeling lonely (7), helpless (16), hopeless (15), frightened (26), sorrowful (22), uncertain (28), empty (29), and depressed (26).

Concern with physical survival. This factor included five items describing bodily concerns during the dying process, such as preoccupation with pain (1), physical symptoms (2), side effects of medication (13), just getting through each day (30), and dying quickly to get it over with (14).

Concern with family. This factor included three items concerned with thinking about family in general and missing them (3), thinking about one's mate (23), and thinking about spending time with siblings (24).

Rancor. This factor included three items describing feelings of anger (8), bitterness (9), and having no feeling of relationship with God (12).

Coping with dying. This factor included four items concerned with hoping for a miracle to save one's life (4), feeling a need for control in the dying situation (10), spending time talking to doctors and nurses (17), and spending time with other patients (18). The latter two items presumably reflected the hope of learning things from others that could help one to survive or to better deal with one's condition.

Seven items did not load on any of the factors. They were: I wonder what will happen to me when I die (5), I think about my past life (11), I experience changes in mood (19), I spend time thinking about ideas (20), I think about my bodily appearance (21), I think about how I am being treated (25), and I don't want to see people now [when dying] (27).

Because the factor scores involved different numbers of items, in order to determine which factors were most favored by the group the mean score for a factor was divided by the number of items included in the factor score to obtain a mean score per item for each factor. From Table 5.2, one can observe that as our participants anticipated going through the dying process, they would think about their family more often than anything else, then concern for their physical survival, followed by their capacity to cope with dying, then their emotional reactions to dying, and finally rancor associated with dying.

Effects of Age, Gender, Ethnicity, and SES

To examine any effects of age, gender, ethnicity, and SES on the way elders anticipated the dying process, analysis of variance was carried out for each of the factors of the Death Meanings Scale.

In the comparisons of three groups aged 70–79, 80–89, and 90–99 (see Table 5.3), the analyses revealed significant age differences in the factors Emotions, Coping with Dying, and Family. The patterns for Emotions and Family were similar. Compared to the 70- and 90-year-olds, the 80-year-olds anticipated greater concern for family relationships and more emotional reactions while dying. The pattern for Coping with Dying was different, in that both the

TABLE 5.2 Mean Scores per Item for Five Dying Process Factors Presented in Rank Order

Factor	Mean per item	No. Items	Mean	SD
Concern with the family	2.85	3	8.55	3.04
Concern for physical survival	2.79	5	13.95	4.67
Coping with dying	2.73	4	10.92	8.55
Emotions	2.44	8	19.55	7.50
Rancor	1.69	3	5.80	2.17

70- and 80-year-olds anticipated more coping with dying thoughts than the 90-year-olds.

In the analyses for gender differences (see Table 5.4), men and women did not differ on any of the five factors.

Finally, analysis of variance was used to determine ethnic and SES differences on the five dying process factors. The three previously defined groups (high SES Whites, low SES Whites, and African Americans) were compared (see Table 5.5). An overall significant *F*-test was followed by planned orthogonal comparisons of both White groups versus the African American group, and the high SES Whites versus the low SES Whites. Significant differences were found for four of the five dying process factors (Emotions, Coping with Dying, Family, and Rancor), with the same pattern of findings in the orthogonal comparison tests for all four factors. That is, the two White groups differed significantly from the African American group, but the high SES Whites and low SES Whites did not differ. The Whites anticipated more emotional reactions, more concern with family relationships and more rancor during the dying process than African Americans. However, African Americans anticipated more coping with dying than Whites.

TABLE 5.3 Summary of *F*-tests for Differences in Five Dying Process Factors for Three Age Groups, With Planned Orthogonal Contrasts

| | Means by Age Group | | | | *t*-test for Contrast | |
Factor	70–79	80–89	90–99	*F*	70–89 vs. 90s	70s vs. 80s
Emotions	18.00	21.37	18.50	2.35*	0.31	−2.03**
Physical survival	13.69	14.08	15.50	0.30	−0.67	−0.37
Coping with dying	10.88	11.13	9.25	0.48	2.05**	−0.30
Family	7.88	9.37	7.75	2.63*	0.57	−2.22**
Rancor	4.90	4.76	4.00	0.32	0.75	0.29

* $p < .10$; ** $p < .05$; *** $p < .01$

Summary

The quantitative findings can be summarized briefly as follows: While dying, the group as a whole anticipated thinking most often about the family, then about concerns for physical survival, coping with dying, emotional reactions, and (least often) rancor. When different age groups were compared, the 80-year-olds anticipated thinking more often about the family and showing more emotional reactions than the 70- and 90-year-olds. The 90-year-olds anticipated less concern about coping with dying than the other two age groups. No gender differences were found. In the comparisons of the three ethnic/SES groups, Whites anticipated more emotional reactions, more concern with family, and more rancor than African Americans, but less concern with coping with dying. Here, ethnicity rather than socioeconomic status seemed to be the important factor.

Overall, the ways in which older adults viewed the dying process varied both by age and ethnicity. However, because use of the Dying Process Scale in quantitative analyses was exploratory in nature, it is of particular interest to examine the qualitative findings.

TABLE 5.4 Summary of *t*-tests for Gender Differences on Five Dying Process Factors

Factor	Men	Women	*t-test*
Emotions	17.58	19.88	−0.98
Physical survival	13.42	14.04	−0.43
Coping with dying	10.92	10.91	0.01
Family	8.92	8.49	0.45
Rancor	5.58	4.67	1.36

* $p < .10$; ** $p < .05$; *** $p < .01$

QUALITATIVE DATA AND ANALYSES

Interview Questions Regarding the Dying Process

In this part of the study, the study participants were asked to respond to several questions about the dying process while we tape-recorded their responses. The basic questions were:

1. What do you think your dying will be like? That is, can you describe the steps that you might go through mentally and physically while dying?
2. Under what conditions would you anticipate dying to be easier or more difficult?
3. Do you prefer having someone with you while dying or would you prefer being alone?
4. What is a good dying process and what is a bad dying process?

As with other portions of the qualitative interview, the open-ended questions were followed with additional probing questions to enable the interviewer to get at the respondent's views more fully. Every effort was made to maintain a relaxed conversational tone in order to put the participant at ease. We sought to elicit as much dialogue as possible relative to the topic, probing in different directions depending on the conversation. We did not attempt to obtain specific responses to each question in a systematic manner, but let topics emerge in a more natural way during the flow of conversation.

TABLE 5.5 Summary of *F*-tests for Differences in Five Dying Process Factors for Three Ethnic/SES Groups, With Planned Orthogonal Contrasts

| Factor | Means by Ethnic/ SES Group | | | | *t*-test for Contrast | |
	High White	Low White	African American	*F*	W vs. AA	Hi W vs. Low W
Emotions	20.46	21.36	17.45	2.30*	2.10**	−0.43
Physical survival	14.38	14.72	13.03	1.10	1.46	−0.26
Coping with dying	10.23	10.16	12.03	2.63*	−2.29**	0.07
Family	9.65	9.16	7.21	6.06***	3.42***	0.61
Rancor	5.31	5.16	4.12	2.80*	2.35**	0.25

* $p < .10$; ** $p < .05$; *** $p < .01$

In carrying out the qualitative analysis, an attempt was made to find themes in the responses of older adults and to integrate them as much as possible with the quantitative findings. Views were also examined for various age groups, the three ethnic/SES groups, and both genders.

To do so, subgroups classified simultaneously on ethnicity/SES, gender, and age were compared. It was hoped that, even if the number of participants was relatively small for certain subgroups, doing so would give us more insight into older adults' thoughts and feeling about the dying process. Based on the availability of the sample for various subgroups, the major categories used were: high SES White men, high SES White women; low SES White women, low SES African American women, and low SES African American men. Within each of these larger categories, responses of 70-, 80-, and 90-year-olds were examined in turn, again depending on the availability of the sample.

High SES White Men

Although none of the men really described the dying process in any step-by-step fashion, some did identify certain physical or psychological events that they expected to occur when dying. Others tended to state their wishes or desires in regard to dying, others indicated prescription of what their dying perhaps should be like, others associated emotions with the dying process, and still others evaluated what a good or bad dying process would be like. A few claimed that they had no knowledge or experience (with friends or family, or their own life-threatening illness) upon which to base any views on dying; and a few simply did not want to think about dying. However, most of these men indicated the conditions under which dying would be easier or more difficult, and whether or not they preferred dying alone.

Some of the high SES White men in their 70s did not want to think about dying or had no imagination of what it would be like. One person stated,

- I don't really think about it, that's one of those things you don't think about.

Others seemed to think that death would be a slow process of declining awareness leading to a peaceful and relaxing state before death. There would be a gradual decline in consciousness, bodily functions, and emotional reactions. The last moments of dying would be peaceful and end in a sleep. Many seemed to use sleep as a metaphor for dying.

- One goes gently into sleep as death comes.
- My general assumption is that I would have a gradual diminution of consciousness, of my perception of bodily functions, and that sometime later, I would be pronounced dead. I doubt that I would feel emotions. Most people I have been with seem to die very, very peacefully. I would say that it is a state of relaxation, a state of impending sleep. That's been such a common experience that I would anticipate such an experience for myself.
- Dying is like going to sleep and you wake up in a different place.

In short, dying itself was likened to going to sleep, with gradually reduced alertness and increasing relaxation. Some felt that they might sense cues while dying that death was coming.

Dying seemed easier for these men in their 70s if there is sudden death, if dying occurs without pain or suffering, if one has lived a long life and the body is worn out, and if one has faith in God. Dying seemed more difficult if: one experiences a long and lingering death, suffers extreme pain, is dying while young, dying occurs without any preparation for it, one has no faith or is doubting God's existence, or if one has lost vision, hearing, or mobility.

The majority of men in their 70s preferred to have someone present with them while they were dying; whereas some did not care one way or another. However, no one preferred dying alone.

The high SES White men in their 80s did not seem to have many ideas about the dying process itself. If anything, they simply evaluated the consequences of dying. A few thought that it might be an adventure in terms of really finding out one's future. As one individual stated,

- I look at dying as some great adventure. I will learn what lies beyond this life. Or, if nothing is beyond this life, I will learn that.

Some felt that dying might be a relief. As one person stated,

- When I think about dying, nothing goes through my mind. I may feel relief.

But it was never clear whether the relief was due to eliminating the process of dying or finally attaining death itself.

The most interesting difference, as compared to the 70-year-olds was the concern of the men in their 80s for disrupting interpersonal relationships. There was a concern for the burden on family if one's dying became long and difficult and also a sadness of being separated from family and friends:

- I wouldn't like to go through a long period of discomfort, both for my own well-being as well as what it would mean to my wife and family.
- I feel that my dying will leave a void in the lives of my family and friends.
- When death is close, I am sure there will be some emotional concerns. I would want to deal with these concern with my family if I am physically and mentally able to do so.

The 80-year-olds did not seem to express views as to when dying might be easy or difficult except in regard to the general theme that it would be difficult because it would disrupt relationships with family and friends. Most preferred having someone with them while dying, but there was some indication that others did not care or would prefer dying alone.

Men in their 90s seemed to make no attempt to anticipate what the dying process might actually be like for them. Instead, they either stated that they did not know, or they evaluated the consequences of dying for themselves. However, one basic theme did emerge. These 90-year-old men stressed that they had lived a long and full life, and therefore they had no fear of dying. Neither fear of dying nor fear of death was reported. For example,

- I don't fear dying. There is no point in fearing it. I think in my case, I'm adjusted to it. I've had an exciting life, a healthy life, a lot of good friends, and a very successful marriage. My wife was truly a partner. I have two sons who have done very well. I've been very fortunate. The thought of dying doesn't bother me.
- As for how I feel about dying, I'll be happy. I'm just thankful for the tremendous opportunities I've had in my many years of existence. I'm very religious, and I'm in conversation with God all day now. And the main thing I do is thank him for the tremendous opportunities that have been placed in front of me.
- I know dying is going to happen but it doesn't frighten me. At 93, I think that I've had it all, so dying isn't going to be that bad.

Although religion was mentioned by some, it was not particularly stressed as the reason for not fearing death. Rather, the most pertinent reason seemed to be the fact that these very old men have lived their expected life span and it was a full and happy one. Second, they did not seem to anticipate a great deal of pain with dying, so they felt more or less ready for it.

However, some did mention that dying would be easier if one had a religious belief, and if it had happened quickly. Beyond this, they did not mention other conditions when dying would be easy or difficult. In fact, they did not seem too concerned with this issue.

The majority no longer seemed to care if someone was with them while they were dying. Over the entire age range, there seemed to be a gradual shift from the 70- to 90-year-olds from those in their

70s wanting people with them while dying to those in their 90s preferring to die alone or being indifferent about it. For example,

- It's immaterial whether I die alone or with someone. If your family is around you and you prolong your illness or death, it's a terrible drain on them. I wouldn't want to do that. When the time comes, I just think I'll fall over.
- I have no preference whether I die alone or have somebody with me. The thought of family being around when I die doesn't give me any great pleasure or any thought that I should die or anything like that. I think that when my time is up my family would recognize that.

It seems that compared to the 80-year-olds, there is a shifting toward detachment from family relationships or perhaps a distancing from the latter. Perhaps, this is a reciprocal process as the expectation of dying increases on both sides.

In summary, high SES White men in their 70s seemed to make more of an attempt to describe the dying process (e.g., as going to sleep), those in their 80s were more concerned in evaluating the consequences of dying for disrupting personal relationships with family and friends, and those in their 90s were more concerned with acceptance of death without fear or concerns for personal relationships as they have a sense of completion of the life cycle.

One fact emerged from interviewing these three age groups of men. They did not seem to be able to anticipate what their dying process might really be like in terms of declining health, physical symptoms, or psycho-social changes over time. One might have expected these highly articulate men to report expectations about the dying process more fully, because at their age, one would expect them to have experienced serious illnesses of their own, or the dying process of friends and family members. Whether they truly are unconcerned about dying, simply do not want to know about it, are going through denial concerning the process, or just cannot imagine what the process will be like is not clear. But it would seem that it is a domain that they should learn more about in order to better cope with the dying process when it comes.

High SES White Women

The 70-year-old White women, like the men, were able to give little description of the dying process itself. For example,

- I don't know what dying is going to be like. I don't know what to expect.
- I can't imagine what it's like. I think of it as being a void.
- I can't figure how I will feel. I think if you had cancer and destined to die in a week, you'd be glad it would be over.
- I really don't know what dying will be like since I have no experience. But I would like to find if there is anything on the other side.

One person did identify what she felt would be an important aspect of dying at the psychological level, i.e., dying will involve a disengagement process.

- I'm sure that there is going to be some feeling of disengagement, getting away from the world and people in order to get to the point of feeling restful enough to accept what's coming. I think you have to separate yourself at some period. Not that you don't want people, but emotionally you have to separate from them.

This was an interesting insight at the psychological level. It implies an important coping strategy, that is, to distance oneself or eventually withdraw from the world to become able to accept dying and death.

Another person also revealed an interesting insight as she related dying to the circumstances of the situation, implying that there is individuality to dying. She said,

- What dying will be like depends upon the circumstances. If I had a heart attack, I don't think I'd feel much. If I had cancer, then I think that I would welcome the end.

These remarks suggest that women may have more insight into the dying process even though they do not describe steps in the process.

As was the case with the men, women did not express any fear of dying although one women did express concern about being disabled. For example,

- For me, dying and death are just another stop on the journey. It doesn't arouse any fears in me.
- Right now, I feel pretty contented. I wouldn't want to be very ill and in pain. Or being immobile, I wouldn't like that at all. I've thought about those things. The time may come when I can't walk up steps, and so on. But I'll keep on going as long as I can.

None of the women in their 70s mentioned being able to control their dying process. Perhaps this was related to their lack of knowledge regarding such a possibility. There was also little mention of separation from others except in one case:

- It's going to be sadness because of my kids, but it is going to be okay, I think. I know where I'm going, though I am not sure what is going to be like.

Similarly, there was no focus on pain, suffering (although a few mentioned that they did not want extended pain or suffering), loss of control, dying as a relief, or disruption of personal relationships. However, the majority wanted someone with them while they were dying.

Like the 70-year-olds, many of the women in their 80s had no idea of what dying is like. They were unable to imagine it, had little experience with dying (even of family and friends), had not thought about it sufficiently to have formulated any ideas, didn't want to think about it, or just wanted to let it happen and accept it. For example,

- You don't know how you are going to feel while you are dying. I know I would follow my mother. She started singing "Shall we gather at the river" as she went into a coma.
- I have no idea or thoughts as to how I will feel when I am dying. I anticipate that I'll have a stroke or some condition in which I have no feeling.

- When I'm dying, I'm prepared to take whatever comes. If I'm aware of things, I think I'd feel happiness that I was going to die. If I'm sick and it's time for me to die, I think I'd die.

Some women used a metaphor to describe dying, with sleep as metaphor occurring frequently.

- Dying will be like putting out a light. I sat by my husband, and I was looking at a magazine, and he was breathing. And I looked up, and he wasn't breathing. It was just that simple.
- I hope that dying is just like going to sleep. I feel that there will come a time when you just slowly lose consciousness, and then slowly stop breathing.
- I have often compared death to anesthesiology. I've had so many. I've been left in the hall, and all at once I'm out of it and then I come to again. I have a sense that it must be like that to die. And I didn't have any pain with it, you just close down.

Others expressed a wish fulfillment regarding the dying process,

- I think dying will involve a vision of Jesus or my son. It would make dying more satisfying.
- I only hope that my dying is simple and quick, and not a problem to other people. I do not want to have to be cared for month after month. My family history suggests that this may not be so. My mother had a stroke and refused to be fed artificially. My father died immediately. My brother died in a few hours. So that the immediate history is one of short periods of illness.

Again, a few women showed sensitivity to the circumstances and individuality of dying. For example,

- As for feelings toward dying, it would depend on what kind of dying you are doing. If it was like [*spouse*], it would be just like going to sleep. But if you have been in an auto accident or something like that, you would have completely different sort of feelings. Can this be happening to me? But I don't think dying is a terrible, terrible thing to experience. No.

This statement not only revealed the individuality of dying, but also a seeming lack of fear.

In general, these women in their 80s did not seem to be frightened by their anticipated dying. They think that drugs exist now to eliminate pain or they feel that they can depend on their God to take care of them, or they are mentally prepared for it through their own living. For example,

- When I'm dying, I don't think I will be frightened. God has taken care of me thus far, and I have no worries when I cross the line.
- Hopefully, when I'm dying, I will be unconscious; then I won't have any pain or have to fear anything. But I don't dwell on this.
- What concerns me about dying is whether I have enough money to keep me going. The medical costs will eat you up now. I hope that dying will not be a long drawn-out affair that will be hard on the family.
- When you die, you give up certain things; it's not going to be a clean-cut thing. But it's inevitable. There has to be a time to die, but I still wish it wouldn't be.

Some woman thought of dying in terms of the popular conceptions of having out-of-body experiences. For example,

- I don't know what dying will be like. I've had people tell me that they've had out-of-body experiences. One friend survived a heart attack, and he said he shot through space. He didn't go down the dark tunnel. But he said his older brother met him and said, 'You go back; it's not your turn yet.' Well, I might wonder who is going to meet me. Whether it would be my husband or my mother, or who?
- Well, you see all these books about how you go through a tunnel and the light comes out. And people who had death experiences say that they had a choice to come back. I have often wondered if I'd get to stay or if I'd come back.
- I like to think that I will know when it's time to die, and just give up and say, Lord take me.

The 90-year-olds did not show any awareness of the dying process, despite their nearness to death. They didn't know what dying would be like, and didn't think about it. For example,

- I don't know what dying will be like. I have no imagination.
- I don't think about dying, period.

However, one woman hoped that the end of the dying process would involve a reunion with family members.

These 90-year-olds did not seem to show any fear or depression regarding death. For example,

- When I was ill, I was up in the Mayo clinic for a month. If I were dying now, I would not be frightened. It would be my time clearly. I would not be sad. I've had a wonderful life.
- I won't be frightened when I am dying. I'll have a feeling that it's time. I'll feel relief and happiness as I will be ready to die.
- I can honestly say that if I went to bed tonight and didn't wake up in the morning, it wouldn't make any difference to me. I'm ready. If God calls me, I'm ready. I've had a good life.
- The idea of dying doesn't bother me particularly. It may be a relief because I won't have to deal with a lot of problems.
- My feelings about dying will depend on the amount of pain I suffer. But in general, I'll be happy, not sad.

In general, women in their 90s know little about the dying process but they feel ready and happy to go when death comes, without having any fear, depression, or sense of loss of control. Perhaps this indifference to dying is related to their age. People in their 90s may not have many close friends or family members left. Most seem to have a sense of having lived their life. Perhaps the lack of fear of dying is related to their lack of knowledge of the dying process, or both lack of knowledge and a true indifference may operate.

These very old women did not seem to identify the conditions under which dying would be easier or more difficult; they didn't seem to feel a need to make that distinction. The majority didn't know whether or not they wanted others to be present while dying. In terms of numbers, approximately 70% preferred dying alone or just didn't care. A minority wanted someone with them. Again, comparing the three age groups, there was a steady increase with age in the preference for dying alone.

Low SES White Women

The low SES White 70-year-old women did not report very much on the dying process itself. They did not feel that they knew much about the dying process or they could not imagine it. For example,

- I can't imagine what dying will be like.
- I can't even imagine dying. I just hope I drop off in my sleep. I hope I don't know about it.

Many woman seem to express a great deal about the consequences of dying, that is, it may involve some pain, but emphasized that they would not have a fear of dying. Also, for many women, there seemed to be a positive outcome to dying.

- I may be dying with more pains than I have now. But I will feel very content and peaceful.
- I'll go quickly. I won't be frightened and I won't have a lot of pain. I'll feel relief.
- I think my death will be quick because of my breathing. I just won't wake up. I'd feel sad about leaving my family. I don't think I'd be frightened. I'd be going to a better life.
- I would like to go to bed some night and not wake up. I know if I am going to die, I wouldn't be frightened.
- I think I would be more happy that I was going to be with God than staying with my oldest daughter. I don't think I be afraid of dying. When I had a cancer operation, I got real peaceful and quiet inside and I thought I was dying, but I didn't. I hope that when the time comes, I feel that way again.
- I feel apprehensive, but I don't think I'm frightened. I'm not going to be in a lot pain when I'm dying, my doctor will shoot me up with something.
- I've thought about death, and it could be very sudden. But I think I may go slowly with a lot of pain. Now, Mom died in her sleep. Dad died a horrible death suffocating in his breathing. Sometimes I think that's the way I'm going to die. I think I'll have a lot of fear, anyone does.

The latter woman had much experience with family members' dying processes, but seemed ambivalent as to how quickly she expected to die. Also, she was one of the very few people who mentioned any fear of dying, perhaps with good reason in view of her experience.

These women did not discuss explicitly under what conditions dying would be easier or more difficult, but seemed to express a general lack of fear of the dying process, and felt that the expected outcome of dying would be something positive, e.g., a sense of relief, of peace, or of being with God.

The majority of women in their 70s preferred having someone with them when dying, although they rarely made explicit mention of family members.

Like the women in their 70s, those in their 80s did not have a clear expectation of physical or psychological changes while dying. Again, many didn't know what it would be like, they didn't want to know, or they hoped or wished the dying process to be a certain way. Some associated certain emotions with dying or evaluated good and bad dying. For example,

- I don't know what it would be like. I think I'll feel sad, but not frightened.
- I guess I'll be like my mother. She went fast. I'll feel sad. I might be frightened. I don't know.
- I just don't quite know. If it was sudden, I wouldn't have time to feel frightened. If I was in a lot of pain, I'd feel relief.
- I don't think anybody knows what dying is like. I could go to bed at night and die at night. I could meet up with family members who have passed on. I think then I would be happy.
- I don't think it is productive to spend a lot of time thinking about this sort of thing. I think that I have tried to prepare myself for those times.

Some women expressed hopes or wishes as to what dying might be like. For example,

- I think I will feel real peace, because absence from the body is being present with the Lord. I couldn't have it any better. And to be in heaven, I'll be happy.

- I would hope that with my faith it would be a happy experience. I don't feel like I would be afraid of dying. It would be something to look forward to. Of course, you won't know until your time comes.
- I have been with people when they died, and there was no fear and no drama, and that's what I expect for me. I would hope that I could die as gracefully as my father-in-law did.
- I just hope my heart gives out and I go to sleep and don't wake up. But I don't think about it now.
- I think we are all a little bit afraid of it. But I know there are lots of times I wish I could die and get it over with; especially when I hurt so badly. I'd feel relief because I wouldn't have to suffer anymore.
- I hope that I wouldn't be afraid to die, but it's something that's going to happen and family and friends aren't going to change anything. I wouldn't be frightened, but I would think about it. I don't think I'll suffer much, but it won't necessarily be fast.
- I hope that I won't be in a lot of pain. I hope I don't have to go through with that. That would be sadness, probably hopelessness.

Approximately half of the women in their 80s preferred having someone present when dying while the other half didn't care or preferred being alone.

The women in their 90s did not seem to think about the dying process itself.

- I don't think that much about it. I don't think I'll feel afraid. My mother just slept away, she just quit breathing, and my husband died suddenly in the hospital.

Some women wanted to predict what kind of condition would kill them. For example,

- I think that I will die from a heart attack, and that's usually sudden. My mother and father both died of heart attacks. But I've lived a good long life. I'd feel happy about going to meet my God.

In short, the 90-year-old women didn't seem to be concerned about the dying process or have any real fear of it. They felt that they had lived their life and viewed dying as no big obstacle. They seemed quite indifferent about whether or not to have someone with them while dying.

Low SES African American Women

For the most part, the 70-year-old African American women did not have many ideas of the dying process or care to think about it. However, some women described it as follows:

- I think you will just go to sleep. Your body is a machine, and when a part of it gets out of orbit, it slows it down.
- I think it would be like going away, or something like that. I won't feel afraid but I don't what to feel.

Others did not know or seem to have any clear idea about the dying process. For example,

- I have no idea. I never think about dying. I think about living. But if I were in a lot of pain, I'd feel dying was a relief from the misery. If I wasn't in a lot of pain, well, I'd think it was time for me to go anyway.
- I just don't know.
- I don't know about that because I don't know when I am going to die. You could go right now.
- When you're dying, I don't think you know whether anyone is around you or not. There is a state of mind you get in when you approach dying but I'm not there yet. So I don't know what to think.
- Dying is an experience. Nobody can know what you will feel until you reach that point. I was with my brother when he died. But he didn't even know I was there. Death is personal so it really doesn't make any difference.
- I think the Lord has all of that in his hands, and I will not know about it. I won't feel bad. I'll feel happiness.
- I don't know. If I am really sick and suffering a lot, I might feel relief. But I don't think I'll ever feel happy.

Other women did not seem to want to think about dying. For example,

- I never think about that. Dying is the last thing I think about. Everyday when I get up, I thank the Lord for letting me get up. And then I plan for what I am going to do that day.
- I don't think about dying. I live day by day, and everyday I ask the Lord to give me strength.

Some of the women expressed their wishes or hopes regarding dying. For example,

- I hope to go to sleep and not have any pain. I don't want to linger a long time. I want to be happy while I'm dying.
- I wish I'd die right off; sleep myself away in my sleep. I don't know if I will be happy or not.
- I feel that death can be a blessing. It all depends on what condition I'm in when I die. I look on death as wonderful. No more bills to worry, or anything. I think I would feel happy. I feel that I would be happy, because I am truly looking forward to being with the Lord. And the way they describe it to be, I think it is going to be wonderful.
- I've got a feeling it will be very peaceful, and I'm not going to suffer. I believe that I'll be happy.
- My preference is go quickly in my sleep. My great fear is having something like cancer and being a lot of pain for a long time. I fear that more than actual dying itself.
- It will be like flying away, a beautiful dream. Nothing to be frightened about.
- I hope that I can keep my mind calm but I don't think that I will be scared.
- I am hoping that things will be all peace, it will be all spiritual . . . that heaven will be there.
- I hope death will be quick. I feel that I'm going to be sad but in another way of speaking, I may be happy.
- I don't think I'll be frightened, I think I'll just sleep away. I'll be happy if I'm going to heaven.
- I don't think I will be sad. I don't think I will be frightened. I don't think I will experience much pain. I don't think it will be slow. At least, I hope not.

Some women seemed indifferent about dying. For example,

- I don't have any feelings about how I would go. I just accept it because everyone has to die.
- It doesn't matter, because I have no control over it. I just accept it.
- Dying is a nature thing so we don't feel too sad about it. If you feel too sad, then you feel more pain. I leave it to God, whatever he will do is good for me.

None of the women responded directly about when they thought death would easier or more difficult. However, there were indirect references to it in some of their previous comments. What is surprising is the relatively few associations between dying and religion or God that were expressed in the interviews. This is in contrast to the strong associations between religion and personal meanings of death.

Approximately two-thirds of these African American women in their 70s would prefer someone with them when dying compared to dying alone. Only a few didn't care one way or the other.

Like the women in their 70s, those in their 80s seemed unable to describe the process of dying. Some felt that they did not know what it would be like but felt that since it was inevitable they just needed to face it. For example,

It wouldn't matter. When you've got to die, you've got to die.

Others did not know what dying would be like but they associated certain wishes or positive consequences with dying. For example,

- I can't say what it's going to be like when I breathe my last breath. But I believe I'll find relief. And where I go, I'll be happy.
- I don't know about dying. But I'm going to try and die like Jesus. I am going to try to be so close to him. I'll be happy at that.
- Since I've never died before, I don't know what it will be like. But I think my dying will be happy; I'll have good feelings.
- I don't know but I hope I'd be ready to meet the Lord, and be happy.
- I'd be glad that I'll be happy, because I'll get to see my mother and father.
- I think it will be nice, just nice. I don't know why I feel that way.

But I'll have a nice feeling, and I am not afraid of it at all. The idea of what might be tough while dying doesn't bother me at all. I think I'll feel okay.

- When the time comes, you just relax and then sleep away, I guess. But I think that I'd feel happiness.
- I'll just pass over to a land of freedom. I hope I won't be sad. I'm quite sure I'll be relieved.

Only about half of the women in their 80s preferred to have someone with them when dying, whereas the other half preferred to die alone.

Among the African American women in general, there was little description of the dying process either in terms of a decline in health, increased physical symptoms, or personality changes. They seemed more focused on perceiving dying as associated with such positive consequences as happiness, relief, or heaven. They seemed to feel little or no fear of dying and no need to control their anticipated dying process.

Low SES African American Men

Although the number of African American men in the study was small, those in their 70s did not spend much time describing the dying process. For example,

- I think it's just like going to sleep.
- I'll feel interested in dying cause I've never died before. I can't imagine it. But I know I'm going to kick off so I'm interested in how I'm going to do this.

Like the women, a few men had certain wishes about dying. For example,

- I would like to die quick. I don't need no pain.
- Dying will bring me relief. The burden of the world and care of everyday life will be gone.

The majority of the men preferred dying alone. As one person stated,

- I want to die alone. What would I want anybody around for?

Although there were a few 80-year-olds in the study, none responded to these questions.

VIEWS OF THE DYING PROCESS: SOME CONCLUSIONS

The older adults taking part in the study were asked to anticipate what their dying process might be like. However, few made any attempt at a literal description of the dying process or described any sequence of decline over time. At most, many viewed dying in a metaphorical rather than a literal sense, often using the metaphor of sleep to represent death. That is, death was depicted as a decline in alertness until a sleeplike stage was attained.

These elders did not seem to recognize a decline in health status, emerging physical symptoms, psychosocial changes during dying, or the physical, social, and emotional needs that may be involved. Some claimed ignorance or lack of knowledge, or could not imagine what dying would be like. Some did not want to know about dying, and some claimed indifference about the dying process. But such a stance seems strange for people of advanced age, many of whom mentioned friends and family members who went through the dying process or who came close to dying of a life-threatening illness themselves. Because dying is a major life event that most people of this age will soon face, one would expect them to think in terms of physical, social, or emotional needs that dying people might have. The fact that these elders did not entertain such thoughts may indicate some denial of the dying process.

If denial existed, possibly it was a way for older adults to experience secondary control over dying (Schultz & Schlarb, 1987–1988) or an indication of searching for meaning regarding the dying process (Marshall, 1980).

Some elders did identify a particular physical or psychological symptom that was expected to occur during the dying process, such as pain or sorrow. But these were isolated symptoms without connection to other symptoms or to particular diseases, and without any indication of a sequence of change in symptoms over time, such as an increase in pain intensity as nearness to death increases.

They were more focused on the outcomes of dying, which were viewed as mostly positive in nature. These outcomes were either expectations, or wishes, or prescriptions of what they felt dying should be.

It was most interesting that the majority expressed no fear of the dying process, contrary to other studies of the advanced elderly (e.g., Johnson & Barer, 1997). Instead, dying seemed like a rather benign process to them. Also, they felt that they had no need to control their dying process. What difference would it make when they were so close to death? Some specifically mentioned that control over one's dying did not seem important when one's life was so near death. In the event that dying was a difficult process, they assumed that they would be sedated and unaware of their passing, or that God would be there to help them. Some sadness at leaving loved ones was anticipated, but extreme emotional reactions were not expected.

A significant omission from participants' statements was any concern for improving the potential quality of their living while they were dying. It seemed foreign to their thinking to be concerned about improving living while they were preoccupied with dying.

Another striking fact was the relative lack of religious comments. When these elders discussed the meaning of death, religion was a central factor for many of them. But in the case of the dying process, it was infrequently mentioned. Some stated that dying would result in their being with God or in a happy afterlife. But no one mentioned other aspects of religion, such as praying to God to relieve pain while dying. Perhaps dying was seen more as an earthly process compared to death which leads to another life.

Also, it seems that not all older people prefer to have a loved one with them when they are dying. Our data seems to indicate that this is possibly age-related, that is, going from the 70-year-olds to the 90-year-olds, there was a decided shift from wanting others present toward dying alone or being indifferent about it. It might be the case that as one gets older, there are fewer close family members or friends available, leading to a lack of concern for having someone present while dying. However, a few participants suggested that there would be a withdrawal from others and earthly concerns as death approached.

Contrary to the literature (e.g., Kubler-Ross, 1969; Pattison, 1977), the older participants in the study did not expect to experience emotions to the extent reported by these authors, nor did they view dying as following some kind of trajectory (Glaser & Strauss, 1968). If anything, there was a denial of death fears, with no notion of trajectories. Contrary to the literature, there was little or no concern with the context of dying (e.g., dying at home, in a hospital, or nursing home, or interacting with family, friends, medical personnel, and so on). In some elders, there seemed to be a slight awareness of the individuality of dying, that is, the nature of the disease or the circumstances of dying which would influence the course of the dying process.

In the quantitative portion of the study, participants were asked to imagine that they were dying of cancer and to rate each of 30 statements on the Dying Process Scale about the kinds of thoughts and feelings they might have while they were dying. Although five factors were identified in an analysis of the item scores, the quantitative analysis did not indicate great concern for these factors related to the dying process. However, there was a tendency for bodily concerns to be greater in the older compared to the younger age groups. Whites showed more concerns about family and more concern for negative emotions and anger compared to African Americans, but less concern about whether or not they could control their life while dying.

Although these older adults were merely anticipating dying and not directly experiencing it, in general they seem to have a rather unrealistic picture of dying, especially in light of their age and experience with the dying of friends and family members and possibly with their own life-threatening illnesses. There seems to be a need to educate older people on what to expect during the dying process so that they can make more realistic plans to better cope with it.

6

The Influence of Religion on Views of Death

FUNCTIONS OF RELIGION

According to DeSpelder & Strickland (2002) religion has a major function within a culture, that is, it can provide a society with a shared set of beliefs, values, and norms that can hold individuals together by giving them a sense of common identity. Such a shared sense of identity is very important for society to function in an effective and efficient manner. At the very least, religion is an important aspect of most cultures. Even in secular societies, the majority of people have some kind of belief in God and some sort of religious faith.

An additional function of religion is its attempt to provide answers to fundamental questions about the purpose of our existence: Does a God exist and, if so, what is our relationship to him? What is the relevance of prayer to such a God? What is the difference between a living being and a living human being, or what is the nature of being human? What is the meaning of life and death? What is the significance of fears of death and dying relative to our inevitable death? Does an afterlife exist and what is its nature? Many different religions seek to provide answers to these and similar questions.

Religious values, beliefs, and norms can also provide the basis for the rules and legal laws by which we regulate our lives. For example, laws of the state may provide for Sunday closings of businesses, banning of liquor sales on Sunday, and a host of other so-called "blue laws." Although this function seems to be most evident in those societies that do not separate church and state, even in societies where church and state are separate, the values, beliefs, and norms manifested in religion act to informally influence the rules and laws of the state.

At the individual level, religion functions as a source of emotional and social support to people, especially in times of crisis. In addition, religion gives people a frame of reference to guide behavior in their personal living, setting up standards for personal behavior and establishing ideals to strive for.

MEANING OF RELIGION

The function of religion and the meaning of religion are different concepts. It is difficult to give a concise definition of the meaning of religion as religion involves several different components. In the research literature, the term religiosity is sometimes used to represent religion, with particular aspects of religion carefully defined. Various instruments have been developed to measure different dimensions of religiosity (e.g., Ainlay & Smith, 1984; Chatters, Levin, & Taylor, 1992; Krause, 1993; Krause & Tran, 1989).

In the present chapter, religion is conceptualized as a multidimensional concept, including some components that others have used in their research and some components that we feel are important to the present study. These components include the following: (a) *organizational religiosity*, which is concerned with religious affiliation and attendance at various church activities; it involves a community of people who belong to the same denomination and follow the religious practices of that denomination; (b) *nonorganizational religiosity*, which is concerned with practices that may be independent of any particular religious denomination, e.g., reading religious books, watching or listening to religious programs; (c) *subjective religiosity* (sometimes called intrinsic religiosity), which is concerned with the person's subjective feelings of intensity and commitment toward religion and God; (d) *religious coping*, which is concerned with the use of religious faith to help in dealing with life's problems; (e) *religious beliefs*, which includes specific beliefs about God, prayer, and an afterlife (including its potentially negative or positive rewards); (f) *ethical standards of right and wrong*, as derived from the religion's conception of God or given to man by God, with such standards to be followed in daily living and perhaps as a requirement for attaining an afterlife; and (g) *spiritualism* (or spiritual experience), which is an emotional reaction to identifying with something or someone greater than oneself (e.g., a God, the universe itself, mankind, science, human rights, human growth, music, art, and so on).

However, it is still difficult to define religion or religiosity. All these components may be aspects of religion, but they do not define an integrated religiosity. For example, a person may attend a particular church for social activities, read religious literature out of curiosity, but have very little subjective commitment to religion. An atheist may have high ethical standards. An agnostic may have spiritual experiences which have nothing to do with organized religion or God.

Also, the previously enumerated core beliefs of religion (God, prayer, and an afterlife) are not defined in an absolute and universal manner. The content of the beliefs may be relative to particular religions, such as Christianity, Hinduism, Buddhism, Islam, Judaism, and so on. Different religions may have different conceptions of God. For some, God may be personal, caring, and forgiving; for others, God maybe indifferent to our individual lives or consider us no better than other species. For still others, God could simply be some grand or intelligent design behind the structure and functioning of the universe, or some invisible connection between individuals. How we define God may influence how we perceive the significance of prayer, the type or existence of an afterlife, the set of ethical standards, the experiences considered spiritual, and the religious practices one implements. These may all vary from one religion to another in degree or kind.

Prayer can be viewed as very formal and recited with others at group meetings, or it can be considered to be a private and personal attempt to communicate with God. The purpose of prayer also varies, e.g., asking for God's help, thanking God for some previous favor, using God as a confidante, trying to gain feelings of closeness to God, and so on (Krause, Chatters, Meltzer, & Morgan, 2000).

The idea of immortality or an afterlife can mean many different things, depending on the particular religion. It may mean rebirth or reincarnation, resurrection from the dead, joining of body and soul and being with God, transformation into some kind of shadowy spirit endlessly roaming the earth, or symbolic immortality (in which one lives on through genetic heritage, achievements, others' memories, financial legacies, and so on). For the atheist, agnostic, or apathist (someone who is indifferent as to whether God exists or not), immortality may mean a continuation of life on earth through such means as genetic engineering, cloning, cryonics, or simply the recycling of one's body chemicals for the continued life of others.

Regardless of how God and the various components of religion are defined, various studies have indicated that people tend to become more religious as they grow older, with a beneficial influence on their morale, well-being, and health (e.g., McFadden & Levin, 1996). It must be remembered, however, that demonstrations of the efficacy of religious beliefs do not provide scientific evidence for the truth of such beliefs. The evidence demonstrates only that holding certain beliefs can have a positive effect on individuals' thoughts, feelings, or behaviors. Even if religious beliefs were totally false, positive effects could still occur if people truly believed them.

The investigation of the truth of religion is a philosophical and not a psychological problem. From a psychological viewpoint and for the purposes of the present study, we were interested in learning whether older adults' religious beliefs and behaviors were related to their personal meanings of death, fears of death, and views of the dying process.

PREVIOUS STUDIES OF RELIGION IN
RELATION TO VIEWS OF DEATH

Although many studies have investigated religion in the lives of older adults (see Levin, 1997, for a review), few have considered the relationship of elders' religious beliefs and behaviors to their views of death. Yet, the importance of religious faith in coming to grips with mortality and coping with impending death are recognized (e.g., Pargament, 1997).

A number of widely shared personal meanings of death stem from religious beliefs (DeSpelder & Strickland, 2002), including such meanings as symbolic immortality and belief in the afterlife. (See also the personal death meanings of study participants in Chapter 3.) In a study of personal meanings of death among college students (Holcomb, Neimeyer, & Moore, 1993), content analysis of free-response narratives on the topic of death revealed that meanings associated with continued existence were among the major constructs used by students in writing about death. Narratives of those with a Christian religious orientation contained such meanings as an afterlife of reward or punishment, a heaven or hell, and transition to a peaceful state allowing them to be with God and loved ones, whereas some narratives of those with other orientations contained different constructs. However, the study did not attempt to relate measures of religiosity to death meanings.

One might expect individuals with stronger religious beliefs to have less fear of death, especially when the beliefs involve the concept of an afterlife. However, the effects of religion on fear of death are complex, depending on whether religious behaviors or intrinsic religiosity (depth of religious belief or commitment) are measured. In general, a weak religious commitment is related to a greater fear of death than a strong religious commitment, but findings vary depending on whether external aspects of religiosity (such as church membership and attendance) or intrinsic aspects (importance of religious faith in daily life) are measured. Thorson and Powell (1990, 2000) found that intrinsic religiosity (religious belief) was negatively related to death anxiety whereas religious behaviors had no relationship. A study by Clement (1998) supported the relationship between intrinsic religiosity and reduced fear of death. In a recent meta-analysis of existing studies of death anxiety in older adults (Fortner, Neimeyer, and Rybarczyk, 2000), 13 studies included religiosity as a variable. In an initial analysis of these studies, the authors found no relationship between religiosity and fear of death. However, a further analysis in which findings involving religious beliefs were separated from findings involving religious behaviors supported the conclusion that stronger intrinsic religiosity was related to less fear of death, whereas religious behaviors were not related. Finally, Tomer and Eliason (2000b), in a study involving college students and older adults, religious attendance and religious devotion (frequency of prayer and reading religious texts) were both found to predict greater fear of nonbeing, although the relationship was stronger for religious devotion than for religious attendance.

A cautionary note is that findings regarding intrinsic religiosity vary depending on the particular content of the individual's religious belief. If the religious belief stresses notions of punishment in the afterlife, then greater religiosity predicts a greater fear of death (Florian & Kravitz, 1983). On the other hand, if the belief stresses love of God, God as a benevolent caretaker, and an idyllic afterlife, then religiosity is related to less fear of death (Rigdon & Epting, 1985). Also, it is possible that the relationship of religiosity to fear of death is curvilinear. Downey (1984) found that men who were moderately religious had more death fear than either those who were strongly religious or those who were nonbelievers.

The little that is known about the influence of religiosity on views of the dying process comes from studies of end-of-life care. Many palliative care programs stress the importance of spiritual needs in terminal care. Although religious behaviors such as church attendance tend to show declines across the last year of life, intrinsic religiosity (subjective religious feeling) did not (Bradley, Fried, Kasl, & Idler, 2001). Those with greater religiosity reported a higher quality of life on a variety of measures, including less depression. One can interpret this finding as indicating that those with greater intrinsic religiosity experience less negative emotionality during the dying process, although more refined studies are obviously needed. Wong (2000) argues that, rather than merely reducing a fear of death, intrinsic religious commitment leads to an "approach acceptance" of death over the period of terminal decline, in which the individual recognizes that his or her mission in life is completed and looks forward to a rewarding afterlife beyond the grave. The theme of acceptance of death during the dying process is also found in the works of Kubler-Ross (1997). Whether such views emerge in the views of the dying process held by older adults not yet in a trajectory of terminal decline is yet to be determined.

THE PRESENT STUDY

Our goals in the empirical study were twofold. First, because religion itself seem to be increasingly an important factor in the lives of older adults, we wanted to increase our understanding of what religion meant for the participants in our study. Second, we wanted to discover any relationships between their religion and their personal meanings of death, fears of death, and views of the dying process.

Study Participants

Our study was an exploratory one, limited by time and money to a relatively small sample of people residing in Central Indiana. As a result, the sample was composed primarily of adherents to Christian religions. However, the sample was sufficient in size to lead to insights and hypotheses for further study, which could then include other religious and nonreligious groups now existing in our multicultural society.

Over 96% of study participants reported some kind of religious affiliation. In terms of religious denominations, their affiliations were: Baptist, 29%; Methodist, 18%; Presbyterian, 14%; Evangelical (Disciples of Christ, Pentecostal, etc.) 9%; Federated Protestants, 7%; Catholic, 6%; Unitarian, 4%; Episcopal, 3%; Lutheran, 3%; Jewish, 2%; and Bahai, 1%. Of the remaining 4% with no reported religious affiliation, 1% indicated not only no affiliation but no belief in God. When religious affiliation was reclassified into major religious types (Roof & McKinney, 1987), 45% of participants were affiliated with traditional Protestant religions and 38% were affiliated with fundamentalist or evangelical Protestant religions. The remaining 17% provided a representation of other religious views.

QUANTITATIVE STUDY OF THE INFLUENCE OF RELIGION ON VIEWS OF DEATH

Religiosity of Study Participants

As previously stated, religiosity is a somewhat elusive concept that encompasses several dimensions, and each of the existing instruments assesses certain dimensions and not others. For the present study, religiosity subscales were drawn from existing sources and other measures were devised to measure five aspects of religiosity.

Organizational Religiosity

The first subscale assessed organizational religiosity (the extent to which an individual participates in organized religious services and activities). It consisted of five items used by Chatters, Levin, and Taylor (1992): how frequently the individual attends religious services (6-point scale), church membership (2-point scale), number of church organizations participated in (exact number), frequency of participation in other church activities (5-point scale), and whether any offices or positions in the church are held (2-point scale). The total score for organizational religiosity could range from 4 to 15, plus the number of number of church clubs or organizations in which the individual participated. A high score indicates greater organizational religiosity.

The results indicated that the great majority of study participants attended religious services; 72% attended weekly or more often and only 5% never attended. Almost 90% were official members of their church or temple; others claimed allegiance to a particular denomination but were not officially members. Additionally, many elders did not always attend the church of their affiliation. Some had mobility problems and attended a church service that was geographically closer, or the church of friends who provided transportation.

There was also low participation in church clubs or organizations, with 59% taking part in no organizations, and another 29% taking part in only one or two. In regard to other church-related activities, 56% never participated and only 20% took part weekly or more often. Only 16% held any kind of office or position at their church. Mean scores for the five items are found in Table 6.1. The mean total score for organizational religiosity was 10.50 (*SD* = 3.44).

Nonorganizational Religiosity

The second measure was nonorganization religiosity (Chatters et al., 1992), consisting of four 5-point items. Items assessed the extent to which an individual reads religious books and other materials,

TABLE 6.1 Means and Standard Deviations for Organizational Religiosity Items and Subscore

Measure	Mean	SD
Attend services	4.48	1.15
Member of church	1.90	0.30
Number of church organizations	0.92	1.56
Other activities at place of worship	2.05	1.33
Hold office in one's church	1.17	0.37
Total organizational religiosity	10.50	3.44

watches or listens to religious programs on TV or radio, prays, and asks someone to pray for him or her. The total score for nonorganizational religiosity could range from 4 to 20, with a high score indicating greater religiosity.

Table 6.2 present means and standard deviations for the items and total score. The results indicated a considerable degree of nonorganizational religiosity behaviors. Only 7% never read religious materials, whereas 68% read such materials at least weekly. Although 26% never watched or listened to religious programming on TV or radio, 51% did so weekly or more often. The frequency at which they prayed was high, with 86% praying at least once daily (many prayed many times a day); only 4% never prayed. The frequency of asking others to pray for them was much lower; 38% never asked others, and only 28% asked weekly or more often. The mean total nonorganizational religiosity score for the group was 14.01 (*SD* = 3.68).

TABLE 6.2 Means and Standard Deviations for Nonorganizational Religiosity Items and Subscore

Measure	Mean	SD
Read religious materials	3.92	1.31
Listen to religious TV/radio programs	3.08	1.50
Praying	4.71	0.87
Asking others to pray for one	2.31	1.33
Total Nonorganizational religiosity	14.01	3.68

Subjective Religiosity

The third subscale was subjective religiosity, which was concerned with the level of religious commitment. It was assessed by three items adapted from the instruments of Chatters et al. (1992) and Krause (1993). Items asked: how religious would you say you are independent of whether or not you go to church (4-point scale), the importance of God in your life (4-point scale), and whether you get comfort and strength from your religion (5-point scale). The total subjective religiosity score could range from 3 to 13. Mean item scores and total score are found in Table 6.3.

Study participants' subjective or intrinsic religiosity was relatively high. When asked how religious they were, 38% were very religious, and another 51% said they were fairly religious. As to the importance of God to an individual's life, 83% said it was very important and another 12% indicated it was fairly important. Finally, 54% felt that they received comfort and strength from their religion all the time, and 31% felt comfort and strength often.

Religious Coping

The fourth measure was religious coping, a measure of the extent to which the person's religion was an aid in coping with life and its problems. A four-item scale was devised for this study, with a 5-point response scale for each item ranging from "not at all" to "all the time." Items asked for the extent to which the individual's religion gave a sense of belonging, helped in dealing with problems, helped to control one's fate, and gave a sense of inner emotional peace.

TABLE 6.3 Means and Standard Deviations of Subjective Religiosity Items and Subscore

Measure	Mean	SD
Feel religious	3.20	0.79
Importance of God in one's life	3.73	0.68
Obtain comfort/strength from religion	4.27	1.06
Total subjective religiosity	11.20	2.08

Total coping scores could range from 4 to 20. Means and standard deviations for the items and total score are found in Table 6.4.

The results indicated that over half of study participants felt that their religion gave them a sense of belonging, helped them to deal with problem, and gave them a sense of inner peace all of the time, with another fourth feeling that it did so sometimes; only a tenth felt that it was of no help in coping. Responses regarding religion's help in controlling their fate were somewhat lower, with 19% feeling that it never helped and only 40% indicating that it helped some of the time. The mean score for religious coping for the group was 16.17 (SD = 4.47).

Religious Change

The final aspect of religiosity was a single 5-point item asking whether the respondent felt that he or she had become more or less religious since middle age. Although the largest percentage of elders, 41%, indicated that they had not changed as they grew older, the remainder felt that they had changed. Only 8% felt that they had become less religious, whereas 25% felt that they had become a little more religious and 26% felt that they had become much more religious compared to when they were middle-aged. The mean score on the change item was 3.65 (SD = 1.01).

Demographic Differences in Religiosity

Scores on the five religiosity measures were examined to determine whether religiosity varied according to demographic back-

TABLE 6.4 Means and Standard Deviations of the Religious Coping Items and Subscore

Measure	Mean	SD
Gives sense of belonging	4.16	1.20
Helps me deal with problems	4.21	1.18
Helps me control my fate	3.66	1.51
Gives me inner sense of peace	4.15	1.18
Total religious coping	16.17	4.47

ground. First, significant gender differences were found for three of the five religiosity scores (see Table 6.5). Women had greater nonorganizational religiosity, greater subjective religiosity, and greater religious coping than did men.

The comparison of religiosity scores for the three ethnic/SES groups (high SES Whites, low SES Whites, and low SES African Americans) is found in Table 6.6. Significant differences between the groups were found for all five religiosity scores. The planned contrasts indicated that, overall, the Whites had lower religiosity than the African Americans When the high SES and low SES White groups were compared, Whites from higher socioeconomic status levels showed more organizational religiosity but less nonorganizational religiosity than Whites of lower socioeconomic status.

Correlations of age, educational level, and marital status with the religiosity subscores are found in Table 6.7. In regard to age, only the correlation with nonorganizational religiosity was significant ($r = -.20$), with nonorganizational religiosity declining as age increased. The correlations with educational level were significant for all but organizational religiosity. For the other religiosity measures, religiosity was lower for those with more education. There was no correlation between religiosity and whether a participant was married or not.

TABLE 6.5 Summary of *t*-tests for Gender Differences in Religiosity Subscores

Religiosity Subscale	Men		Women		
	Mean	*SD*	Mean	*SD*	*t*-test
Organizational	11.12	3.52	10.40	3.44	0.78
Nonorganizational	11.38	3.59	14.47	3.52	3.25**
Subjective	10.19	2.64	11.38	1.93	2.51*
Coping	13.88	4.98	16.57	4.28	−2.27*
Change	3.50	0.82	3.68	1.08	−0.65

* $p < .05$; ** $p < .01$

TABLE 6.6 Summary of *F*-Tests for Differences in Religiosity Subscores for Three Ethnic/SES Groups, With Planned Orthogonal Contrasts

| Religiosity Subscore | Means by Ethnic/SES Group | | | *F* | *t*-test for Contrast | |
	HiWhite	LoWhite	African American		W vs. AA	Hi W vs. Lo W
Organizational	10.28	8.58	11.95	8.93**	−3.92**	2.13*
Nonorganizational	11.43	13.54	16.98	41.99**	−8.10**	−3.05**
Subjective	10.38	11.19	12.05	7.50**	−3.22**	−1.66
Coping	14.76	15.77	17.88	5.64**	−3.05**	−0.94
Change	3.33	3.27	4.22	12.60**	−5.00**	0.28

* $p < .05$; ** $p < .01$

TABLE 6.7 Correlations of Religiosity Subscores With Demographic Variables

Religiosity Subscore	Age	Education	Marital Status
Organizational	–.10	.05	–.03
Nonorganizational	–.20*	.56**	.18
Subjective	.01	–.38**	.08
Coping	–.05	–.39**	.01
Change	–.10	–.29**	.10

* $p < .05$; ** $p < .01$

Summary

Overall, the quantitative data portrayed most study participants as being affiliated with a particular religion, attending church but not necessarily participating in other church activities, actively reading religious material, listening to religious programs, and praying frequently. They seemed to feel a commitment to their religion and felt that it helped them to cope with life. This portrait seemed to be much the same regardless of age, although women seemed to be somewhat more religious than men.

Relation of Religion to Death Meanings, Fears of Death, and Views of the Dying Process

Correlational analysis was used to determine the relationship of the five religiosity subscores to the scores for death meanings, fears of death, and views of the dying process. This analysis, summarized in Table 6.8, revealed some interesting and important relationships.

Death Meanings

With regard to death meanings, organizational religiosity was unrelated to any of the four death meanings. The three religiosity subscores that were more personal in nature (nonorganizational, subjective, and coping) were related to death meanings in a simi-

TABLE 6.8 Correlations of Religiosity With Death Meanings, Fear of Death, and Views of the Dying Process

Variable	Organizational	Nonorganizational	Subjective	Coping	Change
Death Meanings					
Afterlife	.10	.55**	.64**	.58**	.26**
Motivator	-.05	.30**	.34**	.35**	.27**
Legacy	-.06	.29**	.33**	.31**	.13
Extinction	-.08	-.16	-.34**	-.26**	-.01
Fear of Death					
Dying Process	-.12	-.03	-.07	-.06	-.02
Being Destroyed	.10	.34**	.32**	.23*	.32**
Significant Others	.09	.15	.09	.10	.18
The Unknown	-.19*	-.20*	-.26**	-.26**	-.18
Dying Process					
Emotions	-.05	-.14	-.02	-.02	.10
Physical survival	-.40**	-.13	.05	-.01	.18
Coping with Dying	.09	.39**	.29**	.21*	.15
Family	.17	-.17	-.08	-.00	.15
Rancor	-.16	-.50**	-.46**	-.50**	-.19

*$p < .05$; ** $p < .01$

lar way. Those older adults who were high in these forms of religiosity also were more likely to see death as afterlife, as a motivator for certain achievements in their remaining life, and as an opportunity to leave a legacy for others. In contrast, they were less likely to see death as extinction. With regard to change in religiosity, those elders who felt that they had become more religious in their later years were also more likely to see death in terms of afterlife and as a motivator for achievement. One can speculate that at some point as these elders grew older, they came to recognize their own inevitable mortality. This recognition may have been the impetus for an increased interest in the possibility of an afterlife as well for the fulfillment of certain goals before life came to an end.

Fears of Death

None of the five religiosity subscores were related to Fear of the Dying Process or Fear for Significant Others. However, all aspects of religiosity were associated with Fear of the Unknown, with those older adults who reported greater religiosity experiencing less fear after death. Their religious beliefs seemed to give them a greater faith that their spirit would continue on in an afterlife. But strangely enough, for all aspects of religiosity other than organizational, greater religiosity was associated with greater fear of the destruction of their physical body either prior to or after death.

Views of the Dying Process

Those older adults who reported greater nonorganizational, subjective, and coping religiosity expected to use more coping behaviors to deal with the dying process and to have fewer feelings of rancor. Those with greater organizational religiosity expected to feel fewer concerns about physical survival. It is possible that the greater sense of social support experienced through their participation in organized religious groups kept them more outwardly directed rather than preoccupied with their own physical symptoms. Finally, none of the religiosity subscores were related to anticipated emotions during the dying process or to concerns about family.

Summary

The religious views of older people appear to have far-reaching effects on the way they look at death. Their religiosity not only shapes the meanings that death has for them but their expectations of an afterlife help them to face death without fear of what lies beyond. Put another way, their religiosity helps them to accept the inevitability of death, cope with the dying process, and deal with death fears.

QUALITATIVE ANALYSIS: FURTHER EXPLORATION OF THE INFLUENCE OF RELIGION

The remaining part of the chapter is concerned with further exploration of the participants' religious views in order to gain some idea of the implications of these views for the ways they looked at death. Because their religion seemed to be so important for most of the elders who took part in the study, it seems worthwhile to explore their views in more detail. It was hoped that a better understanding of older adults' religious views could lead to the identification of other significant components that might be related to death phenomena in future studies.

In this qualitative part of the study, questions in three general areas were always asked: What do you think will happen to you after death? What are your views about God and the afterlife? If scientific evidence existed that God did or did not exist, how would this affect you? Under what conditions would death be easy or difficult for you? Beyond this, the interview was unstructured, with additional questions introduced as part of a freewheeling dialogue so that new ideas could emerge that we would otherwise miss with only a fixed set of specific questions.

As was the case in earlier chapters, participants' views were examined by subgroups formed by age, gender, and the three ethnicity/SES categories. Each will be presented in turn.

High SES White Men in Their 90s

Views on God and an Afterlife

Although this was probably the most articulate group of the elders we interviewed, we did not always obtain specific answers to our questions. As a result, we did not get a clear idea of their views but often had to read between the lines. The majority seemed to feel that death is just a transition to something else. For example:

• I believe that my physical body is dead but my spirit lives on.

However, these men gave no precise statements as to where this spirit would live after death. In contrast, a nonbeliever stated:

• You go 6 feet under and that is it.

Evidence for the Existence or Nonexistence of God

Many men in this group felt that if they had definite evidence that God existed, it would only reinforce their present beliefs and give them comfort, and if they were presented with evidence that God did not exist, they would simply reject it. It would be unacceptable to them to even consider that such evidence might be accurate.

Death is Easy or Difficult

The majority of these men regarded death as easier when you believe in an afterlife and much more difficult when you do not.

High SES White Men in Their 80s

Views on God and an Afterlife

Interestingly, we found more diversity of views in this group of 80-year-olds, fitting in with our notion that people in their 80s, especially early 80s seem to be going through a transition period with regard to their mortality. For example, some men who professed to believe in God seemed to believe that an afterlife existed but did not feel they knew what would happen to them after they died.

- I don't know. Nobody knows. I believe something lies beyond this life. But what it is, I don't know.
- I don't have any ideas about that. It's a normal process. If there's an afterlife as we have been promised, well, I'll find out.

In contrast, a nonreligious person seemed to have no concern about an afterlife, saying:

- I'd like to be left alone in my grave.

Evidence for the Existence and Nonexistence of God

For the majority, if evidence was presented that God did exist, it would not change anything because it would be consistent with what they already believe. On the other hand, if scientific evidence was presented that God did not exist, it would bother some of them. For example,

- If there were no God, it would upset me considerably; however, there is no possibility that God does not exist. But if I were convinced, I'd be upset.
- If there is evidence that God did not exist, it would mean existence would be like a black night, and I would simply disappear in body and spirit.

The latter statement seems to imply that life would then be meaningless.

Death is Easy or Difficult

For the majority, death was seen as easier when you have faith and/or prepared for it and difficult when you don't have faith or have made no preparation to face death.

High SES White Men in Their 70s

Views on God and an Afterlife

Those men who were more traditionally religious felt that when they die they will go to heaven:

- When I die, I think that I will go to heaven and meet the great architect of the universe.
- My body will be put into the ground; my soul will go to heaven, if you want to use that expression.
- When I die, I'm going to heaven because it defeats my sense of justice that the whole purpose of living is to end it all and that's it. To me, it is illogical; we are human beings with emotions. If we weren't created by someone loving, how does the option come about that we love so much, and that we are concerned with love.

Some of the men were concerned about the fate of their body even though their soul might be going to heaven. For example,

- Assuming that my body is in any kind of shape at all, the local mortician is going to contact the College of Medicine to render a judgment of whether there is going to be enough left of me to be useful in the laboratory. I don't intend to be put under the ground. I intend to be cremated. I don't think God is going to be particularly involved or perturbed about it one way or the other.
- When I die, my body will be cremated, releasing part of the components of which I'm made. And the rest of what's remaining will be put back into circulation, so that I will become part of the atoms of some other living forms.

The highly educated men in this group (which included some Unitarians and nonbelievers) were more concerned with the nature of God than what he does for people. For example, some saw God as the universe, and one might meditate to experience a rejuvenation of energy. Understanding God and the universe may motivate one to explore religious freedom, ethical standards and practices, political beliefs, and one's own social advancement. The universe is governed by laws, with God the agency behind the laws.

God is within all of us as he is the universe and we are part of that universe.

Some saw God is a vehicle for self-actualization or self-empowerment. They don't believe in God as a force for which sacrifices have to be made; God doesn't punish people for misdeeds.

Evidence for the Existence and Nonexistence of God

Again, for the majority of men in this age group, definite evidence that God existed would only reinforce their existing views. However, some felt that definite knowledge would give them further comfort. For example,

- If I had definite evidence of God's existence, I'm already sure I'm going to a better place, and meet all my friends and family. It wouldn't change my feelings but still I might feel a little better.
- If I had evidence that God existed, it wouldn't change things, because I believe that now. I've read those about life after death, and for the most part they know what they're talking about, and that gives me emotional support.

However, one agnostic disagreed,

- If I had definite evidence that God existed, it would make a difference in your views but I doubt if it would make a difference in mine. If I were convinced of a personal God with whom I would have to converse, I could imagine myself saying, "Well, it's been a good show, God. I'm grateful for the lease that you accorded me the time and space in my body. And my demise is your decision. So go."

If one could provide scientific evidence that God did not exist, these men might reject such evidence, accept it, or react with emotional turmoil:

- If there was no God, I would feel bitter, afraid, nasty.
- If God did not exist, you can't convince me. I reject that entirely. I am not willing to accept that assumption. It's a false premise and I reject that totally.

- If there was no God, I don't think it would change things very much. It's just a matter of that, if you have consciousness at the time that death occurs. If you have continuing consciousness, there are other kinds of knowledge and experience you will have. I would be happy no matter which is true, God or no God. I'm a determinist in that respect.
- If death were the end of my identity, extinction, the end of everything, I guess I'd have to use the word indifferent. Death means nothing beyond my present life. When I'm dead, it's not going to make much difference to me.
- If there were no God, I think that, more than the meaning of death, it would influence the meaning of life. I would feel that life had no purpose. Full of sound and fury, signifying nothing. I would honestly feel that way, especially in view of today's headlines. There would be no purpose to anything. Life would be just a meaningless bad joke.

Death is Easy or Difficult

The 70-year-olds did not seem to include God or an afterlife in their ideas of when death would be easy or difficult. Only one man expressed a traditional religious viewpoint:

- Death is easier when there is a faith in a loving God and difficult when there is no faith.

The others seemed to be concerned with the conditions under which one might die or the type of life one lived on earth.

High SES White Women in Their 90s

Views on Existence of God and an Afterlife

The majority of this group of 90-year-old women expected to go to heaven after death. However, some were uncertain or vague about what heaven would be like and others mentioned other hopes for the afterlife. For example,

- I think there is an afterlife. I can't imagine what it's like when I think of the millions of people who have died. I would hope I could go some place where I could be with loved ones.
- I think that I will go to heaven and visit God, but I can't envision heaven. So I don't think about it.
- What is important is to live now in the way that God expects us to live.
- I have no idea what will happen to me when I die. But I wish that I could see my loved ones again.

In short, the 90-year-old White women had traditional expectations of going to heaven but, compared to men their age, they seem to express more qualifications about how to get there and what it would be like.

Evidence for the Existence or Nonexistence of God

The prevailing viewpoint of these women was that if proof of the existence of God reinforced their existing beliefs, then it would not affect them. If it affected them in any way, it would give them feelings of comfort and security. For example,

- If God existed, I don't think I would change since I already believe there is a God.
- If there is evidence of God, it would take away any lingering fear of what would happen to me.
- If God existed and cared about me, yes, it would make death easier with his help.
- If God existed, death would mean transferring to another existence and find someone to take care of me.
- If God existed, it would make a difference; it would make me feel sure.

In regard to definite evidence that God did not exist, many participants rejected any such idea. Examples of comments were:

- If there is no evidence of God, I can't imagine that.

- If God did not exist, there would be no incentive to live in such a manner that I have lived.

Other participants felt that nonexistence of God would leave them in emotional turmoil:

- If God didn't exist, that would make me afraid of death.
- If God did not exist, then death would be hard.
- If there is no God, that would be terrible.

None of the women in this group were willing to accept and live with the idea that God does not exist.

Death is Easy or Difficult

Most of these older women gave explicit conditions under which death would be easy or difficult, but only a few of the women expressed religious themes:

- Death is easier when you have faith in God and difficult when you don't.

High SES White Women in Their 80s

Views on the Existence of God and an Afterlife

Women in this age group expressed a great diversity of views. Some held traditional religious beliefs about an afterlife with God:

- I figure that I'll be going to heaven.
- I think there will be an afterlife with God.

Although most of these women were from traditional religious backgrounds and believed in an afterlife, it did not seem that their primary or only motive was to be with God. Some mentioned a desire to be with family again:

- I think you live in spirit after death. This will give me a chance to talk to my husband after I die.
- I don't think death will be the end personally. I hope I will get a chance to see my mother and father.

Others seemed to be more concerned with the style in which they would leave this earth than with where they would be going. For example,

- I want to have a funeral in church. I want to be cremated. I want to have a memorial service, and then a bunch of Methodist hymns, and I want someone to sing "Going Home" and I've altered the words to that.
- I think that I will go to heaven, my soul will. I want angels to escort me. I have faith they will.

Still others felt that having an afterlife would provide the opportunity to clarify the meaning of one's past or present life. For example,

- I will have memories of my past in my afterlife.
- I would like to be able to experience another dimension that would be what I call a meaning dimension. I might find out what the meaning of this life had been.
- I just wish there could be respect for me and what I have done in my life.

In other cases, there was some degree of doubt or uncertainty about the existence of an afterlife or what it would be like:

- I think I have a soul that will head for wherever souls go, hopefully with God.
- I would like to think that after awhile I would go to heaven and find out what are all the things that you don't really know about are about.
- Supposedly, I will be in heaven, or hope I am.
- I know that I will be embalmed and put in the ground. Death has no fear for me. It will be a wonderful ending. I'm not anx-

ious for it to happen, but I don't worry about it at all. I think I will go to heaven, at least, I hope so.

- I have no idea, I suppose what is to be, will be. And as with other steps of life, accept it.
- I wish I could believe like I'm supposed to believe, a Christian afterlife. But I'm not sure anything will happen after I die.
- I don't know. But I would like to find out if there is something on the other side.
- I'm just a blank on that. I think this is the life I'm living, and that's it, and it's all done. If you think I'm going to experience walking around seeing my grandparent and so on, no, I don't. I'm sorry.

It was surprising, given their age and religious backgrounds, that many of these women did not express certainty about going to heaven to be with God, or even show great enthusiasm. More importantly, many showed considerable doubt regarding the existence of an afterlife with God.

Evidence for the Existence or Nonexistence of God

Many women felt that definite evidence that God existed would merely confirm what they already believed. For example,

- If evidence for God were demonstrated, I already have evidence of that, so it wouldn't change anything.

For others, such evidence would enhance their comfort:

- If God exists, I'd then have God with me all the time.
- My death would then be a happy ending.
- If God existed, I would look forward to being cared for or being given the opportunity of having another life or so.
- I think it would be amazing. I think it would consummate what I did believe.
- Life has been a great mystery, and if God existed, I'll think I'm finally going to find out what it is.

- I think your belief in God certainly affects your feelings toward death. If God exists, I guess I would be thankful to be taken. I would have happiness.
- If God exists, it makes it more certain that you would live on after death. To me, it would make it more palatable to think that this is not the end.
- If God existed, then death would be more meaningful. I would be more contented.

Elderly women in this age group responded in different ways to the notion that scientific evidence indicated that God did not exist. Many completely rejected the idea:

- If God did not exist, I can't believe this. I've grown up with my beliefs and I can't be changed at the very end. If necessary, I would go on playing like there is a God.
- If God did not exist, I don't think you could convince me of that.
- If God didn't exist, it would mean the end of experience. But you'd have great trouble convincing me. I'd never accept it. It would be hard on me.
- If God didn't exist, I would say you are mistaken.
- If God did not exist, Oh you couldn't convince me of that. No one could convince me. No way. Not you, not anyone. I can't possibly imagine what it would be like to know there was no God.

Others would accept the nonexistence of God and try to make the best of it:

- If God did not exist, I don't believe it would affect me at all; I would take it in stride.
- Well, if there is no God, they'd just bury me, and I'd go back to earth, right to dust. I don't think I'd have any feeling.
- If God did not exist, I think it would be the end of it.
- If I had lived all my life believing there is a God and an afterlife, that has done me a lot of good . . . just to believe that. It helped me live to the best of my abilities. But if at the end of it, there is no God, so what. I'd just say, well, that's it. I'd have to accept it.

- If God did not exist, I don't know if there would be anything I could do about it, but just accept, because every one has to die.

Some women felt that they would be very emotionally upset. For example,

- It would make me furious. If I were on my deathbed, I would punch you in the nose.
- If God did not exist, it would be very upsetting; it frightens me. I would be upset about it.
- If God did not exist, the disappointment would be tragic. My whole entire life depends on religious belief. I would be petrified. I would absolutely fall apart.
- If God did not exist, I would be frightened. If you knew there was no afterlife, it might take away some of your motivation. You would live a lot more recklessly.

Death is Easy or Difficult

In regard to questions of when death would be easy or difficult, only a few individuals related their answers to religion. For example,

- Death is easier when you believe in God.
- Death is difficult when you have not fulfilled God's calling.

High SES White Women in Their 70s

Views of the Existence of God and an Afterlife

One might expect 70-year-old White women from a traditional Christian background to indicate that they were going to be with God in heaven after death; surprisingly, only a few did. For most, there was no direct mention of being with God in heaven. There was more of a feeling of uncertainty of what might happen after death, which sometimes led to apprehension and other times to acceptance. This seems somewhat contradictory to Christian beliefs in God and heaven. For example,

- There is a great deal of controversy in theology about what happens, and nobody knows, so it is a mystery. I could accept just being happy no matter. I'm not particularly anxious to meet loved ones and those things. Just suppose we believed in reincarnation, we don't remember who we used to be. So I feel very comfortable with the thought that wherever I'm going, it will be all right.
- I'm putting my bets on heaven, but I don't know, really. I know I'm far from perfect. I wish I could spend part of my years in sainthood or whatever.
- I have no idea what will happen to me after I die.
- I cannot imagine what death will be like. I think it's just like going into a void. My mother was visiting just when she died in the hospital. She said hallelujah and then she said that she saw bursts of light and angels. But she was conventionally religious and active in the church. I will never know but I think that she may have had a subconscious expectation. I don't have any trouble with angels, but I'll never know.
- I think I'll go to heaven. At least, I hope I will.

Evidence for Existence or Nonexistence of God

The responses to this question followed patterns noted for other age groups of women. Some women indicated that proof of God's existence would make no difference to them because they already knew God existed:

- If God existed, it would have no influence on me since I already believed he existed.
- If God existed, there would be no change in my view.

Other women would welcome scientific evidence, as it would increase their sense of happiness and comfort. For example,

- If God existed, it would mean a lot for me to know for sure. It would give me comfort.
- If God existed, I think it would give me a happy death.

- If God existed, it would give me more to look forward to.
- If God existed, it would make it more acceptable.
- If God exists, I would be so astonished, it would take me awhile to understand. But I think it would be a comfort.

Similarly, if evidence showed that God did not exist, the pattern of responses was either to reject such evidence, accept it, or react with emotional turmoil. Examples of rejection were:

- I don't think that there is any way one can know that he doesn't exist.
- I just wouldn't believe it, even if you tell me. I just can't fathom that.
- I don't think you would know what you are talking about.

Examples of accepting the nonexistence of God were:

- If there was no God, it probably wouldn't affect me at this point in my life.
- If God did not exist, I would see it as a release from the care of this world.
- If God doesn't exist, it wouldn't matter anyway, since I don't believe that he does exist.
- If God does not exist, then death is the end of life.

Some women reacted in an emotional manner, for example,

- If God did not exist, life would then be a wasteland. What would be the sense of trying to live with other people and help others if there isn't a sense of unity for all of us to go to afterwards?
- I would feel helpless, hopeless. I would feel fear, empty. If there was no God, I wouldn't know what to do. I wouldn't know which way to turn.
- I would make me sad, maybe frightened, give me an empty feeling.

Death is Easy or Difficult

No one in this group associated religious themes with death being either easy or difficult.

Low SES White Women in Their 90s

Views of the Existence of God and an Afterlife

A few women mentioned being with God in the afterlife, although there was some degree of uncertainty that this will occur:

- I don't know. I think that I will live to see my family, friends and God in the afterlife. I think it will be pleasant.

Others seemed to focus on God's help to them prior to death. For example,

- God helps me to deal with my problems. He takes away bad feelings. God is there.
- In time of trouble he'll come to help. If I pray sincerely, the Lord looks after me.
- God helps me through rough times, e.g., losing my mother and father. God is physical and spiritual. But more important, he helps me out.

Evidence for the Existence or Nonexistence of God

If scientific evidence showed that God existed, it seemed to reinforce these women's existing views and also give them greater comfort, similar to the high SES White Women in their 70s.

If scientific evidence showed that God did not exist, the responses followed the typical patterns of either acceptance, rejection of such evidence, or emotional upset. Examples of these three viewpoints follow:

- If God did not exist, I don't think I would believe it; you couldn't convince me.
- If God did not exist, I don't think it would upset me. I would accept it because who wants to stay on this earth all the time.
- If God did not exist, I would feel helpless, hopeless. I would feel fear, emptiness. If there was no God, I wouldn't know what to do. I wouldn't know which way to turn.

Death is Easy or Difficult

None of these 90-year-old women responded with religious themes as to when death was easy and difficult.

Low SES White Women in Their 80s

Views of the Existence of God and an Afterlife

In regard to being with God in an afterlife, there were diverse views. Some women felt great certainty that there would be a hereafter. For example,

- I'll be in heaven.

  An interesting variant of this theme was:

- I have tried to prepare myself for that time. I love that program "Touched by an Angel," and I have said so many times that if the angel of death, Andrew, comes and takes my hand, I'll go away with him because he is beautiful. I know that show has prepared a lot of people. It is definitely Christian based.

Even among women who felt that there is a hereafter, there is some uncertainty as to whether they will be with God in such an afterlife as indicated by the following comments:

- I hope and I'm sure that there will be a hereafter.
- I hope I'll go to heaven.
- I hope I'll be in heaven with Jesus.

Other participants did not mention being with God in such an afterlife. For example,

- I think that your spirit goes on forever.

Some participants did not explicitly deny the existence of an afterlife but they did not seem to have any idea of what it will be like, or whether it will involve being with God:

- I don't know. Nothing is going to happen.
- I know what I would like to believe, but I am just not sure about the spiritual part.
- I don't know what the afterlife will be like.
- I think at some time that none of us knows, we are going to be judged for the afterlife. I'll either go to heaven or hell.

Evidence for the Existence or Nonexistence of God

If scientific evidence showed that God existed, many women felt that it would reinforce their previous beliefs:

- If God existed, it wouldn't influence me as I understand all of that very clearly at this point.
- It wouldn't change anything. I already know that he exists.
- God exists, I just think that everything is in God's hands.

Others felt that proof of God's existence would being greater happiness, comfort, or even a sense of relief. For example:

- If God existed, it would mean a lot. It would give me great comfort.
- It would make me very happy.
- I would have real peace in my heart.
- I think it's just a relief to have evidence if you are very uncomfortable about it. If you have a personal God, he knows what's best for you.

Others who were nonbelievers would find it difficult to accept evidence, but feel that they might gain from the situation. For example,

- I think it would be wonderful if there was a heaven, but I really don't believe it.

If scientific evidence showed that God did not exist, many participants would reject the evidence:

- I believe in God, even if science cannot prove it. I don't need to delve too deeply into it.
- If God did not exist, it would not influence me as I know better. There are umpteen people writing the word of God and they all agree, and how many lawyers today agree?
- If God did not exist, I don't think you could convince me.
- You wouldn't convince me. I couldn't even entertain the thought. I've had the same religion for 86 years and I am going to stay with it.

Other participants would accept it if God did not exist. Examples of such comments were,

- If God did not exist, I don't think it would change things much. I'd be disappointed but accept it. I'd have no fears.
- I have never been afraid of death and I don't think it would make any difference.
- Whatever will be, will be. Why would you have fear, you're just going to be put in the ground.
- If God did not exist, It wouldn't change the meaning of death. If that's the end, that's the end. If you could prove to me there is no afterlife, then I think you have to move on and out. There is too much population anyway.

Other participants would be emotionally upset. For example,

- If God did not exist, I think it would make me sad. Maybe frightened, an empty feeling. Then I think about being cremated.
- If God did not exist, I would feel nothing. Death would have no meaning. If I didn't exist, nobody else would either.
- If God did not exist, I'd be very, very angry.
- I would feel awfully bad. I'd feel sad, betrayed. I've tried to live a good life all my life you know.
- If God did not exist, I would feel disappointed, frightened, disappointed.
- If God did not exist, it would scare me. It would be a kind of emptiness.

Death is Easy or Difficult

Only a few women associated religious themes with considering death as easy or difficult:

- Death is easier when you die in your sleep and difficult when you have nothing to look forward to if you don't believe in eternity.
- Death is easier when there is a strong conviction of life hereafter and a loving God and difficult when you suffer.
- Death is easier when you have peace in your heart and difficult if you don't know the Lord.

Most of the remaining women associated the conditions of death itself with whether it would be easy or difficult.

Low SES White Women in Their 70s

Views of the Existence of God and an Afterlife

There was a great deal of diversity in the views of these women about God and the afterlife. Some participants gave direct answers:

- I'm going to heaven.
- My soul is going to heaven.

These women made no explicit attempt to assert the existence of an afterlife or God; it was more of an implicit acceptance and decision that they would be with God after death.

A few women revealed ambivalent or potentially negative feelings about meeting God. For example,

- I feel God is waiting for me. I am going to be apprehensive but I don't think I'll be frightened.
- I'll go to heaven or hell.
- I think I would be more happy that I was going to be with God than staying with my oldest daughter . . . I don't think I would be afraid to die.

Some women focused more on being with loved ones in an afterlife than being with God. For example,

- I am going to climb a steep staircase to up above, and meet all my friends.

Some women seemed to be focused on the dying process rather than the possibility of an afterlife with God. Others did not deal with the question of an afterlife, but simply expressed positive views about God. For example,

- God is a forgiving person.
- God is someone who cares and helps others. He gives me the strength to take care of myself.
- God is with me all the time. I can see over the years that he has guided my life.
- God is all powerful, forgiving, loving . . . he's just God.
- God gives loves, forgives, cares about me, protects me, gives me the good things in life and when the bad things come, he gives me a source of strength to get through the situation.
- God gives me the peace I asked for. He keeps me sane. He helps me when I ask for it.
- God provides miracles; he protects me.
- God is loving, caring. If I do something wrong, I don't expect him to forgive me immediately. I now know that he is there. He is the only thing you can trust in.
- God takes care of people; takes care of all.

Evidence for the Existence or Nonexistence of God

For most people in this group, scientific evidence of the existence of God would not change anything because they are already convinced that he exists. For example,

- If God existed, it wouldn't change anything. I already know that he exists.
- If God exists, there would be no difference.

However, for some women, proof of God's existence seemed to give them a greater sense of certainty, and greater happiness or comfort:

- If God exists, it would absolutely influence the meaning of my death. I would have a strong feeling of what to expect.
- If God exists, I'd be happy.
- I'd feel more comfortable about dying.

If scientific evidence showed that God did not exist, the same patterns of response observed for previous groups were found: that is, acceptance, rejection of evidence, or emotional turmoil. However, in this group, there were only a few women either rejecting the evidence against God or accepting it. For example,

- If God did not exist, nothing could prove that to me.
- If God did not exist, I don't know; I guess that I would just have to live with it.

Most of the women expressed emotional reactions to the possibility that God did not exist:

- If God did not exist, I would feel that life is over. It would be like Santa Claus and the Easter Bunny, you've been lied to all your life. I would feel this is it. You probably should make better use of your life.
- If God did not exist, it would be a big difference. I wouldn't want to go. I would not know what to expect.
- If God did not exist, it would make me feel real mad and betrayed. I've had my religion all my life, and it would be terrible to find it wasn't true.
- If God did not exist, I would feel emptiness, probably. I don't think I'd feel scared. I'd probably feel "Why in the hell did I have to be good?" Think of the things you've not done in your life because you thought they weren't right. Now you can just go ahead and do these things. I didn't have sex when I was a kid. God was watching me. I might as well have.
- If there was no God, I'd feel betrayed that I'd spent all this time obeying God's laws. I think I'd be frightened.

- If God did not exist, I would feel bitter, but not frightened. I'd feel betrayed in terms of what I thought was coming.
- If there was no God, I'd wonder what was going to happen to me. I think I'd feel betrayed and lost.

When Death is Easy or Difficult

Only a few women in this group mentioned God or religious themes. One said,

- Death is easier when you have faith in God to carry you through and difficult when you have suffering and pain.

Low SES African American Women in Their 80s

Views on God and an Afterlife

Responses of the African American women in this age group, as compared to the White women, were characterized by feelings of confidence and a somewhat more complete depiction of what would happen after death. For example,

- I believe I'll feel relief when I breathe my last breath. Whereever I go, I'll be happy. I'll go where the Lord has a place for me.
- God died for each and everyone of us on the cross. They beat him all night long and did nasty things to him, and he died anyway. That's the way I see it . . . After I die, I'll lay dead in the ground until judgment day, and the angels will tell each of us where the Christians go.
- I'm hoping to be with the angels.
- I hope to go to heaven. I don't know what will it will be like but God will be like a spirit.
- I think I will live forever in the afterlife, as a spiritual being.
- After I die, I hope that I go to heaven. I go to church and pray for that.
- I'm just passing to a land of freedom. I hope I won't be sad. I'm quite sure I'll be relieved. After I die, I will go to see my maker.

- After death, you have to stay in the earth. Then I know I'm going to heaven.
- After I die my soul is going to a resting place, and they are going to put me in the grave. I don't worry about this. I'll just take it as it comes.

Like the lower SES White women, many of the African American women focused on the positive aspects of God:

- God has helped me with my health and family. He is forgiving and loving.
- God is good to you. He keeps you alive.
- God is great. I depend on him. If nobody wants to talk to me, I can always talk to him. I think he is wonderful.
- I see God as powerful, loving, watches over us. He's helped me by just keeping me alive.

Evidence for Existence or Nonexistence of God

If scientific evidence could prove that God exists, most of the women felt that their beliefs would be confirmed. For example,

- It doesn't change anything because this is what I have always believed.
- If God exists, well, if I know for sure that I'm going to be with the Lord, I'd be happy.

If, on the other hand, scientific evidence showed that there was no God, many women would reject such an idea. For example,

- If God does not exist, I don't believe it because I know there is a God. I never thought about anything else.
- If God did not exist, I wouldn't believe it. I'd just go on being the same way.

A few comments implied acceptance of the nonexistence of God:

- If God does not exist, I wouldn't be frightened of dying. I'd just have to accept it.

- If God didn't exist, I don't know what I'd do. But I wouldn't change the way I live because it's still a good, clean, honest life, so I would still live the same way; what I learned from believing in God is still a good way to live.

However, the majority of the comments indicated that the women would be emotionally upset at the thought that there might be no God. For example,

- If God did not exist, I don't know. It would make me feel bad about dying.
- I think that I would be frightened and lost because I always believed that there was a God ever since I was a baby. If they said there wasn't, I'd be awfully unhappy.
- If God does not exist, I'd be completely lost.
- I would feel bad. It would feel that it had smashed my hopes of a better life.
- I don't know how I'd feel because I have in my mind that there is a God. I just think I'd feel very upset.
- If God does not exist, I would feel awful bad and sad, and I'd go to hell.
- I would feel betrayed, to think there is no God is frightening. I would be real afraid.
- I would be frightened of no God because I'd have nothing to look forward to.

When Death Is Easy and Difficult

In response to the question as to when death is easier and difficult, some women mentioned concerns with illness and suffering, but the majority mentioned religious themes. Some of their comments were:

- Death is easier when you are going to heaven and difficult when you have done so many things wrong.
- Death is easier when you are a Christian and difficult when you are not a Christian.
- Death is easier when you are going to meet the Lord, and difficult when you don't think you've got any chance to meet the Lord.

- Death is easier when you are prepared to meet the Lord and difficult when you are not prepared.
- Death is easier when you know the Lord and difficult when you don't do as he wanted you to do.
- Death is easier when you believe in God and difficult when you don't.

Lower SES African American Women in Their 70s

Views on God and the Afterlife

In this younger group of African American women, the majority felt that there was an afterlife and that they would be with God. Only a very few had any doubts. However, many expressed a certainty that they were going to attain an afterlife and be with God, but did not reveal what the afterlife would be like. For example,

- I hope to go to heaven. I hope to be out of my suffering and misery.
- My understanding of the Bible is that heaven is a place of peace and happiness. The body will decay and you'll have a spirit.
- I am hoping that things will be all peace; it will be spiritual and heaven will be there.
- I'm going to go to my resting place and just be there until Christ comes again. I wish Christ would come right away so that I don't have to lay there in the ground for too long.
- I think we're all spirits, and we have a being. I don't believe that dying is the end, because we have a spirit and a soul. How these things are going to interact, I don't know, but I have this faith that it is going to happen, and I will be in heaven.
- I'm going to be with my maker. The body is only a temple, and when you are looking at it, you're not looking at me. The real me is the inner person. So when your body goes, your soul don't die . . . you go back to the one that made you.
- I feel that death will be a blessing. After I die, I think that I will be in a spiritual like atmosphere, where everything is milk and honey, and you won't have to worry about nothing, and you will be happy. I hope so.

- I hope that I will be going to heaven, and not down. I think it will be glorious, because I have so many friends and my family. I believe they're all up there. I believe we'll have a joyful time. I believe my spirit will be floating around. I don't think I'll have another body.

As with the older group, some women commented on the positive aspects of God:

- God helps me. He cares about me. He love you. He is the only thing I can count on.
- God is up there. He cares and loves you. I can depend upon on him. If it wasn't for the Lord, I would be lost.
- God is understanding. He overlooks any faults. He loves and forgives you. He takes care of our needs.
- God has supernatural power. He brought me through when I couldn't get help from anyone else. He is the only real support that I have.
- God is someone who can do things for you. He is the light of my life. He is powerful. He answers my prayers. He loves me. I put him first.

Evidence for the Existence or Nonexistence of God

If scientific evidence could prove that God existed, most felt that the evidence would be consistent with their beliefs. At most, it increased their sense of security. For example,

- If God existed, it wouldn't change anything. I already believe in him.
- I already know that, but if somebody reassured me, that might comfort me.

Although many religious elders rejected such evidence, one woman responded in an interesting manner. She believed in an afterlife and God but did so on the basis of faith, and rejected any attempt to provide scientific evidence. She stated:

- If science stated that God existed, I'd still resist evidence from researchers because my belief in God is a matter of faith.

In response to the possibility that scientific evidence could demonstrate that God does not exist, patterns were noted similar to those found with other groups: rejection of such evidence, acceptance of such evidence, or reacting with emotional turmoil. Examples of comments rejecting scientific evidence were,

- I couldn't even pretend that. I can't believe there is no God.
- If God did not exist, it wouldn't influence me because it would never be true. They have been trying to disprove God for centuries. But listen, if there was no God, why are we here, why are the trees here, why the water, why the air?
- No one could convince me of that. I think I'd have to feel like a fool. What difference does it make if there is no God? I just can't get my mind to accept that.

Examples of comments accepting scientific evidence were,

- If God did not exist, I think it would just be something that we have to work out for ourselves as best as we could.
- If it was true that God did not exist, I'd just have to accept it.

Examples of responses revealing emotional turmoil were,

- If God did not exist, it would be very bad. I'll feel sad, disappointed, and nothing to look forward to.
- It would make feel bad. I would feel like there was a lot of time wasted on religion.
- If God did not exist, I would feel terrible. I'd feel betrayed. I think I'd just want to give up the ghost right then . . . it would be a terrible illusion.

Compared to the 80-year-olds, many more of the 70-year-olds rejected the notion that God did not exist, whereas more of the 80-year-olds showed emotional turmoil over such a thought.

Death Is Easy and Difficult

Again, there were many religious themes in response to this question. For example,

- Death is easier when you believe in God, and difficult when you don't believe in God.
- Death is easier when you have prepared your life to meet your maker and difficult when you know you haven't lived right and you are scared.

Low SES African American Men in Their 80s

Views of God and an Afterlife

There were only a few African American men in our sample, and their comments could be summarized in a general statement that one would be going to a better place in heaven and being with God.

Evidence for the Existence or Nonexistence of God

If scientific evidence proved that God existed, it would simply fit in with these men's existing beliefs and it would not change anything. However, some men resisted the idea of scientific evidence that God did not exist, For example,

- If you say there isn't a God, something is wrong.

No participant accepted the idea that God did not exist, but a few reacted with emotional turmoil:

- If God did not exist, it would make me upset.

Death Is Easy and Difficult

None of the men used religious themes to describe when death would be easy and difficult.

Low SES African American Men in Their 70s

Views of God and an Afterlife

Most of the men in this small group felt that they would go to heaven and be with God. For example,

- I think my body will be buried and my soul will go back to God.

Evidence for the Existence or Nonexistence of God

If scientific evidence for the existence of God was presented, most men felt it supported what they already believed. For example,

- If God existed, it wouldn't change anything since I already believe this to be true.

   However, one man disagreed,

- I wouldn't believe your evidence since I don't think God exists.

   But an interesting and third point of view was represented by another man:

- If God does not exist, religion has made me a better man, and made me treat my fellow man better, and try to live a good life. So whatever happened, I lived a better life because of my belief in God.

Death Is Easy and Difficult

None of the men mentioned religion or God in response to this question. Instead, they focused on conditions surrounding the dying process and things in life they would be leaving.

Summary of Interview Data

God and Afterlife

The great majority of the older adults taking part in the study held a belief in some kind of afterlife following death. However, there was considerable diversity of views as to what the afterlife might be like, both between the various subgroups (by ethnicity, SES, age, and gender) and between individual members of these subgroups.

The number of White men in the sample was not large, with most of them well-educated and of higher socioeconomic status. Their views on God and the afterlife tended to be more philosophical and abstract. The 90-year-olds seem to feel that death was a transition stage to something beyond, but they offered no clear definition of an afterlife and little mention of God. The 80-year-olds more frequently mentioned God's existence, but seemed uncertain as to the existence and nature of an afterlife. The 70-year-olds made a more definite assertion regarding God and going to heaven after death. A minority of the high SES White men did not hold a traditional Christian view of God and heaven. Whereas most atheists and agnostics were indifferent to the existence of a God or afterlife, a few viewed God as the universe or as the agency behind the laws of the universe; their conception of the afterlife involved recycling of the atoms of the body for use by others in the universe.

In regard to the high SES White women, most of the 90-year-old women expected to go to heaven, but hoped for a reunion with loved ones as well as with God. Some had difficulty envisioning heaven, and some were concerned about following God's rules in order to gain admittance to heaven. The 80-year-old women were quite mixed in their views. Some felt certain that they would be with God in an afterlife; many were concerned about a reunion with family in such an afterlife. Others expected and hoped to be in heaven, but expressed some degree of doubt about its existence. Still others were quite doubtful, almost to the point of being agnostic, and did not show any great enthusiasm for an afterlife with God. A few hoped that an afterlife would provide an opportunity to understand the meaning of life on earth. Although some of the

70-year-old women hoped to go to heaven, others did not directly mention God or heaven. The underlying theme of this age group was uncertainty and apprehension of what awaits them after death. It was quite surprising to find such a wide diversity of views among women from traditional Christian backgrounds. Perhaps such views are related to higher socioeconomic status levels.

The high SES men and women were all relatively well educated, which may account for their departures from traditional religious views and the doubts and uncertainty about the existence and nature of an afterlife which many revealed. The men seemed to be more philosophical than the women, whereas the women seemed more concerned about reunions with loved ones after death.

In contrast to the high SES groups, the low SES White women generally affirmed the existence of a personal God who cared about them; the majority felt that they would be in heaven with him. However, some had doubts about being with God in the afterlife, whereas others were concerned about whether they would experience heaven or hell after God's judgment. Others were vague about the nature of an afterlife, although the 70-year-olds were less vague than the older groups. Like many of the high SES women, some were concerned with reunions in the afterlife.

Among the low SES African American women, there was little difference between the age groups in their views concerning God and the afterlife. In nearly all cases, there was an expression of great love for God, who was viewed as caring, forgiving, and loving. These women voiced no uncertainty about going to heaven after death. Many were quite definite about remaining in the grave for a period until they were called to be with God at judgment day; some seemed anxious about this part of the process. Compared to both the high and low SES White women, the African American women differed in their certainty about the afterlife and in the intensely personal nature of their relationship with God.

Views of the low SES African American men differed little by age group; most had little doubt that they would be with God in heaven. However, they did not attempt to describe to any extent the nature of that afterlife, nor did they display the same enthusiasm regarding the afterlife as the African American women.

Scientific Evidence for the Existence or Nonexistence of God

The questions probing elders views on the existence of God yielded responses that were particularly interesting. On the one hand, if evidence showed proof that a God existed, the majority felt that their views about God and the afterlife would not change because such evidence would merely be consistent with what they already believed. Yet, some elders felt that having the weight of scientific evidence supporting their existing beliefs would make them feel more secure about their beliefs and lead to greater happiness. Those who were nonreligious were indifferent to any scientific evidence.

On the other hand, if scientific evidence indicated that God did not exist, responses fell into three main groups. The majority of believers would reject such evidence completely; another group would accept the validity of the scientific evidence and adjust their lives accordingly; and the third group would feel emotionally upset by such a finding. The few nonbelievers were either indifferent or glad to have support for their views.

Although all subgroups manifested the three main types of response, the relative frequencies of the types differed. For example, African Americans were more likely to feel increased comfort and security when the evidence was consistent with their belief in God and feel more emotional turmoil if the evidence indicated that God did not exist. Whites were more likely to reject the evidence if it did not agree with their beliefs.

Conditions When Death Is Easier or Difficult

In examining responses to this question, we were primarily concerned with whether participants would attribute an easier death to their religious beliefs and a difficult death to lack of such beliefs or a failure to behave in accord with their religion. In other words, we were interested in whether they felt that their religion helped them deal with death. (Many elders responded regarding conditions during the dying process, social concerns and so on, but such responses were not of interest here.)

Some differences between subgroups were found in the relative frequencies with which religious themes were mentioned.

Among the high SES White men and women, frequencies of religious themes were relatively low, but were higher among the older two subgroups than among the 70-year-olds. In contrast, the low SES White women rarely mentioned religious themes at any age, and the low SES African American men did not mention religion at all. However, the African American women responded in terms of religious themes with the highest relative frequency of all groups. This seemed consistent with their strong religious orientation overall.

CONCLUSIONS AND INTERPRETATIONS

Many of the findings of the study are not surprising, given what is known from previous research. The high proportion of elders who see death as meaning some form of afterlife is typical of Americans in general, where approximately 80% hold such a belief (Hood, Spilka, Hunsberger, & Gorsuch, 1996). Higher percentages of believers in an afterlife are found among Protestants, women, older adults, the less educated, and the lower class. Results from our study supported the differences by gender, education, and class level, but not by age. However, we did not find significant age differences. This may be due to the fact that all elders in our study were over age 70, whereas data reviewed by Hood et al. pertained to younger groups.

Our findings regarding fear of death support findings in the literature (e.g., Fortner et al., 2000) that subjective or intrinsic religiosity is related to less death fear. Here our quantitative findings were bolstered by the qualitative results. The qualitative findings go beyond existing literature, however, by presenting the diversity and richness of older adults' views on death.

Finally, our findings of the relationship of religiosity to coping with the dying process are consistent with Pargament's (1997) views of religious coping. In both cases, intrinsic religious faith appears to be a mechanism to help in dealing with the vicissitudes of life as well as the dying process.

Some Theoretical Interpretations of the Influence of Religion on Death Views

Terror Management Theory

Terror management theory was discussed earlier (see Chapter 4) as one explanation for phenomena surrounding the fear of death. One tenet of this theory is that the individual's participation in the culture and adherence to its norms aids in facilitating the suppression of fear of annihilation (Greenberg, Solomon, & Pyszczynski, 1997; Solomon, Greenberg, & Pyszczynski, 1991a). As an important part of the culture, belief in religion and adherence to religious norms offer a promise of immortality, which would act specifically to lessen fear of death. When norms of the culture are threatened, including religious norms, the individual reacts to defend the cultural worldview, particularly under conditions where death is more salient to the individual.

Findings from both the quantitative and qualitative analyses of the study support predictions from the theory in several ways. First, those elders strongest in religiosity had less fear of annihilation (Fear of the Unknown), and affirmed their expectations of an afterlife. Second, when their religious views were threatened by assertions that God did not exist, many reacted vehemently to defend their "cultural worldview" (religious beliefs in this case), completely rejecting or denying any scientific evidence of God's nonexistence. One elderly lady went so far as to suggest punching the interviewer in the nose for suggesting such a thing. Those who even considered the possibility that God did not exist were emotionally upset; many stated that they would be afraid to die under such circumstances. Thus, terror management theory seems consistent with older adults views of death in many ways.

Religion as an Attachment Phenomenon

Another theoretical position that helps to explain the influence of religious beliefs on older adults' views of death is the conception of religion as an attachment phenomenon (e.g., Kirkpatrick, 1998; 1999). Briefly, the concept of attachment refers to the infant's relationship to the mother (or other caregiver) and is an internal state within the individual that is inferred from the child's propensity to seek proximity and contact with the mother (Bowlby, 1979, 1980; Ainsworth, 1989). The mother (or other attachment figure) is seen as stronger and/or wiser and is associated with feelings of security. The child manifests distress when separated from the mother, and shows joy and elation upon reunion. The mother provides a secure base when the child leaves the mother for exploration, but any threat causes the child to return to the mother for security. When the mother is responsive to the child's needs, the child gains feelings of security and comfort and develops a secure attachment. If the mother is not reliably responsive, an insecure attachment results, with feelings of anxiety or ambivalence toward the mother. Gradually, the child forms an internal working model of attachment that acts as a template for future relationships.

Research evidence has demonstrated that attachment does not end after infancy, but continues (although in a different form, including symbolic attachment when the attachment figure is not physically present) throughout life in relation to new attachment figures (Ainsworth, 1989; Rothbard & Shaver, 1994) as well as to the mother (Cicirelli, 1991, 1995a). After childhood, an additional attachment behavior develops in which the individual acts to protect and defend the attachment figure in order to preserve that figure's existence (Bowlby, 1979, 1980; Cicirelli, 1991, 1995a).

The relationship of the individual to God can be viewed as an attachment relationship (Kirkpatrick, 1998, 1999; Pargament, 1997). According to Kirkpatrick, in Christianity and other monotheistic religions, believers maintain a personal, interactive relationship with a powerful, wise, and loving God. All the criteria for attachment are present in such a relationship. The desire for proximity and contact is satisfied through communication with God in prayer and participation in religious services and activities; God is viewed as a source of security and comfort who is always available. Additionally, religious beliefs offer the promise of a complete reunion with God in the afterlife. When believers are threatened in some way (by alarming events, by loss or threatened loss of loved ones, or by illness, injury, or fatigue), they turn to God as a haven to regain a sense of security and comfort. God provides a secure base for activities, as believers feel that God is watching over and protecting them. The threat of separation from God causes anxiety in believers. Individuals will attempt to protect the existence of God as an attachment figure by vigorously defending their beliefs when outside forces threaten these beliefs. Obviously, not all individuals develop a secure attachment to God. However, some individuals who were insecurely attached as children and into adulthood can become converted or "get religion" and develop a secure attachment to God. The relationship to God offers them a security that they were unable to find in earlier relationships with others.

The conception of God as an attachment figure can be seen as particularly applicable to older adults. Many older adults hold the traditional Christian core beliefs in the existence of a personal, helping, and caring God who watches over them in life and whom they will be with in an afterlife, and in the importance of prayer to communicate with God. In addition, they are likely to have lost other attachment figures (e.g., parents, spouse) who gave them security throughout life, leaving God as a main source of comfort and security. Finally, illness and recognition of vulnerability to death lead to a greater need to gain security and comfort. Many turn increasingly to religion as they grow older, and if not already securely attached to God, can "get religion" in their later years and become attached. In this sense, God can be seen as an "ultimate attachment figure" for older adults. From a psychological viewpoint, such an extension of attachment theory would explain older adults' increased interest in God and the afterlife.

Many of the older adults in our study, especially the African American women, appeared to regard God as an attachment figure; at least this can be inferred from their statements. They saw themselves as having an intense personal relationship with God, achieving proximity to God in their interactions with him through prayer. They viewed God as someone they could rely on for help, who watched over them, and who knew what was best for them. God gave them protection, security, and comfort by helping them deal with the fear of death and problems of everyday life now and offering the promise of reunion for an everlasting life in the future. When threatened with the loss of their attachment figure (scientific proof that God did not exist), they sought to maintain the existence of the attachment figure through vigorous denial of any evidence of God's nonexistence, or they experienced emotional distress (including a resurgence of the fear of death).

The conception of God as an attachment figure is given further credence by the flocking of people to religious rituals and services in the wake of some kind of disaster (such as the recent World Trade Center crash and collapse), seeking a sense of comfort and security. This is a typical attachment phenomenon arising in childhood. When the child leaves the attachment figure for exploration, any kind of threat can send the child fleeing back to that attachment figure for protection, comfort, and security. Similarly in adulthood, some kind of threat can cause a resurgence of attachment behavior.

The conceptualization of God as an attachment figure is not without problems. One is its lack of universality. Conceivably, it could apply to most religions with a monotheistic conception of a personal God. Some religions with multiple Gods would not seem to fit this category, nor would Buddhism. Also, this conception of God would not apply to agnostics, atheists, and apathists who don't believe in God or are indifferent to the God's existence. Those with impersonal conceptions of God, for example, God is the universe, would not seem to fit the conceptualization. The concept of God as an attachment figure does seem to fit many people in various religions, and possibly could explain the sense of security, protection, and comfort these people obtain from their religious beliefs.

Another difficulty is that only some older adults may have a secure attachment style that they can then transfer to God as an attachment figure. A study by Webster (1997) measured the attachment styles of older adults and found that not only did only 33% of the older adults manifest a secure attachment style (in comparison to 47% for young adults) but that 52% were characterized as having a style that was dismissing (compared to 18% of young adults). That is, they believed that one does not need an attachment figure in later life. Webster concluded that a dismissing style is consistent with the reality of widowhood for large numbers of elders.

Although attachment to God seems to provide an explanation for the positive benefits of religion for those who are securely attached, it also has negative aspects for those who initially had insecure attachments (Pargament, 1997). When traumatic events or severe illnesses occur and such individuals perceive that God fails to provide help, they may feel that God has somehow abandoned them, with accompanying feelings of great anger, resentment, disappointment, hopelessness, and despair. Pargament terms these feelings "religious struggle." In such circumstances, religion is no longer an aid to coping. The findings of our study that those weaker in religiosity anticipated greater feelings of rancor in the dying process would fit in with such a view.

A recent longitudinal study (Pargament, Koenig, Tarakeshwar, & Hahn, 2001) investigated effects of some of these negative aspects of religious attachment. In a survey of some 500 hospitalized elders, Pargament and colleagues found that those elders who initially reported such indicators of religious struggle as feeling abandoned by God, questioning God's love, feeling punished by God, and feeling the devil was responsible were more likely to have died over an approximately two-year period. Although the study needed further controls over other possible influences on mortality, the conclusion was that struggles with religious faith led to poorer ability to cope with illness in old age.

Some Implications

According to existing literature and our own findings, older adults tend to become more religious and have a stronger belief in God, prayer, and the afterlife. These beliefs are associated with less fear of death and a greater ability to cope with the dying process. Many elders consequently have an attitude of positive acceptance toward death.

However, it must be reiterated that although many studies show a positive (and sometimes negative) impact of religion on the daily lives of many people, they do not provide any evidence for the truth of religion. From a scientific perspective, they only provide evidence of the influence of beliefs about religion on a person's life.

As our study also found, there is a great deal of diversity in older adults' views of religion and in the influence of religion on views of death. Some elders are nonbelievers in God and others have idiosyncratic conceptions of God. Even among those with a traditional belief in God and the afterlife, the content and strength of such beliefs varies considerably. Associated with such differences in religious belief are differences in personal meanings of death, fears of death, and expectations about the dying process.

Anyone attempting to study the influence of religion on older adults' views of death or attempting to counsel older adults in coping with death as they go through the dying process must take this diversity of religious traditions and beliefs into account. An essential first step is to try to understand just what kinds of beliefs the individual holds in order to place his or her views about death and dying in appropriate context.

7

The Influence of Health on Views of Death

WHAT IS KNOWN ABOUT HEALTH AND DEATH VIEWS

In earlier chapters, we have seen that older adults' views about death meanings, fear of death, and the dying process change as they grew older. One might expect that as an elder's health declines, views about death would also shift as the possibility of death becomes more likely. Whether or not this is the case is the question addressed in this chapter.

Aging and Health

The fact that aging tends to be accompanied by declines in health and vigor is well-known. Although many octogenarians and nonagenarians retain good health despite advancing years, most indicators of health show declines with age.

Before discussing this question further, it is important to clarify what one means by the term health. According to a medical model, health can be defined as the absence of acute and chronic disease and impairments (Deeg, Kardaun, & Fozard, 1996), with illness being the presence of such disease or impairment. A second definition of health arises from a functional model. In this case, functional health consists of the ability of the individual to engage in activities that are necessary, expected, and personally desired in the society (Verbrugge, 1994), with disability arising primarily from the effects of chronic conditions (although disability can also arise from effects of acute conditions, accidents, and other causes) on people's ability to engage in such activities. In this case, an underlying physical pathology is manifested in an impairment in some bodily system which in turn leads to certain restrictions in basic actions which are reflected in the inability to perform needed activities of daily life. A third model of health, the growth model, defines health as a state of complete physical, mental, and social well-being (Birren & Zarit, 1985). In such a view, a healthy person is one improving in bodily and mental functioning in order to adapt more effectively to the environment.

A variety of indicators of health according to the medical model exist, such as the incidence of certain chronic conditions. Not only are older adults increasingly likely to die from any cause as age increases, the top five causes of death among older adults (cardiovascular disease, cancer, chronic obstructive pulmonary disease, pneumonia/influenza, and diabetes) all show an increase with advancing age. For example, the percentage of adult men reporting various heart conditions rose from 16% in the 45–64 age group to 32% in the 65–74 age group to 43% in those aged 75 and over. For women, the percentage with heart conditions rose from 11% in the 45–64 age group to 25% in the 65–74 age group to 36% in those aged 75 and over (U. S. Bureau of the Census, 1997). Similar age increases in prevalence are found for many other chronic conditions. Despite the fact that many older adults suffer from more than one chronic condition, about one-fifth of those over age 65 reported no chronic conditions (Guralnik & Kaplan, 1989). It must also be remembered that incidence of chronic conditions among older adults varies by gender, socioeconomic status, and ethnicity, with minority groups and those of low socioeconomic status typically reporting more chronic conditions. There are no consistent gender differences, with men having a higher incidence of some conditions and women having a higher incidence of other conditions.

Functional health in the elderly has been studied in some detail, usually in terms of those needing help with basic activities of daily living (ADL) such as bathing, dressing, eating, walking a short distance, rising from bed or chair, and toileting, or those needing help with various instrumental activities of daily living (IADL) such as preparing meals, shopping for personal items, doing light housework, doing laundry, using transportation, telephoning, handling finances, and taking medications when needed. Existing studies have found a general decline in functional health with age. For example, Kunkel and Applebaum (1992) found that 91% of men and 89% of women aged 65–74 had little or no disability (at most having problems with only one ADL or IADL activity), but that by age 85 and over only 58% of men and 50% of women had little or no disability. In regard to severe disability (problems with two or more ADLs), only 4% of men and 5% of women aged 65–74 had this level of disability, but 22% of men and 32% of women had severe disability by age 85 and over. Similarly, Crimmins, Saito, and Reynolds (1997), in an analysis of data from the Longitudinal Study on Aging and the National Health Interview Survey, found a clear increase in the percentage of older individuals disabled in either ADL, IADL, or both from age 70 to 94. Similar findings have been reported by Dunkle, Roberts, and Haug (2001) for the oldest old. There have been suggestions that the incidence of disability has declined among more recent cohorts of older adults as a result of better health practices. A recent national study of the prevalence of disability (Schoeni, Freedman, & Wallace, 2001) found some evidence that routine care disability (IADL) showed a decline in the population aged 70 and above over a 15-year period, particularly among the well educated, but personal care disability (ADL) was essentially stable.

Self-ratings of health (subjective health status) are typically made on a single 5- or 6-point rating scale. Such a global self-rating of health represents physical, emotional, and social aspects of health and well-being. Verbrugge (1989) reported that 52% of adults aged 45–64 rated their health as excellent or very good compared to only 35% of those aged 65 or over. At ages 45–64, only 12% rated their health as fair or poor compared to 22% of those aged 65 or over. This indicator of health seems deceptively simple, but a number of studies have found self-rated health to be correlated with measures of functional health (e.g., Ferraro, 1985) and with judgments by physicians (e.g., LaRue, Bank, Jarvik, & Hetland, 1979). Further, those elders who rate their own health as "poor" have been shown to be more likely to die within the succeeding few years than those who rate their health as "excellent" (Schoenfeld, Malmrose, Blazer, Gold, & Seeman, 1994). In a review of more than 45 studies of the prediction of mortality from self-rated health, Benyamini and Idler (1999) found a highly consistent relationship between self-rated health and mortality. A more recent study (Ferraro & Kelley-Moore, 2001) using multiple waves of data from a national sample over a 20-year period, demonstrated that self-rated health was quite sensitive to declines in health, especially those declines occurring in the terminal drop period. After controlling for a large number of health-related and status characteristics, changes in self-rated health were found to be the best predictors of mortality, especially for African Americans. They concluded that elders appear to take the general trajectory of their health into account when making ratings, thus helping to explain the relationship of such ratings to mortality. This conclusion is particularly relevant for the present study, in which self-rated health was examined in relation to older adults views of death.

Regardless of how health is defined, there is a significant association between health and age, with health likely to become poorer with advancing age. However, it must be remembered that poor health is not an inevitable accompaniment of aging. The studies cited above indicate that a substantial number of elders at every age remain in good health. Also, once chronic health problems are encountered, the trajectory of decline is different for each individual. In this sense, it is important to examine how health influences older adults' views of death independently of any effects of age.

Effects of Health on Death-Related Attitudes

It seems reasonable to hypothesize that one's views of death may be influenced by perceptions of the state of one's own health, inasmuch as declining health can render death much more salient in one's thoughts. Considerable data exist to support this hypothesis.

One might expect that elders in poor health would have greater fear of death than those in better health. As health declines, the inevitability of one's death becomes more difficult to suppress or deny, leading to greater fear among those unable to accept such a prospect. However, research studies have yielded mixed findings. On one hand, Mullins and Lopez (1982), in a study of nursing home patients, found that fear of death was greater among an older, sicker group than among those who were younger. They concluded that when older people are actually closer to death, they may have more fear than they had when in better health. Work by Viney (1984) and by Kureshi & Husain (1981) supports this finding. Conversely, Robinson and Wood (1983) found no difference in fear of death between ill patients and healthy controls, emphasizing the controversial nature of existing findings. Yet, in the Fortner et al. (2000) meta-analysis of fear of death studies involving older adults, greater physical health problems were found to predict higher levels of death anxiety. Thus, the preponderance of the data supports a general conclusion that poorer health is associated with greater death anxiety. Such a general conclusion may not apply to all cases, however. A recent in-depth longitudinal study in which several older patients were followed throughout their terminal illness to the time of death (Staton, Shuy, and Byock, 2001) emphasized the great individual differences in the ways in which these patients approached their impending deaths. Some, in their 80s, seemed to deny or to be unable to grasp the fact that they had a terminal diagnosis, and just continued living serenely until the end despite the effects of their illness. One insisted that she was fine and in good health. Others manifested a quiet acceptance of the coming end of life, gained through religious faith or a general philosophy of life. At the opposite extreme, one woman with a lifelong history of fear of death (refusing to talk about people dying or to attend the funerals of friends) appeared to have such high death anxiety that she refused to even speak about death, and at night would be too frightened to lie down.

For example, declining health near death has been found to influence elders' attitudes of acceptance of death. In a study of over 500 elderly patients with congestive heart failure judged to have no more than 6 months to live (Levenson, McCarthy, Lynn, Davis, & Phillips (2000), acceptance of death, as indicated by completion of a "do not resuscitate" (DNR) order, increased as illnesses became more severe. Whereas only 33% of patients had such orders between 6 months and 3 months before death, 47% had completed

DNR requests at 1 month to 3 days before death, with the frequency of such requests increasing as patients' conditions worsened and death approached. However, such a finding does not tell the whole story. When terminal patients were assessed repeatedly over a period of days preceding death (Chochinov, Tataryn, Clinch, & Dudgeon, 1999) their attitudes fluctuated wildly between a strong will to live and a low will to live (suggesting an acceptance of death). These findings suggest that death-related attitudes may undergo considerable change once death is perceived as quite close.

Studies have also indicated that those adults who have been revived after having a close brush with death (e.g., cardiac arrest) and who have had a "near-death experience" have reported a nonexistent or greatly reduced fear of death as compared to those who did not have such an experience (Greyson, 1994; Moody, 1975; Sabom, 1982). A "near-death experience" typically includes at least some of the following: extreme cognitive clarity, a life review, a tunnel leading to strong light, strong positive affect, out-of-body experience, and a sense of being in a nonearthly dimension. Those with such an experience tended to report dying and death as a benign, if not pleasant, experience and many gained a strong confidence in the existence of an afterlife.

Relation of Health to Fear of Death

Some older studies probing the relationship between illness and fear of death yielded mixed results. Robinson and Wood (1983), studying five subgroups of elders varying from being in good health to suffering from cancer, found no difference between the groups on three different measures of fear of death. However, subgroup sizes were small. In contrast, Mullins and Lopez (1982) found that nursing home patients with worse self-reported health had a greater fear of death regardless of age. Similarly, Viney (1984) found that more seriously ill patients had a greater fear of death than those who were less seriously ill or those who were in good health. A study of HIV-infected gay men (Hintze, Templer, Cappelletty, & Frederick, 1994) found death anxiety to bear a strong relationship to measures of the severity of their condition, although there was considerable overlap with the effects of depression.

In a reanalysis of data from a study of nearly 400 older adults attending senior centers in the Midwest (Cicirelli, 1995b, 1997), those elders who had poorer self-rated health also had greater fear of death on the Multivariate Fear of Death Scales (Hoelter, 1979; Neimeyer & Moore, 1994). Correlations were weak but statistically significant, and remained so when statistically controlled for age, socioeconomic status, and ethnicity. Not only was poorer health related to greater Total Fear of Death, but also to greater Fear of Being Destroyed and Fear for the Body after Death.

A recent meta-analysis of 49 existing studies of fear of death in older adults (Fortner, Neimeyer, & Rybarczyk, 2000) reviewed 12 studies in which physical health was a variable and 8 studies in which mental health was included. In regard to physical health, there was a small but significant linear relationship ($r = .17$, $p < .05$) with fear of death, such that poorer physical health was related to greater fear. Only a global measure of health was used in reaching weighted average correlations across studies, however, so one doesn't know whether greater fear of death is associated with certain types of illness or treatment settings than with others. For example, Fortner and colleagues cite study findings by Hendon and Epting (1989) that patients in hospice care had less fear of death than patients in general hospitals. In regard to psychological problems, greater depression and general anxiety were related to greater fear of death. Unfortunately, other types of psychological illness were not included in the studies reviewed. The link between depression and fear of death is not surprising, given the well-known association between depression and mortality in old age (Schulz, Martire, Beach, & Scheier, 2000). Certainly these effects need to be disentangled.

To explain the puzzling mixed findings regarding the relationship between health and fear of death, Tomer and Eliason (2000a) have proposed a comprehensive path model in which the influence of salience of death on fear of death is mediated by six factors. A person's eventual death can take on greater or less salience in his or her thoughts, depending on that person's age and state of health, as well as a variety of environmental stimuli. According to the model, the individual will experience greater death anxiety to the extent that he or she has past-related regrets, future-related regrets, and perceives death to be meaningless. Past-related regrets refer to the person's feelings of guilt or remorse over having failed to accomplish what he or she expected to accomplish in life, whereas future-related regrets refer to feelings of frustration and disappointment that he or she will be unable to fulfill expectation or meet goals important to his or her identity in the future. A self-actualized person has low past- and future-related regrets because he or she has been able to meet important goals in life; hence, that individual would be expected to have an attitude of acceptance of death rather than fear of death. Viewing death as meaningful, in contrast to viewing death as meaningless or absurd, is related to death anxiety; when the person sees death as the beginning of an afterlife or immortality, as some kind of transcendence of the self, as some kind of cosmic unity, or even as an escape from an unbear-able life, death takes on meaning. In the Tomer and Eliason model, these three factors (past-related regrets, future-related regrets, and death meaningfulness) are influenced in turn by beliefs about the self (e.g., self-concept, self-esteem) and the world (e.g., nature of one's culture, concepts of justice) and by the coping processes available to the self (including life review, life planning, and gen-erativity and self-transcendence). A model such as this can help to explain why the salience of death in a person's thoughts engen-dered by his or her declining health does not automatically lead to greater fear of death. Instead, the nearness of death is reinter-preted, both cognitively and emotionally, by examining past and future life in terms of complex belief about death, the self, and the world. More simply, the way that death is conceptualized and accepted influences the extent to which fear of death will be expe-rienced.

Relation of Health to Views of the Dying Process

It is to be expected that a person's state of health would influence his or her views of what the dying process is like, particularly if he or she is suffering from a terminal illness. Ideas about the dying process are gained from physicians and health care professionals, from the media, from fellow-sufferers in support groups, and from one's own experience as a terminal patient.

Those individuals far from death and still in relatively good health have no direct experience with the dying process, and must rely on vicarious experience of deaths of family members and others, information in the media, and so on. People apparently do gain some ideas of what the dying process will be like (whether short or protracted, painless or painful) and many use these ideas as a basis for formulating advance directives in an attempt to gain some control over the dying process. For example, elders who are concerned over the possibility of experiencing a dying process that may be protracted by various forms of futile life-extending medical treatments are likely to prepare directives explicitly refusing such forms of treatment as cardiopulmonary resuscitation, tube feeding, ventilator, and intravenous fluids, preferring to be allowed to die with only comfort care. Similarly, those already in a terminal phase of illness often refuse such treatments when offered by physicians, or insist that treatments already begun be withdrawn. As noted earlier, Levenson et al. (2000) found that as patients' health deteriorated and they grew closer to death, the percentage completing "do not resuscitate" orders increased.

Lawton (2000) also found that elders' rejection of treatment near the end of life was influenced by the severity of their illness. Similar results were found in a study using hypothetical severity of illness. Schonwetter, Walker, Solomon, Indurkhya, and Robinson (1996) elicited preferences of older adults regarding cardiopulmonary resuscitation under several illness scenarios: 34% would refuse resuscitation under current health conditions, 67% would refuse if acutely ill, and 92% would refuse if terminally ill.

In interview studies investigating older adults reasons for refusing life-prolonging treatments (Everhart & Pearlman, 1990; High, 1993b; Moore & Sherman, 1999; Zweibel & Cassel, 1989), among the most common reasons included not wanting to live with physical limitations or loss of mental acuity, avoiding pain and suffering, not wanting to be on life supports, the impossibility of a cure, and feeling that it was one's natural time to die. Such reasons reveal a mostly negative view of the dying process. Although such views were typical of older adults living in the community, a study of the views of terminally ill elders (Steinhauser, Christakis, Clipp, McNeilly, McIntyre, & Tulsky, 2000) includes many of the same concerns. From 70% to 99% of terminal patients wanted to be free of onerous symptoms (e.g., pain, shortness of breath) and to be kept clean and comfortable, to have treatment preferences in writing (e.g., not be connected to machines), and to feel prepared to die. Like participants in the present study (as reported in Chapter 5), they were also concerned about such aspects of the dying process as communication with medical staff, closeness to family, and emotional concerns (e.g., anxiety).

Only a few studies have considered elders' views of the dying process independent of end-of-life decisions. Fry (1990), in an interview study of death-related concerns of homebound older adults in poor health, found that elders were concerned about pain and suffering and fears of sensory loss that they felt likely to experience in the dying process. In a longitudinal study of the very old (those beyond 85 years of age), Johnson and Barer (1997) observed that as elders' health declined and they became increasingly frail and fatigued, most had thought about and made practical preparations for death. Such preparations included making a will, planning burial arrangements, and leaving instructions regarding other practical matters. They became increasingly aware of the finitude of life and seemed prepared to die, taking death into account in their everyday lives and becoming detached from everyday practical and social concerns. Many became philosophical, ruminating on the meaning of life and death. Whereas their symptoms seemed to be those of increasing fatigue and vague medical complaints, rather than more acute manifestations of illness, their greatest fears were of an extended and painful dying process. This is somewhat surprising in view of a study (Moss, Lawton, & Glicksman, 1991) that found that although most elders experienced pain in their last year of life, the oldest old reported less pain than those somewhat younger. According to Johnson and Barer, some elders worried about dying alone and who would find them after they had died.

The few studies available indicate that older adults' views on death do indeed change as their health declines and they perceive themselves to be getting closer to death. They seem to have a philosophical acceptance of their approaching and inevitable death. In addition, they appear to have less fear of death itself but perhaps more fear of the dying process. Although this latter point may seem at odds with the more benign conception of the dying process voiced by study participants in Chapter 5, most of our studying participants were still in relatively good health.

THE PRESENT STUDY

Using data gathered for our study of older adults' views on death, we explored the relationship of their health status to quantitative measures of death meanings, fear of death, and views of the dying process, as well as to their qualitative views in the open-ended interviews. In so doing, we made comparisons between elders in different states of health, that is, we sought to determine whether individual differences in health were related to different views on death. It is hoped that such a strategy will give us some clues as to how an individual's views might change as his or her health changes over time on the long trajectory toward death.

QUANTITATIVE DATA AND ANALYSES

Health Status of Study Participants

Health of study participants was assessed in several ways: a self-rating of health, the number and severity of chronic conditions, the number and frequency of symptoms, instrumental activities of daily living (IADL), mobility, and general well-being. Each of these indicators of participants' health status will be discussed in turn.

Self-Rated Health

A six-point rating scale, ranging from "excellent" to "very poor," was used to elicit study participants' judgments of their own state of health. They were asked first to rate their health in comparison to others of their age, and then to rate their health in comparison to younger people. In comparison to others of their own age, their rating were overwhelmingly positive: 18% rated their health as excellent, 32% rated it as very good, 42% rated it as good, 6% rated it as not so good, none rated it as poor and 2% rated it as very poor. The mean rating was 4.58, with a standard deviation of 0.97. As might be expected, ratings in comparison to younger people were lower: only 5% rated their health as excellent, 14% rated it as very good, 39% rated it as good, 30% rated it as not so good, 8% rated it as poor, and 4% rated it as very poor.

Chronic Conditions

To assess the incidence of various chronic conditions among study participants, a checklist of 20 frequent chronic conditions of older adults was used. In each case, participants were asked whether they had this condition and, if so, whether it was minor, moderately severe, or very severe. A minor condition included cases where a condition was present but was managed satisfactorily through medication (e.g., hypertension). Table 7.1 presents the percentages of participants reporting each condition and the percentages experiencing the condition at a moderately severe or very severe level. The most frequently occurring conditions were arthritis (82%, with 51% at more severe levels), hypertension (60%, 7%), eye diseases (59%, 15%), and back problems (48%, 30%). There was also an open-ended "other" category for conditions not on the checklist, with 24% of participants reporting an additional condition; osteoporosis was most frequently mentioned. An overall score for the severity of health conditions was also obtained by summing over the number of conditions reported. This severity of chronic conditions score ranged from 0 to 30 ($M = 8.61$; $SD = 4.86$).

Many elders suffered from multiple chronic conditions (see Table 7.2). The number of chronic conditions reported at any level of severity ranged from 0 to 13 ($M = 5.47$; $SD = 2.45$). Fewer conditions were reported at the moderately severe or very severe levels, with the number ranging from 0 to 9 ($M = 2.18$; $SD = 1.73$).

Symptoms

To assess the degree to which these elders were troubled by various symptoms, a checklist of 42 common symptoms reported by elders in an earlier study (Cicirelli, 1982) was used, determining

TABLE 7.1 Percentages of Study Participants With Various Chronic Conditions

| | Percentage of Study Participants | |
| | Has the condition | Severe or very severe condition |
Condition		
Arthritis	82	51
Hypertension	60	7
Glaucoma, cataracts, etc.	59	15
Back problems	48	30
Loss of hearing	37	16
Heart disease	35	11
Allergies, asthma	32	14
Gastritis, stomach problems	26	15
Diabetes	23	6
Bursitis	19	5
Crippled limbs	16	12
Cancer	15	4
Hemmorhoids	15	2
Skin growths, rashes	15	3
Kidney disease	10	6
Stroke	10	6
Emphysema, COPD	9	6
Hernia	8	0
Ulcers	6	1
Liver disease, cirrhosis	1	0
Other	24	11

first whether the elder had experienced a particular symptom and then how frequently it was experienced (on a 5-point scale ranging from "0 = never" to "4 = almost all the time"). The percentages of participants reporting each symptom on the checklist at two levels of frequency are shown in Table 7.3, with the percentages reporting the symptom either "frequently" or "almost all the time" greatest for overweight (49%), frequent urination (34%), trouble walking (31%), swelling of extremities (26%), lack of energy (23%), joint pain (20%), and feeling tired (20%). An overall score for the frequency of symptoms experienced was obtained by summing over the 42 symptoms; scores ranged from 1 to 80 ($M = 26.41$; $SD = 17.66$).

TABLE 7.2 Percentage of Study Participants Reporting Different Numbers of Chronic Conditions

	Level of Severity of Condition	
Number of Conditions	Minor Severity or Greater	Moderately to Very Severe
0	1	12
1	3	29
2	6	25
3	8	16
4	18	9
5	16	5
6	18	2
7	12	1
8	6	1
9	3	1
10	3	
11	3	
12	1	
13	1	
Mean	5.47	2.18
SD	2.45	1.73

As was the case for chronic conditions, many participants experienced multiple symptoms (see Table 7.4), with the number of symptoms experienced at least "occasionally" ranging from 0 to 27 ($M = 8.37$, $SD = 5.92$) and the number of symptoms experienced "frequently" or "almost all the time" ranging from 0 to 21 ($M = 4.39$, $SD = 4.15$).

Instrumental Activities of Daily Living

The Instrumental Activities of Daily Living scale (Lawton, 1972) was used to assess the functional health of study participants. The amount of help needed to carry out a task (rated on a 4-point scale) was obtained for each of eight activities: use of telephone, shopping, meal preparation, housekeeping, laundry, managing medications, managing finances, and grooming: The IADL score was

TABLE 7.3 Percentage of Study Participants Experiencing Various Symptoms

Symptom	Percentage reporting symptom	
	Occasionally or more often	Frequently or most of the time
Muscular, skeletal		
Trouble walking	36	31
Joint pain	37	20
Backache	34	18
Stiffness	36	17
Leg cramps	25	9
Foot pain	19	8
Paralysis	2	2
Digestive system		
Constipation	14	14
Lack of appetite	17	10
Indigestion	25	12
Heartburn	17	9
Stomach pain, cramps	7	3
Nausea	8	2
Diarrhea	8	0
Trouble swallowing	5	0
Vomiting	2	0
Circulatory		
Swelling of extremities	36	26
Rapid heartbeat	10	3
Chest pains	5	0
Respiratory		
Sinus congestion	27	15
Coughing	25	9
Urinary		
Frequent urination	48	34
Painful or difficult urination	2	2
Sensory		
Trouble seeing	24	15
Trouble hearing	19	14
Trouble speaking	3	3

(continued)

TABLE 7.3 *(continued)*

Symptom	Percentage reporting symptom	
	Occasionally or more often	Frequently or most of the time
Energy		
Lack of energy	34	23
Feeling tired	46	20
Loss of strength	24	12
Feeling weak	25	3
Miscellaneous		
Weight problems	51	49
Trouble getting to sleep	29	17
Shortness of breath	25	14
General pain	14	7
Itching	17	5
Hot flashes	12	4
Dizziness	25	2
Headache	17	2
Cold sweats	5	2
Fainting	2	2
Sore throat	2	2
Fever	0	0

the sum over the eight items, with a high score indicating poorer functional health. Most study participants had good functional health, with scores ranging from 8 to 28 ($M = 10.30$; $SD = 4.12$). Areas in which the greatest percentage of elders needed some degree of help were shopping (22%) and laundry (24%), and areas in which the smallest percentage of elders needed some degree of help were use of telephone (1%) and managing medications (8%).

Mobility

To assess functional health in terms of mobility, a 6-item mobility instrument was used (Lawton, 1972) in which a 5-point item response scale was used to indicate the degree of help needed. A high score corresponds to poorer mobility. Percentages of partic-

TABLE 7.4 Percentage of Study Participants Reporting Different Numbers of Symptoms

Number of Symptoms	Frequency of Symptoms	
	Occasionally or More Often	Frequently or Almost Always
0	7	17
1–3	22	34
4–6	14	20
7–9	17	17
10–12	15	8
13–15	14	2
16–18	8	0
19–21	2	2
22–24	0	
25–27	2	
Mean	8.37	4.39
SD	5.92	4.15

ipants reporting some degree of difficulty in the six areas were: climbing stairs (57%), walking outside (35%), walking at home (21%), rising from chairs (10%), use of wheelchair (9%), and getting in and out of bed (3%). The total mobility score ranged from 6 to 23 ($M = 8.46$; $SD = 3..42$), indicating relatively good mobility for most of the older adults taking part in the study.

Well-Being

A quantitative assessment of psychological well-being was obtained using the Bradburn (1969) Affect Balance Scale. The 10 items in the scale are asked as a series of "yes-no" questions about feelings in the previous few weeks. Items include feelings of interest or excitement, restlessness, pride, loneliness, accomplishment, boredom, elation, depression or unhappiness, that things were going one's way, and upset by criticism. Each "yes" response is scored "1" and each "no" response is scored "0," and separate subscores are obtained for positive and negative affect items. The affect balance score is 5 plus the difference between the positive and negative affect scores; it can range from 0 to 10, with high scores reflecting a more positive feeling of well-being. Bradburn reported satisfactory internal consistencies for the positive and negative subscores, as well as evidence for stability and validity. For study participants, scores ranged from 1 to 10, with a mean of 7.48 and a standard deviation of 2.10. With scores of 6 and above on the scale indicating an overall positive affective mood, 80% of study participants could be considered as having a positive sense of psychological well-being.

Relationship of Health to Views on Death

The real question of interest here is whether older adults' state of health influenced their views on death. Therefore, we correlated the self-rating of health (in comparison to others their age), severity of chronic conditions, frequency of symptoms, IADL, mobility, and psychological well-being with the death meanings, fear of death, and dying process variables. The effects of age, gender, ethnicity, and socioeconomic status were statistically controlled.

Death Meanings

When the health measures were correlated with the four death meanings (death as afterlife, death as extinction, death as a motivator, and death as legacy), there were only a few statistically significant relationships. The self-rating of health was related to death as extinction $(r = -.31)$, with those elders in poorer health holding stronger views of death as meaning extinction. Additionally, psychological well-being, as assessed by the Bradburn Affect Balance Scale (1969), was related to death as a motivator $(r = .21)$ and death as legacy $(r = .30)$. That is, those elders with a greater sense of well-being were more likely to see death as legacy and death as a motivator.

Fear of Death

Of the four MFODS subscores used in the study (Fear of the Dying Process, Fear of Being Destroyed, Fear for Significant Others, and

Fear of the Unknown), only Fear of the Dying Process was related to the health variables. Fear of the Dying Process was significantly related to the self-rating of health ($r = -.24$), frequency of health symptoms ($r = .38$), mobility ($r = .20$), and well being ($r = -.21$). Those study participants with poorer self-ratings of their health, more frequent symptoms, poorer mobility, and a poorer sense of well-being had a greater fear of the dying process. It is interesting that neither the severity of chronic conditions nor the need for help with instrumental activities of living were related to fear.

Views and Expectations of the Dying Process

As discussed in Chapter 5, elders' views and expectations about the dying process were expressed by five factors: emotional reactions, concern with physical survival, concern with family, feelings of rancor, and coping with dying. Four of the five factors were significantly correlated with health variables; concern with family was the only factor showing no relationship.

First, emotional reactions were related to frequency of symptoms ($r = .44$), with those elders more troubled with frequent symptoms tending to view the dying process in terms of more negative emotional reactions. Second, feelings of rancor connected with expectations about the dying process were related to both the severity of chronic conditions ($r = .22$) and the frequency of symptoms ($r = .25$). Those elders with more severe chronic conditions and with a greater frequency of troubling symptoms were more likely to expect the dying process to be accompanied by such rancorous feelings as anger and bitterness.

Second, feelings of concern with physical survival and expectations of coping with dying were both related to the self-rating of health and mobility. Those seeing themselves in better health expected to have less concern with their physical survival during the dying process ($r = -.25$) and less coping with dying behaviors ($r = -.21$). Those with greater mobility problems, in contrast, expected to have greater concern with their physical survival during the dying process ($r = .23$) and more coping with dying behaviors ($r = .21$).

Summary

In summary, older adults' reports about their own health were found to be related to the ways in which they viewed death. Their self-ratings of health were related to their conception of death as extinction, fear of the dying process, and their anticipated concerns with physical survival and coping during the dying process.

Second, the overall frequency with which they experienced a variety of troubling symptoms, although unrelated to their death meanings, was associated with their emotional reactions to death: fear of the dying process, expectations of negative emotions during the dying process, and expected rancorous feelings associated with dying. It would seem that whatever the severity of chronic condition or functional health disability may be, these health problems are experienced in terms of a variety of symptoms, with the overall impact of these symptoms reflected in the emotional reactions to death.

Third, the severity of chronic conditions was related only to expectations of rancorous feelings during the dying process, and not to death meanings or fears. One might interpret the association of severity of chronic conditions with rancor as a "why me?" response, that is, feelings of anger and bitterness that they were afflicted with these conditions in contrast to other elders who were not.

Fourth, the first of two indicators of functional health (IADL) was associated only with expectations of feelings of rancor in the dying process. Inasmuch as the great majority of elders in the sample had few problems with instrumental activities, those who had greater problems in comparison may have experienced anger and bitterness that they were dependent on others for certain activities of daily living while their age peers were not.

Fifth, the second indicator of functional health (mobility) had no relationship to death meanings, but was related to fear of the dying process as well as expectations of concerns with survival and coping behaviors during the dying process.

Sixth, a positive sense of psychological well-being was associated not only with less fear of death, but with a tendency to see death in positive terms as a motivator for the fulfillment of certain goals in life and an opportunity to leave some sort of legacy for others (loved ones and mankind in general).

QUALITATIVE DATA AND ANALYSES

In the open-ended interviews, no specific questions were asked about how the elders' state of health influenced their views on death, and only a few spontaneously referred to their health while responding to other questions. As a result, we used a different strategy in attempting to tease out any influence of health on study participants' views. We identified two groups of elders. The first group consisted of those elders who had the poorest self-rated health (not so good, poor, or very poor) and/or who reported the greatest frequency of symptoms and/or a very low sense of well-being. The second group was a mirror opposite of the first, consisting of those who had the best self-rated health (excellent) and/or who reported the smallest frequency of symptoms and who felt a very high sense of well-being. Simply put, we identified one group of older adults at the extreme of very poor health and another group at the extreme of very good health. Then we compared the comments of both groups to find out whether they differed in their views of death in any discernible ways.

Older Adults in Very Poor Health

Beginning with the group of participants identified as being in very poor health, we examined their comments regarding death fears and the dying process. Some saw life as a burden with death as a release:

- Death doesn't frighten me. All I see of life is more pain and suffering.
- I don't want more [*life*] like this. Death will be a relief.
- We're all just a little afraid of it. There are lots of times I wish that I could die and get it over with, especially when I hurt so badly. I'd feel relief, because I wouldn't have to suffer any more.
- Life at my age is limited. I think dying will be frightening at first, the idea of pain and coping with illness. But I think it will be a relief.
- My own illness taught me to value life. A great deal of regret has to come at the end, regret at leaving life. But you might welcome death if you're in a great deal of pain.

- Sometimes I think about dying in my bed. Dying will be a relief.
- The closer I get to death, the less it worries me. Probably relief, the burdens of the world will be gone.
- Sometimes at night when the lights have all gone out, I think about it. I hope to go to sleep and not have any pain, not have to linger a long time. I think I'll feel some relief.

Other elders seemed to see death as more fearsome and were concerned about what they might experience during the dying process:

- I broke these hips, that's the start of my incapacity. I know death is getting closer. I can honestly say that if I went to bed tonight and didn't wake up in the morning it wouldn't make any difference to me. I'm ready. The one thing I'm afraid of is having to know that I'm suffering an awful lot.
- Death is something to fear.
- I think about death day and night. The thought of what I'll go through bothers me sometimes. I'm going to try to be so close to God he'll let me die easy. I'll be happy at that.
- I'll be ready to die. I wouldn't want to be ill and in pain. I guess I have a little anxiety.
- I think my death will be quick, because of my breathing. I just won't wake up. I don't think I'll be frightened, but not exactly happy.
- I just hope that I drop off in my sleep. To know that you are dying is a very tragic thing.
- I hope dying will be quick. I feel that I'm going to feel sad.
- I think I will have some feelings of fright, because it is unknown . . . My greatest fear is having something like cancer and being in a lot of pain for a long time. I fear that more than actual dying itself.

Only a few saw death as a positive experience:

- I think I'll have a happy death. I'd have good feelings.
- I have a feeling it will be very peaceful and I'm not going to suffer. I believe I'll be happy.
- Knowing that I'm eventually going to have to face death, I try to live so I have a reasonable hope of the hereafter . . . I don't think I'll feel afraid.

Older Adults in Very Good Health

Some of the elders who manifested very good health looked upon death in positive terms, as some kind of glorious experience or adventure:

- I believe that there is something that lies beyond. Dying will be an adventure.
- I've got good health. I have no fears of death. My soul will go to heaven.
- I think dying will be beautiful. I think I'd feel happy.
- Dying is a promise of glory. It's an experience.
- I look on death as wonderful.

Others were simply unconcerned about death or minimized any possible fears or discomfort associated with dying:

- I feel like I'm going to live forever. I'm not afraid of death.
- I'm in good health. There's no point in fearing death.
- I don't think about death. It doesn't arouse any fears in me.
- When I was close to dying [*an earlier serious illness*], I gave it no thought, no emotional reaction.
- I think about death, but don't worry. I'll be like my mother, she went real fast.
- I wouldn't be frightened, but I would think about it. I don't think I'll suffer much.
- No, the thought of death doesn't bother me. My idea is that your heart is going to stop . . . you wouldn't have time to feel frightened.
- It's a natural thing, so we don't feel too sad about it.
- I don't think I'm frightened. I'm not going to be in a lot of pain . . . my doctor will shoot me up.
- I wish I could die right off, sleep myself away.
- I've had dreams of dying and I slept through it. I don't think I'd be scared.

A Comparison of Views on Death

In comparing the views of those older adults who were in very poor health with those who were in very good health, one is struck by certain differences. Those who were in very poor health tended to see life as a burden with death as a relief or release from pain and suffering, whereas none of those in very good health voiced such ideas. Those who were in very poor health expressed fears about dying and what they might go through during the dying process, whereas those who were in very good health seemed relatively unconcerned about the dying process or minimized any fears or discomfort associated with dying. Finally, some of the elders in very poor health viewed death in positive terms (e.g., happy, peaceful), whereas some of those in very good health viewed death not only in positive terms but as a great, glorious, wonderful adventure.

CONCLUSIONS

Evidence from all three sources of information about the influence of health on older adults fear of death appears to converge in many respects. Findings from existing literature, from the quantitative empirical study, and from the qualitative analysis of the interview protocols point to several conclusions.

Those in poor health are more likely to accept and welcome death, regarding it as a relief or release from the pain, suffering, and struggles they face in their daily lives as a result of their health conditions. Those who are besieged by various life-threatening chronic conditions, loss of mobility, increasing dependence on others, and frequent onerous symptoms, including those accompanying their increasing frailty, see death as an escape from a life that is no longer rewarding.

Additionally, those in poor health are more likely to fear the dying process. This makes sense intuitively, for individuals who deal with pain and suffering resulting from their poor health have little basis for believing that the dying process will miraculously end their woes. On the contrary, many expect dying to result in increased and prolonged pain and misery. Although some previous research (e.g., Greyson, 1994) has reported that those individuals who survived a "near-death experience" had a reduced fear of death, this does not seem to be the case for the great majority of elders who may be in poor health but who have not had a near-death experience. At the other end of the health continuum, those in good health appear to have less fear of the dying process. One might speculate that, without the negative experiences endured by those in poor health, they have little reason to anticipate a difficult and prolonged dying process. Instead, they rely on vicarious experiences of death, often derived from the sanitized depictions of death as presented in film and television. In the media, deaths of older people are relatively benign, often a quiet passing away in sleep without prolonged suffering. It is easy, therefore, for those in good health to regard death as glorious, wonderful, or an exciting adventure.

Various aspects of the quantitative relationship of health variables to death meanings are of interest. First of all, there were few relationships between the health variables and the death meanings dimensions. This is not surprising in that an individual's personal meanings of death are developed from childhood on; by adulthood, one would expect them to be relatively stable. They may not be influenced greatly by late-life illness. The only death meanings dimension related to self-rated health was death as extinction. Those in poor health were more likely to view death as meaning extinction. On the one hand, this might imply that at least some sufferers have lost faith in God and a promised afterlife as a result of their misery. On the other hand, this finding may suggest that those elders who see death as meaning extinction may have little hope for a future; negative feedback from such a lack of hope could exacerbate health problems. Finally, more positive psychological well-being was related to the meanings of death as legacy and death as a motivator. Positive psychological well-being would fit into a growth model of health, in which there is further improvement in bodily and mental functioning. From this perspective, a person with greater psychological well-being would be more likely to see death as a motivator for continued activity and growth, making the most of opportunities to leave a legacy for the future.

Further research in this area needs to examine how other variables (e.g., personality variables) may moderate the relationship between older adults' health and their views of death. For example, dispositional optimism has been related to positive physical health outcomes in addition to subjective well-being (Salovey, Rothman, & Rodin, 1998). At the very least, it might have an indirect effect on death meanings, death fears, and views of the dying process. Another possible influence on the relationship between older adults' health and their death views is the process of social comparison. Downward comparisons with those who are worse off has been associated with better coping and adjustment to illness (e.g., Wood, Taylor, & Lichtman, 1985). Again, such comparisons may have an indirect effect of views of death.

Also, further research is needed to determine how older adults' views are shaped by earlier experiences and contextual factors. Longitudinal studies could trace any changes in views of death accompanying ill health during the aging process, particularly during the years of terminal drop. Explorations of death views using a model such as that proposed by Tomer and Eliason (2000a) would be desirable in order to gain a fuller understanding of the factors and processes contributing to death meanings, fears of death, and views of the dying process in later life.

8

The Influence of Family Relationships on Views of Death

It is quite reasonable to suppose that older adults who have close and supportive relationships with a circle of family and friends will view death in a different way from those individuals who are relatively alone late in life. As Nadeau (1998) has pointed out, the meanings that an individual attaches to his or her own death or the deaths of family members are related to his or her feelings about the family as a whole as well as about individual members. Given that the family is a fundamental institution of society, one can hypothesize that the nature of that family has a great influence on older adults' views of death.

MEANING OF FAMILY AND AGING FAMILY

A standard definition of family sets a boundary, making it clear which individuals are included or excluded as family members, thus identifying a family unit. In past years, a standard definition of family was accepted by society as a whole. As defined by the U.S. Bureau of the Census (1991), a family consists of two or more persons residing together, and related by birth, marriage, or adoption. A family as so defined assumes certain obligations important to its functioning as a social unit, such as maintaining a household, dividing household tasks, supporting and protecting children, and providing a legacy for the family. Legal privileges include such things as tax breaks, family medical insurance, Social Security benefits, rights of inheritance, right to consent to medical treatment for family members, and so on.

In the 1990s, it became increasingly difficult to agree upon a standard definition of the family. Rapid advances in science and technology, economic and industrial changes, and social and cultural changes have produced a fragmented and heterogeneous society with multiple conflicting values and norms. In such a society, the emergence of many new family forms requires a new definition of the family if one is to determine the boundaries of families as well as the obligations and legal privileges of family members. Such a definition (Cicirelli, 1998a) is as follows: The family as a group of individuals exists when (a) two individuals are legally married, or (b) two or more individuals are genetically connected, or (c) one or more individuals are legally adopted by an adult, or (d) unmarried and unrelated individuals share a household and living arrangements of long duration and exclusivity with a relationship characterized by love and commitment, or (e) unmarried and unrelated individuals share a relationship with love and commitment but without sharing the same household, or (f) an individual lives alone but interacts, participates, and communicates in a committed relationship with one or more individuals who have a genetic commonality.

Such a broad definition of family allows one to regard various groupings as specific family types (albeit diverse ones), and provides a common ground for dealing with them. It eliminates the necessity of talking about households, living arrangements, and alternate lifestyles as separate from families. Instead, one can use the latter to help define specific types of families, such as the multigenerational family, the single parent family, the heterosexual cohabitant family, the reconstituted or blended family, the childless family, the singlehood "family," the homosexual family, the communal family, and so on.

However, the participants in our study represent an older generation that follows more traditional family patterns, that is, either an extended family, modified extended family, or a single career or dual career nuclear family. Although relatively rare among our study participants, an extended family involves family relatives of more than one generation living in the same household. A modified extended family is one where relatives live relatively near each other but in different households. Finally, a nuclear family is one where mother, father, and children live in the same household with one or both parents working. Extended and modified extended families include the phenomena of not only three- but four- and five-generation families. In its most general sense, the family becomes almost synonymous with the kin network. Thus, a wider conception of a traditional family may include members who have more remote blood relationships to the nuclear members. In short, our position is that traditional families may go beyond the nuclear family or the typical members of an extended family to include any type of kin that family members view as included in the family, for example, even a second or third cousin.

A traditional family that is also an aging family has some additional attributes. Family members belonging to the older generation are beyond childbearing years (or are childless couples beyond the age of 65); older family members are influenced by and influence various generations (siblings, children, grandchildren, nieces and nephews, grandnieces and grandnephews, cousins, etc.); family members share a lengthy family history (a large memory reservoir of shared companionships, conflicts, etc.); and older family members have dealt with and shared events unique to later life (retirement, widowhood, chronic illness and concomitant dependencies, loss of ascending and many contemporaneous family members, and so on) (Brubaker, 1983).

EXISTING STUDIES OF THE RELATIONSHIP OF FAMILY TO OLDER ADULTS' VIEWS OF DEATH

A large literature exists regarding caregiving provided by family members to older adults during their declining years and the dying process. However, few studies have explored the influence of family relationships on older adults' personal death meanings, fears of death, or views of the dying process.

Family relationships in later life involve a different composition of family members than was the case earlier in adulthood. By the time they reach old age, most older adults have already lost their parents, aunts and uncles, and other ascending kin. Many have also lost some of their contemporaneous family members, such as a spouse, sibling, or cousin. Their experience with such losses tends to give older adults a greater awareness of the finitude of life and their own vulnerability to death (Marshall, 1980).

Some researchers have observed that older adults' loss of family members and awareness of vulnerability is accompanied by a gradual disengagement from relationships with others and an increasing acceptance and decreasing fear of death (Johnson & Barer, 1997; van Doorn et al., 1999). Although Johnson and Barer's conclusions were drawn from a study of the very old (those past age 85), others have reached different conclusions. Tobin (1996), who also studied the very old, found that elderly mothers who still assumed the responsibility of caring for a mentally retarded son or daughter did not manifest such an acceptance of death. Additionally, when Lang (2000) studied some 200 men and women aged 70–103 over a 4-year interval, he found that when these older adults felt near to death, their emotional closeness in relationships with family members did not decrease although there was diminished closeness to others. Whether or not elders' relationships with family members decline with nearness to death, family members are taken into account in elders' views of death. Some see death as a positive opportunity for reunion with family members who have gone before (particularly a deceased spouse or parent); some are motivated to accomplish certain family-related goals or fulfill certain responsibilities toward family members before death; some view their own nearness to death in terms of the life spans of significant family members; others view death as more acceptable than becoming a burden to family members. Not wishing to become a burden to family members was found to be one of the most common reasons for enacting advance directives to refuse medical treatment near the end of life (High, 1993b; Moore & Sherman, 1999).

According to the Moss and Moss (1989) study of sibling death in old age, about a third of the elders studied found the loss of a sibling extremely hard to bear, whereas about half were not bothered by the loss. Those most upset by the loss were those who had had the closest relationship to the sibling. They reported a sense of existential incompleteness in the family, loss of emotional and (in some cases) instrumental support, and shifts in family relationships. For many of the surviving siblings, there was an increased sense of vulnerability to death; some were concerned about their own life expectancy and others took steps to put their affairs in order. Cicirelli (1989, 1995c) interviewed 99 older adults regarding sibling relationships, finding that sibling death was related to feelings of loss of family togetherness, as well as feelings of depression and loneliness. Studies of sibling loss in later life are few in number, but tend to converge in their findings of family incompleteness, loss of emotional support, and personal vulnerability to death. The strong feelings associated with sibling loss are perhaps more understandable in the light of White's (2001) recent findings in a national study of the sibling relationships of 9,000 individuals aged 16–85. Sibling contact and proximity remained essentially constant from middle age on, whereas exchange of help actually increased from age 70 on, particularly for those whose siblings lived within 25 miles. It is evident that many elders seek to maintain and even strengthen their ties with siblings in old age, with sibling relationships contributing to their sense of well-being. With a lifetime of shared history, siblings can play a major role in the life review process. Also, the relationship with a sibling is one for which no other family member can substitute (Connidis, 2001).

Widowhood is also increasingly common in old age. Feelings similar to those experienced in sibling loss are experienced by those who have lost a mate with whom they have had a close relationship (Cook & Oltjenbruns, 1998). The increased vulnerability of the recently widowed to death and to suicide is well-known (Kastenbaum, 2000b).

Other studies have considered effects of supportive family relationships and relationships that are dysfunctional on fear of death. Older adults who have more support from family members and close friends reported greater fear for significant others and less fear of the unknown on the Multivariate Fear of Death Scale (Cicirelli, 2000). Poor or dysfunctional relationships between family members have also been related to greater death anxiety (Heckler, 1994).

No studies were found linking relationships with adult children, grandchildren, and other descending kin on older adults' views of death. However, previous results regarding social support would suggest that those elders with close, warm, and supportive relationships with their adult children would be less likely to have a positive acceptance of death. Rather, they would be more reluctant to leave life on earth.

In sum, there are few studies of family relationships in relation to elders' views on death, but the limited information available suggests that close family relationships may indeed influence the way that older adults look at death. It is hoped that our present study will provide some basis for hypotheses to guide future studies in this area.

THE PRESENT STUDY: NATURE OF FAMILY RELATIONSHIPS

The findings of the present study will be presented in two separate sections of this chapter. The first section will give the reader some idea of the kinds of family relationships reported by our 109 older adult study participants and the second section will consider the connection between study participants' family relationships and their views of death.

Quantitative Description of Family Relationships

To gain some idea about older adults' family relationships, we asked study participants about their marital status and about each of their siblings and adult children. In regard to the siblings and adult children, we asked whether this family member was still living or had died, as well as how close the elder felt toward the family member (assessed on a 4-point scale). Although we were aware of White's (1998) caveat regarding the counting of half-siblings and stepsiblings, we accepted as a sibling whichever family members the elder named as siblings without attempting to distinguish more complex family relationships. However, this occurred rarely. The same procedure was used for adult children, so that stepchildren, adoptive children, and fictive children were not distinguished if the elder considered them as children. Again, this occurred rarely. From responses to these questions we were able to get measures of the total number of brothers in the respondent's family of origin, the number of living brothers, the total number of sisters, the number of living sisters, the total number of siblings, the number of living siblings, the number of deceased siblings, the proportion of deceased siblings, and the mean feelings of closeness to siblings. Analogous measures were obtained for adult children. (Admittedly, all these measures are not independent of one another; however, they were retained due to the exploratory nature of the study and because it is possible that certain measures could yield information not obtained with other measures.) Table 8.1 presents the range, mean, and standard deviation for each of the sibling and adult child variables.

Marital Status

The majority of study participants (63%) were widowed. Of the rest, 16% were still married and living with their spouse, 16% were divorced, 2% were separated, and 4% had never married. Overall, more women (89%) than men (56%) were not married and living with their spouse (widowed, divorced, separated, or never married). Although marital status (married, not married) was uncorrelated with age, it was related to SES/ethnic group membership, with the high SES White subgroup more likely to be married than either the low SES Whites or the African Americans.

Siblings

As can be observed from Table 8.1, the number of siblings reported by study participants ranged from 0 to 15, with 2 siblings the most frequently reported (23%). On average, participants reported 3.5 siblings in the original sibship. Only 73% of participants reported having living siblings, with an average of 1.8 living siblings. The percentage of deceased siblings increased from a low of 40% for the 70–74 age group to 74% for the over age 90 group. There were no gender differences, but the high SES Whites came from smaller sibships and had a smaller percentage of deceased siblings than either the low SES Whites or the African Americans.

TABLE 8.1 Variables Describing Participants' Siblings and Adult Children, With Range, Mean, and Standard Deviation

Family Variable	Range	Mean	*SD*
Siblings			
Total number of brothers	0–7	1.81	1.65
Number of living brothers	0–5	0.79	1.01
Total number of sisters	0–8	1.69	1.63
Number of living sisters	0–5	0.95	1.22
Total number of siblings	0–15	3.54	2.73
Number of living siblings	0–9	1.76	1.86
Number of deceased siblings	0–10	2.01	2.05
Proportion of deceased siblings	0–1	0.43	0.36
Mean closeness to living siblings	1–4	3.27	0.91
Adult children			
Total number of sons	0–6	1.33	1.14
Number of living sons	0–6	1.18	1.12
Total number of daughters	0–6	1.29	1.24
Number of living daughters	0–6	1.18	1.17
Total number of adult children	0–22	2.80	2.66
Number of living adult children	0–22	2.53	2.61
Number of deceased adult children	0–2	0.29	0.54
Proportion of deceased adult children	0–1	0.11	0.22
Mean closeness to living children	1–4	3.65	0.62

In general, the average feeling of closeness to living siblings was high, with a mean of 3.27 on a 4-point scale. Approximately 78% felt close or very close to their living siblings, on the average. Overall, the data regarding siblings indicate that the sibling relationship is still viable for the majority of elders in the study.

Adult Children

The number of adult children reported by study participants ranged from 0 to 22, with 9% of the elders being childless. About 80% of elders had from 1 to 4 children, with the 2-child family the most frequent. Only 11% had more than 4 children. The average number of children was 2.8, with an average of 2.5 still living. The number of deceased children ranged from 0 to 2, with an average of .29. The percentage of deceased children was only 11%. There were no significant differences in the adult child variables by gender, age, or SES/ethnic group.

The average feeling of closeness to children was quite high, with a mean of 3.65 on a 4-point scale. Approximately 91% reported feeling close or very close to their children, on the average. In sum, most of the study participants had living children and reported feeling close to them.

Qualitative Description of Family Relationships

The open-ended interviews provided a great deal of detailed information about the family structure and family relationships of study participants. During the interviews, they talked about their extended family relationships in childhood and adolescence as well as during the adult years. In a broader sense, they talked about ascending kin (family members who were of an older generation than the participant and represented the family of origin, such as parents, grandparents, aunts, and uncles), collateral kin (those in the same generation, such as siblings and cousins), and descending kin (family members younger than the participant and in younger generations of the family, such as children, grandchildren, nieces, and nephews). They talked about family members who exerted considerable influence on them earlier in life (i.e., the degree that other family members changed the views, thoughts, feelings, or behavior of the participant), about their feelings of closeness (or lack of it) toward various family members, and the degree to which certain family members were important to them now for emotional and tangible support if needed. However, these aspects of family relationships could be quite independent of each other. The participant could feel very close to a family member but never receive any help or be influenced by that person.

This material is too voluminous to include in full here, but excerpts from representative protocols are included to give the reader a better idea of the full variety of family backgrounds and relationships of study participants. We will look at broad groups of study participants categorized by gender and SES/ethnic membership. It is hope that by doing so, some questions for further study will be suggested.

High SES White Men

In this group, the fathers typically died much earlier than the mothers. Although both parents had somewhat different kinds of influence (father the disciplinarian, mother the nurturer), the mother's influence was usually the strongest. For example,

- I grew up with my father, planted corn together, fished together, hunted rabbits together. My father was a stern disciplinarian, a churchman. I learned self-discipline from him. From my mother, I learned tender loving care. And she was concerned about my education.
- My mother had the most influence on me. This was partially due not only to the fact that my father died early (age 59) but my parents went through a divorce when I was only 8 years old. This further compounded the fact that my father had a negative influence on me. But I still felt that he loved me. He was a physician and probably had some influence on me becoming a doctor. My mother gave a me great sense of support and comfort.

A considerable variety of sibling relationships was revealed by these high SES men:

- I talked to my sisters but they went their way. I had conflict with them, especially my older sister. She tried to boss me; she was always unhappy.
- There was no sibling rivalry that I could discern or describe. We were brothers. Maybe we had little differences, but nothing that bothered us. We minded our own business and made our own decisions.
- I was somewhat influenced by my brothers. I think I learned perseverance from my brother Russell, From my other brothers, I got affection and learned how to give affection. As far as help is concerned, I had only to ask them. And if they were able to supply it, they would.

- I was much older than my siblings so I didn't get too close to them although I became closer later in life. We never asked each other for help. We were all independent and on our own.
- I didn't feel close to my siblings when growing up. They didn't have the same interests but I did feel closer to them as adults. We helped each other if needed, but we really didn't have much influence on each other.
- We are not close but we do maintain contact. I do feel closest to my sister because her husband is dying of cancer and needs help.

Overall, these high SES men tended to regard their mothers as more influential, focusing on religious training and personal relationships, whereas the fathers tended to focus on discipline and career achievement. Their views of siblings were mixed. Some, particularly the younger men, felt close to their siblings but did not provide help or influence. Some had a history of rivalry and conflict, but had drawn closer in later years. Others went on to lead independent lives. The younger men seemed to discriminate between particular siblings, feeling close to some and not to others. Most of these men had adult children and grandchildren but spoke little of them, except to say that they took pride in their children's accomplishments, felt close to them, and could rely on them for help if needed.

High SES White Women

Like the men, most of these women regarded their mothers as having the greatest influence. However, the women viewed their mothers as emphasizing a strict upbringing with adherence to rules, religious training, and training in household tasks. In some cases, the father seemed more compassionate and understanding, and had more influence in motivating them to go to school and achieve. For example,

- I was very close to my father as he was very understanding. My mother was more demanding.

- They both influenced me equally. Mother wanted me to be a nice Southern lady, and my father wanted me to do the right thing. Their influence on me was in different ways.
- My father was away on business during the week, but he came home on weekends and he was very hard on us. I didn't realize it at the time. You just took it for granted that he was like that. He was a cold person. My mother was more positive; she was wonderful.
- Both my parents had influence on me but my mother had the greatest influence. She made sure that I finished high school, and went to college to become a teacher.
- My dad had the most influence on me. He held me and hugged me and kissed me. My mother never did that.
- It was hard for my father to show affection while my mother was more of a confidant.

In some cases, circumstances of life altered the balance of parental influence:

- My mother died at 38 and my father at 65. Both had a big influence on my life. However, since my mother died so young, my father had the most influence.
- They both had much influence on me. However, I became closer to my father when my parent split during my high school years.
- My mother had the most influence on me. My father left the family when I was 12.

Most of these high SES women felt that there was a certain degree of sibling closeness, help, and influence, but it varied with the particular brother or sister involved. For example,

- My older siblings all went to college so I imitated them. My oldest sister was the one who taught me to play the piano. But I was closest to my youngest sister. We were not wealthy so we couldn't help each other in big ways . . . just little things.
- My brother and sister never helped me, but it's comforting just to know they were there; they did give me emotional support . . . a feeling of closeness.
- I didn't feel close to my brothers. I couldn't get any emotional

support from them. I do feel that I could ask them for help but I never did.

- We had more in common when growing up, and as we became older, we became even more close.
- I was closest to my older sister. She bossed me around but I did appreciate her more. However, I do miss all my siblings terribly. We always did things together. We never had any rivalry or fights with each other. We could expect help from each other and we did help each other. But they are all dead now.
- I always felt closer to my brother because he had a sense of adventure. I'm afraid that I followed him.
- I spend more time with my younger sister. Brothers and sisters satisfy different needs.
- My brother went to the university first. I didn't get any help from him. We developed along our own lines. When we were growing up, we did play and study together. He married later, and went his own way while I did graduate work. We kept in touch but he really had little influence on my life, and vice versa. Just a social relationship.
- I can depend upon my brother for help. If I ask him, he comes. He's always sending me presents about every six weeks. We used to get together often when I could drive.
- At one time I felt closer to my younger brother, then later I felt closer to the older one. But they didn't influence me much. However, I could have depended on them for help but I never did ask.
- We'd all help each other if needed. We're in frequent contact now and we do things together. My sisters played a big part in my life. I am close to them but I'm also different.
- We were fairly close growing up. We never fought or had bad feelings. We wrote each other every other week for years, and in later years, we always called each other every Saturday morning. We never asked each other for help most of the time. But, she had two hip operations and an operation for carotid artery, and at those times when she asked, "Can you come," I immediately dropped everything and went. And when I broke my wrist several years ago, she was here the next day to take care of me.

An opposite viewpoint was voiced by other participants:

- I didn't get along with or care for my siblings. They were too bossy, didn't show much affection, they lived a different lifestyle, and I could never depend upon them. I never asked them for help and never received any emotional support from them. We just don't have enough in common.
- I had some sibling rivalry with my sister. We irked each other but it never went too far.
- I realized when I had children of my own that my sister was jealous of me. Mother had centered on my sister when she was a baby. I don't think she ever outgrew it.
- I guess for a while I was jealous of my brother, but I got over it, and we got along all right. But my sister and brother really had sibling rivalry. They fought like cats and dogs. My sister was very aggressive. She scratched him bloody.
- As a child, my older sister did not want me there, she pushed my carriage off the porch. That rivalry lasted my whole life. But my younger and older sister were always close. I was always excluded . . . I couldn't depend on them for help.
- I was not influenced by them. I am the opposite of them. I don't think they would ever help me. I wish that we could have been closer. I feel regret and sadness, no indifference.

In regard to descending family, the adult children and grandchildren were the basic kin members that were close to the participants and could be depended upon for help, if needed. For example,

- If I need help, any of them would come running.
- We are very close, and we talk to each other on the phone. If I needed help, she would be right there to help. We are all close and all work together to help each other. It's a very supportive family.
- If I needed help, they would come. They are very devoted.
- I am very close to my family. I keep up my health with exercise and my religion, and they help give me my energy to enjoy my family.

- I get financial advice from my son and loving words of comfort from my daughter. I sometimes help them with money.
- I am close to the whole kit and kaboodle.
- My son constantly calls me. I'm amazed. My daughter calls me often, but she is in Florida. If I need anything, I just call one of them or one of my grandchildren.
- When I raised them I wanted to make sure that I was an important of their lives, but not to interfere. But I encourage their independence. You can love, and be close, but still be independent.

Another participant was unhappy with her children:

- They're not even working. I'm disgusted with them. My daughter is only two hours away but she can't give me help. Right now, I'm self sufficient but I don't know what happens later. That's what worries me.
- I have some difficulty with one daughter. She doesn't want to take me on errands when she comes to visit and that hurts me. But in general, I suppose I could depend on her if the chips were down.
- I'm not as close to my oldest son as I could be. I'm closest to my middle son. We understand each other. My daughter is more independent in temperament. The oldest son is very serious-minded. But they would all help if needed.

Overall, the relative influence of the mothers and fathers of the participants varied, depending on circumstances and personalities. Sometimes the mother showed greater affection and in other cases, it was the father. They were more able to talk about personal things with their mothers. Neither parent seemed concerned with achievement or occupational advancement in life.

As was the case with the high SES men, the women seemed to differ in feelings regarding siblings. Within the same family, there could be closeness to one sibling, rivalry with another, and indifference towards still another. In a large number of cases, the women felt close to all of the siblings. A great deal of variability existed regarding degree of sibling influence and helping.

With few exceptions, study participants felt close to adult children and grandchildren and felt that they could depend on them for help if needed.

Low SES White Women

The women varied in their judgments of which parent had the most influence; for some it was the mother, for others the father, but rarely did they have equal influence. For example,

- My mother left me when I was a very small child; she ran away. Mother put all three of us in a children's home. After a year, my father gave my oldest brother to a family in another town, and he took my youngest brother to the farm with him, and I was like Topsy. I just grew. I was shoved from pillar to post. I lived with an aunt for awhile and then a stranger. And until I was 14 years old, I didn't have a home. Then some people took me in and put me through high school. That was the first home I ever had. But still I felt close to my dad. He was all I had; I didn't really know my mother.
- My mother had a strong negative influence on me. She was a very cold person. My father would kiss me goodnight but I can't ever remember my mother doing it. My father was a warm, loving person. However, my mother and father were always fighting and I had to raise myself in many ways.
- Everyone had to mind my father. He was always extreme about everything.
- I was closer to my mother but neither of them had much influence on me.
- My mother had the most influence on me because she lived longer (father died at 34 and mother at 94), and because of her religious influence.
- Both influenced me. My mother taught me things like ladies never go without a hat and gloves when they go out. My father used to read stories to me all the time, e.g., Horatio Alger and adventure stories a lot.
- Mother had the greatest influence. Dad never paid much attention to us children.
- I didn't like my mother at all; she wouldn't take care of the younger children. They were taken away because of neglect. She was a horrible person. My stepfather left first, and I left at 16. I was glad that my siblings were taken away from her.
- My mother taught me about life.
- She was fun and we were also friends. I missed her tremendously

after she died. She taught me lots of things. Dad was more stern and more strict. Mom was Irish through and through. I had a good childhood.
- My mother taught me everything. I was closer to her.
- I always looked to my mother. If I asked father, he would send me to my mother.

Relationships with siblings were mixed. Some women had close relationships with siblings, whereas others had grown apart. Some had sibling rivalry early in life but there was a shift to closeness by adolescence. For example,

- I had three sisters and one brother. When we were children, I had a rivalry with my sister, but later on we got along well. After we became close, we didn't have any real rivalry or fighting. In fact there was no fighting among all my brothers and sisters. My parents would not allow it. We were close and could always ask each other for help and get it whether it was from brother or sister.
- I had two brothers; one died at 82 and the other at 55. But I didn't grow up with them so there was no feeling of being close, or helping each other . . . I think that if we had lived in a different time, a different atmosphere, we all would have had something great.
- I had one older sister who died at 54 years of age. I have a younger brother who is still living here in town. I was moderately close to my sister but not close to my living brother at all. I had helped him in the past, and when I asked for help, he wouldn't do anything for me.
- I am not really close to her. We had sibling rivalry when growing up. However, we did help each other in the past but I probably will never see her again.
- I have one sister who lives in California. I don't keep in touch; we are not close and have no influence on each other.
- We were all very close to each other; we helped each other when we could, and we had an influence on each other's lives.
- I'm the baby. I'm close to them as there are no rivalries. I have tried to imitate them in some ways so they do have an influence on me. We would help each other, but haven't had to.

- We got along all right growing up, but these younger sisters didn't influence me. Our relationships became less close over the years. They have not asked me for help. If they did ask, I'd help if I could. I have asked them for help, but they would not help me.
- My sister and I fought quite a bit; she thought she was grown up and I was a tagalong. We got pretty close when we were grown up. When we get together, once or twice a year, we talk mostly about our own children and what we're doing right now. I could depend on them for help, but I never asked, I did help my younger brother a time or two.

In regard to adult children, there were also mixed responses. Some women had adult children and grandchildren to whom they felt close and upon whom they could rely. Others had more difficult relationships, and in some cases they were estranged. For example:

- I'm extremely close to both of them and they would help me if I needed it.
- I have one son and three daughters living. I feel extremely close to all of them, but some of them live out of town and don't come back often. However, I feel very close to a son who is here in town. However, I can count on any of them for help, even the ones from out of town.
- I don't help or depend upon my daughter. I don't help because she is old enough to take care of herself.
- The youngest daughter would help, but you'd have to drag it out of her. I still love them all and I have taught them well about responsibility.

In summary, the family relationships of this group of low SES White women were notable for their diversity. There was variation in the degree of influence of each parent and on the extent of closeness to parents. Although the general trend was to feel close and influenced by at least some siblings, there were numerous exceptions. Many had lost touch and others had conflict-filled relationships. Most of the women felt close to their adult children and grandchildren and could depend on them for help. However, there were again exceptions as to how many of the adult children and/or grandchildren that they feel close to and can depend on for help. Many of their children and grandchildren were separated by distance, and were at best an occasional source of support.

Low SES African American Women

It was interesting to see if African American women from the lower socioeconomic status level showed any different patterns of family relationships from the White women. Let us begin with the women's relationships with their parents.

Whose influence predominated as well as the type of influence varied from family to family, but it was primarily concerned with everyday living rather than long range aspirations for education or occupational advancement. For example,

- Both of my parents influenced me. They influenced me to stay in church and to live a good life.
- My father influenced me the most. He trained me. He was a good father.
- My mother died at 97 and my father died at 90. But they both influenced me. Mother taught me how to sew. She also taught me to cook. She worked hard and I took care of the house. My father just loved me to death. He tried to teach me pride.
- They taught me right from wrong, to go to church, to go to school, and they taught me to help our neighbors and other things.
- My mother influenced me the most. Mother was around children all the time, and taught me how to love people, how to be a good woman, how to cook, keep house, and take care of children.
- My mother had a great deal of influence on me. My mother would say to me, "Baby, don't you be going out there and getting into trouble. You hold yourself like a lady, act like a lady, and if you see trouble coming, you leave."
- Even though my mother died in her 40s, she influenced me much more than my father. My mother was kind, good, patient, and understanding. She tried to teach me about life, and how to treat people the way that I wanted to be treated.

- My mother had the most influence. My father was never around. He deserted the family when I was a child.
- My mother had the most influence on me by her teaching and the life she lived. My father was a great person but he was busy making a living while he was always there to help my mother.
- Both of my parents influenced me. My father taught me to stand up for myself and my mother taught me to be a good wife and mother.
- Both my parents influenced me, especially in regard to church life. I was not allowed to play any games on Sunday.
- I felt close to my parents but they had little influence on me. I was really raised by aunts and uncles.
- I lost my mother when I was two years old. My father was in his 50s when he died. He didn't take much interest in children but he did influence me to some extent.

As for sibling relationships, many participants felt close to all their siblings but the siblings did not help or influence them in most cases. Even though many of their siblings are now dead, they still feel close to them. In some cases, there was a moderate degree of sibling rivalry and conflict. Often relationships changed as they grew older, sometimes improving and sometimes worsening. Examples of the variations in sibling relationships, both between and within families are as follows:

- I had three sisters and two brothers who are now all dead. When we got older, the relationship got better. But I never gave them help, because I wasn't able to. But I got no help from, and I couldn't depend on them.
- We squabbled among ourselves but no one else could touch us. When we grew up, we all went our separate ways. And then later, when we came together for reunions, we didn't fight any more. Then, when we would get together we talked about the squabbles we used to have and how senseless they were. Some have asked me for help in recent years and I gave it. But I never asked them for help. I guess because I thought the oldest should know better.
- They both are in town and I am extremely close to them. We do whatever we can to help each other but we don't influence each other much.

- I don't remember my older sister teaching me anything, and my older brother would boss me around. I do feel close to my younger brother who is still alive, we help each other and I'm somewhat influenced by him.
- I was very close to all of my brothers and sisters. Sometimes we squabbled when were coming up but it's not that way now. They didn't ask me for help but I asked them. They gave me financial support. But then I would help them if I was able.
- We had some rivalry when growing up but we changed. We get along well; we're close now. At this time of my life, I can depend on my brothers and sisters for help and they can depend on me. But we never ask each other for help. We do things together. We influence each other because we learn a lot from each other.
- My oldest brother had a great deal of influence on me. My brother would tell me to get up and try. If things don't work, then try something else. We were all close when growing up but we don't visit much now since mother died.
- My older sister kind of took me under her wing a little bit. I wasn't as outgoing as some of the others. We're all pretty close. I could depend on them for help if needed, but never needed to ask. When we get together we just enjoy one another.
- When we were young we used to fight but as we grew up, we developed a bond for each other. As grownups, we all helped each other. I cared for one of my brothers who had diabetes for almost two years, and I cared for another brother in a nursing home. Now I am helping my sister. But in the past, they helped me.
- I feel very close to them. We'd get along fine. But we never did help each other or influence each other.
- We did a lot of fighting until I got big enough to whip my older sister. Once I pushed her off the porch and that stopped her. Over the years, we became closer. I never asked for help. I could have, but I would never have heard the end of it. But I would help her. As for my brother, I couldn't depend on him. When I would ask for minor things, I never got them.

In regard to their children and grandchildren, some of the participants felt very close to their adult children but only a few could depend on them for more than limited help, if needed. For example,

- We all help each other out. I watch their house when they travel and they help me a lot in taking care of my house.
- I don't need money especially. My daughter here in town takes me to the doctor, gets my medicine, takes care of paying my bills. I can really count on her.
- My son would help if I asked him, but I never asked. He is always wanting money, money, money.
- I feel very close to both my sons. I am very close to my grand-children. But we all help each other, including me, my children and my grandchildren.
- I can depend on my daughter for help. My daughter has never been married and has no children. I miss grandchildren.
- I stayed with my older son in Carolina for two years after I had this stroke, and whenever I get ready to come there, he'll come and get me. I am not as close to the younger son. He goes on his merry way, but if I needed help from him, he'd be there. I give them help too, financially.
- I love my son, but he has so many problems. I could depend on all my children but that one. For example, my daughters came and stayed with me about two months last year when I had my surgery.

In summary, the low SES African American women displayed even more diversity in their family relationships than did the low SES White women. In addition to varying influence of mother and father, many were also influenced by grandmothers, aunts and uncles, and sometimes cousins (although this information is not presented here). Sibling relationships ranged from being very close to being estranged, often within the same family. Most of the participants felt close to their adult children and grandchildren, and they felt that they could depend upon them for help if needed. With some exceptions, most seemed to have a strong relationship with their adult children and a great sense of family; they felt that they could depend on at least some of their children for help. However, when families were separated by distance, it was not always clear how that help would become available.

Low SES African American Men

There were only a few African American men who participated in the study, but these few showed an extreme range of variation in their family relationships. For example, with regard to relationships to parents, the following statements offer a marked contrast:

- My father had just a little smoking and no vices, and he didn't encourage his children to have vices, and since we respected and loved him, we tried to do what he wanted us to do. Mother was gentle, never raised her voice, never hit any of us. She had a giving attitude which I think rubbed off on the children.
- My father didn't teach me a damn thing. He let me go do what I wanted to do, and when they [*his siblings*] told on me [*for doing something wrong*], he'd get mad.

Relationships with siblings also offered a contrast:

- They all influenced me by teaching me how to live. They taught me to live right and get along. We all helped each other but I depended on my younger brother the most.
- We never fought each other; instead we fought for each other. We are just as close now as we ever were. I can ask them for help and get it, and I do the same for them.
- When we get together, we talk about what I'm doing and what they're doing, and we talk about our life roles. I even visit some of their children. But they did not influence my own lifestyle.
- I'm not close at all. I hate the sons of bitches, the ones alive and the ones dead. I couldn't depend on them.

The pattern of either close or difficult, conflict-filled family relationships carried over to their relationships with adult children: For example,

- I feel real close; she is everything. If I need help, I go to her first; she is my salvation. My granddaughter cleans up for me every week and my grandson cuts the grass.
- I feel very close to all of them. After their mother died, the only one they have is me. I could count on them for help if I need it.

- I can't depend upon my son for any help, and there are no grand-children.
- It don't take long to make a baby, especially with different women. I don't feel close to any of them [*his 22 children*].

Global Rating of Family Support

The data presented thus far regarding the family relationships of study participants illustrates the point that having a large kin net-work by itself doesn't guarantee love, closeness, influence in devel-opment, or help in old age. Some families appeared to be extraordinarily close and caring, whereas others appeared to be either too limited in size, availability, resources, or closeness of feeling to function effectively to support the participant in old age. Indeed, some families appeared to be severely dysfunctional.

To try to capture this overall variation in family relationships, we rated each protocol on a 5-point scale. A rating of "5" was assigned when the participant had close family relationships with members in three generations (siblings, adult children, grand-children) of the family, with at least some members living nearby and acting as a source of immediate help if needed. A rating of "4" was assigned when there were close family relationships but only two generations of family were involved. A rating of "3" was assigned when there was a close relationship with only one or two family members, not necessarily living locally, and with other family non-existent or having drifted away. A rating of "2" was assigned when there was some conflict or estrangement within the family involv-ing siblings or adult children. Finally, a rating of "1" was assigned when the participant had severely dysfunctional relationships with family members, or when the participant had no family to count on. (Two raters judged all protocols independently, with an inter-rater reliability of .80.) As might be expected, the global support rating was significantly correlated with the quantitative measures of numbers of siblings and adult children and feelings of closeness to them.

The frequencies of the global support ratings of participants was as follows: 14% had a rating of "5" indicating a highly functional family system, 20% had a rating of "4," 34% had a raging of "3,"

20% had a rating of "2," and 12% had a rating of "1" indicating a highly dysfunctional family system. The global support rating was unrelated to gender or to SES/ethnic group membership, although it was related to age. It appeared that the oldest participants had the least viable family supports, not surprising given their greater loss of family members through death.

Summary

A goal of this portion of the chapter was to gain some understanding of the structure of the existing families of the older adults who participated in the study, and to explore the nature of these family relationships for men and women in the three SES/ethnic subgroups. It was felt that this undertaking would provide insights into family variables that might be related to personal meanings of death, death fears, and views of the dying process.

Most of the older adults we studied had positive relationships with family members, although the loss of siblings through death seemed to leave feelings of incompleteness. Most felt close to their adult children and either received help from them at present or felt that they could call upon them if needed. For many, the emotional support of their children seemed to be a lifeline into the outer world. However, help was a two-way street, as many older parents were still helping their adult children (and grandchildren) in some way.

Siblings seem to have a greater impact on the participant than expected, although the results were mixed and did depend on the particular sibling involved, that is, the age and gender of the sibling, the degree of interaction with that siblng, and the circumstances of their lives. Close relationships with siblings, when they existed, were much valued for the emotional support they provided. There was little sibling rivalry evident in these older adults. Whatever rivalry existed had occurred in earlier in life and had either been resolved or had led to conflict and estrangement in some cases. These elders felt that they would give help to siblings if asked, and would receive help from siblings if needed. But in most cases, they neither gave help nor asked for it.

THE PRESENT STUDY: RELATIONSHIP OF
FAMILY TO VIEWS OF DEATH

Quantitative Analysis

The set of family structure and family relationship variables described earlier in this chapter were correlated with the measures of death meanings, fear of death, and expectations about the dying process measures. These correlations are presented in Tables 8.2, 8.3, and 8.4.

Death Meanings

Only a few of the correlations of the family variables with the older adults' death meanings were significant (albeit rather weak), but

TABLE 8.2 Correlations of Personal Meanings of Death With Selected Family Variables

| Family Variable | Personal Death Meanings | | | |
	Afterlife	Motivator	Legacy	Extinction
Marital status	.00	−.07	.13	−.05
Total number of siblings	.09	−.00	.03	−.03
Number of living siblings	.04	.10	.11	−.04
Number of dead siblings	.10	−.11	−.05	−.04
Proportion of dead siblings	.11	.00	.12	.10
Mean closeness to living siblings	.24*	.17	.16	−.06
Total number of children	−.16	.06	−.00	.07
Number of living children	−.21*	.05	−.01	.10
Number of dead children	.10	−.11	−.05	.04
Proportion of dead children	.14	−.08	−.05	−.23*
Mean closeness to living children	.10	.08	.25*	.08
Global rating of family system	−.02	.21*	.15	.07

* $p < .05$; ** $p < .05$

**TABLE 8.3 Correlations of Fears of Death With Selected
Family Variables**

| Family Variable | Fear of Death | | | |
	Dying Process	Being Destroyed	Significant Others	Unknown
Marital Status	−.14	.14	−.04	−.02
Total number of siblings	−.04	.27**	.07	.15
Number of living siblings	.14	.06	.10	.23*
Number of dead siblings	−.10	.33*	−.02	−.16
Proportion of dead siblings	−.21*	.31**	.04	−.07
Mean closeness to living siblings	−.06	.08	.31*	−.09
Total number of children	−.05	.06	.09	.06
Number of living children	−.04	.03	.07	.05
Number of dead children	−.08	.21*	.31*	−.09
Proportion of dead children	−.05	.26**	.04	−.01
Mean closeness to living children	−.07	−.07	.21*	−.16
Global rating of family system	.09	−.10	.14	.01

* $p < .05$; ** $p < .01$

they formed an interesting pattern. Those elders who had fewer
living children and who felt closer to their siblings were more likely
to view death as meaning afterlife. In a similar way, those with a
higher proportion of deceased children were less likely to view
death as extinction. That is, those who have experienced the death
of their loved children were less likely to feel that death was the
end of everything.

TABLE 8.4 Correlations of Views of the Dying Process With Selected Family Variables

Family Variable	Views of the Dying Process				
	Emotion	Survival	Coping	Family	Rancor
Marital Status	−.12	−.08	−.04	−.39**	−.05
Total number of siblings	.04	.01	.13	−.07	−.01
Number of living siblings	−.00	−.00	.19*	.01	.08
Number of dead siblings	.10	.01	−.03	−.16	−.11
Proportion of dead siblings	.01	.07	−.00	−.15	−.21*
Mean closeness to living siblings	.03	.12	−.00	.21*	−.29*
Total number of children	.14	.02	−.08	−.04	.49**
Number of living children	.15	.06	−.06	−.02	.45**
Number of dead children	−.10	−.20*	−.16	−.11	−.06
Proportion of dead children	−.14	−.17	−.16	−.13	−.13
Mean closeness to living children	−.22*	−.12	.10	.09	−.42**
Global rating of family system	.01	−.05	.13	.17	−.00

* $p < .05$; ** $p < .01$

Those elders who were rated as having a more effective family support system tended to view death as a motivator to fulfill certain goals before death, and those who felt closer to their children were more likely to view death as an opportunity to leave a legacy.

Fear of Death

In looking at the correlations of the family variables with fear of death, several correlations are of interest. Those elders with a higher proportion of dead siblings tend to have less fear of the dying process. We can speculate that this is another instance of the "pioneering" function of siblings often observed in sibling studies of children and adolescents (Cicirelli, 1995c), where other siblings will more readily follow in an activity after one sibling has done it (whether it is a positive activity such as going on to college or a negative activity such as smoking). With regard to dying, once an elder's sibling(s) have gone through the dying process, it may be perceived as less fearsome. The finding that fear of the unknown is greater the more living siblings an elder has can be regarded as another instance of the same phenomenon.

Fear of bodily destruction after death was related to a number of family measures, with this fear greater among those who had more siblings in the family, more dead siblings, a higher proportion of dead siblings, more dead children, and a higher proportion of dead children. It would seem that an elder's greater experience with the deaths of close family members sensitized them to aspects of bodily destruction after death and led to greater fear.

Finally, greater fear for significant others (either the effects of one's own death on loved ones or the effects of the deaths of loved ones on oneself) was related to elders' greater closeness of feelings toward their living siblings and adult children, as well as to the number of deceased children they have. It is not surprising that the closer one feels to family members, the more one might fear the sense of loss and sorrow that one's own death or the death of a loved one might bring. This fear would be felt more keenly by those who have already experienced the deaths of their children; they know what a sense of devastation the loss of a child can bring.

Views of the Dying Process

As was the case with death meanings, there were relatively few significant correlations with the measures of elders' views of the dying process, but they also form an interesting pattern. Those who felt closer to their living children expected to feel less negative emotions (such as loneliness, sadness, depression, and helpless) during the dying process; they also expected less feelings of rancor (such as anger or bitterness). Those who felt closer to their living siblings and had a smaller proportion of deceased siblings also expected less feelings of rancor. However, those elders who had a larger number of children and a larger number of living children expected greater feelings of rancor. It is possible that simply having more children, if one does not feel particularly close to them, can lead to feelings of anger and bitterness over one's failure to achieve close and satisfying relationships with them in life.

Having more deceased children was associated with fewer expectations of concern with one's physical survival during the dying process. It's as if those elders who had outlived their children felt that there was little left to stay alive for.

Those older adults who had more living siblings also expected to have more concerns about coping with the dying process (gaining control over their dying in some way). That is, the more siblings they still have, the more concerned they are about being able to deal with events during the dying process.

Finally, those elders who were still married and those who felt closer to their living siblings expected to have more thoughts and concerns about family during the dying process. It appears that having stronger ties to those family members in one's own generation means that thoughts and feelings about family are expected to be prominent during the dying process.

Summary

The quantitative analysis carried out was limited but nevertheless interesting in that it indicated the effects that family relationships can have on the way that older adults think about various aspects of death and dying. Those who had closer family relationships viewed approaching death as a motivation to carry out further activities in their remaining life with their families; additionally, those who felt closer to their children viewed death as an opportunity to leave a legacy. Overall, those participants who felt closer to their families perhaps perceived limited time left in life to carry out meaningful activities with them and for their benefit in the future. Those who had closer relationships with their remaining siblings and who had fewer living children (also a greater proportion of children who were dead) looked at death more in terms of an afterlife and not as extinction.

The older adults' fear of the dying process and fear of being destroyed appeared to be related to the losses of siblings and children that they have suffered in their lives, whereas the fear for significant others was related to their feelings of closeness to those siblings and adult children who are still living. These death fears make sense if the participants are sensitive to the possible loss of their remaining family members.

Finally, the closer the elders felt toward their siblings and adult children, the fewer negative feelings (e.g., anger and bitterness) they expected to feel when dying. Those closer to their living children also expected to feel less emotions such as sadness and depression. It would seem that having close relationships with family somehow would allow these elders to go through the dying process with greater peace of mind. In any event, relationships with family do seem to influence the ways that older adults look at death.

Qualitative Analysis

The qualitative portion of the interview dealing with family was quite limited, in that we sought elders' views only in relation to one central question: What will your death mean to your family? If we could carry out the interviews again, we would surely include other topics as well. Nevertheless, we will consider participants' responses to the question we did ask, again looking at the various subgroups in turn.

High SES White Men

Many of these men viewed what their death would mean in terms of a legacy, that is, how well they were able to provide for their family members after death. For example,

- I have two sons and six grandchildren. They know it's coming, I've discussed it with them. They know that financially I've set things up for them as best I can. I think they'll accept my death with pride. I think they have pride in the kind of father and grandfather I've been. And I think that's the attitude they'll take.

- I think that my family know that in a number of ways I have prepared for my death and to some extent to die. I have a health care power of attorney, insurance to provide for care during the dying process, and so on. I'd like to think that my family will miss me to some extent . . . I don't think there will be wild celebrations that I'm going to leave them a humongous estate. I'm not. As far as I know, they will have a philosophical view of my demise which will be in harmony with my own views.
- I'm pretty well off and I have my affairs in pretty good order. I've given a lot of stuff to my children, they will get more. Most don't need it; one daughter who needs it is a profligate spender so she won't have it for long when she gets it . . . I always looked at death in the same way before I ever had a family.

Others spoke in terms of the memories their family members would have of them and that they expected to be missed, at least for awhile:

- I hope they will be kind and think of some of the good things I have done. Family would have remembrances of things past. My daughter was with me when my wife died, and we have been pretty close ever since.
- They'll miss their father, grandfather, companion. I think I'll remain in people's memory for awhile.
- I think they will miss me. I figure I will miss them. I think they will all feel deeply.
- They will mourn. [*He became overcome with emotion at this point.*] My children have become more important to me since my wife died.
- I think my family will feel badly that I have died. But I don't think they will mourn my death for too long. I hope they feel that I have lived a good life.
- I'm gone. They'd probably miss me for awhile, and then they'd probably go on with their lives.

High SES White Women

In contrast to the men, only a few of the women viewed their deaths in terms of a legacy for their family members. When they did, they spoke of the transmission of ideals, values, and family history rather than a material legacy. For example:

- I think they [*grandchildren*] are going to realize what Grandma tried to do for them. They ask me so many questions because they realize that I'm the only one who knows these things. I would like to make a tape like this, all about their mother who died. Let them know the foundations of our family and the principles we had.
- I have a sense that I will be missed. I am very close to my grandchildren, and I have three great-grandchildren. But the grandchildren are very affectionate and I think I would be missed. My own illness taught me to value life. I want to be an example to my children of the way to live.
- I think that we have prepared our sons to accept life's changes. They've seen grandparents die and they've seen that we accepted that and took care of the remaining grandparent. I think they will do the same for us and continue to live. I hope that we have cleared up any misunderstandings they may have had with us and they have no guilt. I think they will accept our death with dignity.
- I suppose they will feel sad about me. I hope that I will be able to leave them something, something that will help them live better.

A few women felt that family members would feel their loss keenly when they died:

- I think my girls are going to cry. They are going to lose a great friend and supporter.
- I think they are going to be sorrowful. We have a pretty close-knit family. At the age I am now, I think my family will feel very badly.
- It will be hard on my two sons.
- I think they are going to have an empty place. You can't love somebody and not have that as a result.

The majority of the women felt that they would be missed, but took a realistic, philosophical position that the initial grieving would pass and that family members would be able to get on with their lives. They felt that family members would have some pleasant memories of them, but didn't want them to mourn for any length of time. For example:

- I feel that I'm appreciated. I hope that they would remember me kindly for whatever contribution I made to their lives. I wouldn't want them to grieve. I have one child who would, more than the others. I wouldn't want anyone to be sad when I'm gone. When you're gone, you're gone.
- With older family members it will be a "well, at least she didn't have to suffer" kind of thing. With my kids, it will be a loss because I've been a stronger influence on them . . . I think most people come to a realization shortly after someone has died that they are gone and life will go on. Not that you don't think about them, but unless you want to be morbid, you don't dwell on it.
- I think they'll all miss me for awhile, but they'll get used to it. And they may think of the fun we had together. But they'll get over it eventually.
- They'll miss me, but I don't think they're going to be too tragic. I think somebody else will take my place.
- I would think they would miss me, but I don't think they will grieve. I've asked them not to. I've had a good life, satisfactory in every way.
- They will be sad for awhile. I'm their mother and grandmother. I have input in their lives. But they're grown up now. They will remember me.

Only a few felt that their death would be a relief to their families or that they wouldn't be missed:

- They'll probably be happy that I don't have to suffer any more. That's the way I feel about other people.
- Probably a relief to the family. I don't have any regrets about the way I've lived.
- My son will be glad to have my estate.
- I'm a survivor. There's nobody left in the family. I've outlived them all.
- I have only my brother's children left. My death would not have any major impact.

Low SES White Women

Like the high SES White women, these women responded in diverse ways to the question of what their death would mean to their families. However, only two women suggested a kind of personal legacy for their children:

- My prayer is that my life will be a testimony to my children and my family. It will be a loss to my children.
- I feel like my death will have a very telling effect on my children, because I've tried to be involved in their lives. And I'm a springboard for a lot of their questioning [*about family history*] and I do a lot of research for them.

Some of the women felt that their passing would be a great loss for their families:

- I'm very close to my family and I think they'll miss me terribly.
- My family will feel a big loss.

Like the high SES women, the majority of the low SES group took a more realistic, philosophical view of what their death would mean. For example:

- They will feel the loss, but they are not going to be all broken up because they'll say she lived a good full life. We wish we had her a little longer, but God decided to take her now.
- I think that they would mourn, but death is one of the facts of life. You just accept this.
- I think they'll say she had a beautiful life. There won't be any resentment that I was taken too young when I die, as there was when my son died.
- They will be sad for a couple of days. My family is very realistic. When we lost my mom, dad, brother (all very close to me), grief comes and then it goes.

Finally, some of the women expressed mixed messages about what death would mean to their families. In some cases, they felt that some close family members would care and others wouldn't.

In other cases, they contradicted themselves about how much a family member would care. For example,

- To some, it won't make too much difference. Although my daughter tells me it's been proven to me which ones really care. . . . As for my daughter, it will break her heart, but she knows that day will come.
- Oh, thank God I've got some money. They won't miss *me* a whole lot. My death won't mean much to any of them, except for my son. We love each other, but it's not that kind of close. He's got his life and I've got mine.
- My adopted children will miss me and hate to see me go, but I don't think anyone else really cares.
- A big loss, especially since their father has nothing to do with them. I'm the only one they have. They might miss me for an hour, but that would be it.
- I think that my son would be devastated. But I have a daughter that I have no contact with since my husband died . . . she also closed contact with the grandchildren

Low SES African American Women

This group of African American women produced a greater variety of responses to the question of how their death would affect family members than any of the other groups. Only one women spoke in terms of a legacy, and even then it was unclear whether these items were things that she wanted to give or were things that her family members were eager to take possession of after her death:

- One daughter wants my crystal collection, another wants my organ, another wants my bedroom suite, another wants to live in my house. Other than that, they'll miss me.

Some other women felt that their family members would miss them for the particular roles they filled in the family:

- Well, it will be hurtful to them [*granddaughters*] because when they go out of town or go places, they leave their kids with me.

- I know that because I have helped them through so many things, they'd feel that my death would mean that I wouldn't be there for them.
- They are going to miss me in a lot of ways, me being around and helping them and encouraging them to do this and that.
- They are really going to miss me because we have five generations in our family and I'm the last girl.

Some of the women felt that their family members wouldn't mourn their deaths because the family knew that they would be with God, or that it would be only a short while before they would meet again. For example,

- They'll miss me and miss my love, but they'll be happy for me because they'll know where I'm going.
- I'd tell them, don't worry because I'm going to a place where I'll be well taken care of.
- They'll miss me, but not too long, because I'll only be gone for awhile.

Others felt that their death would be difficult for their family members to deal with:

- I think they'd take it hard. If I'm sick they just collapse, you know.
- I know my children will be very unhappy . . . my grandkids will be upset.
- My daughter will probably take it really hard.
- It will be very upsetting, because there aren't that many of us.

The majority of the women in this group felt that their families would be sad and miss them, but many took a more philosophical view. For example:

- My family loves me so much and I love them very much. It will be hard to leave them here. But I know they will get through the loss because this day will come for everybody. Time will heal everything.

- They'll be sad and miss me, but they'd get over it. Time heals all wounds. In time, even my children would get over it.
- I think they would be upset for awhile, but then they would adjust.
- I tell them to accept it. We've all got to die, so accept what you can't change.
- Well, everybody will accept it, except my younger son. He's too attached to me. I'm trying to remove myself from him a little bit.

Finally, one woman felt that there would be a mixed reaction to her death, and a few others felt that no one would care:

- I really don't know if they'd care. Some would, some wouldn't.
- If I die, I die. That's it.
- They'll probably just keep going.
- Nothing! Just another person passing on.
- Well, the way children are nowadays, I think some of them would be glad if I would go and get out of their way.

Low SES African American Men

Only two of the African American men in this group responded to this question and they represented two extremes. One felt that the example of his life would be a legacy that his children could profit from, and the other felt that no one would care when he died:

- I think that they will miss me, but I believe it will help them if they follow in some of the things that I did and didn't do.
- Nothing! Hell no, they won't feel sorry.

Summary

The qualitative data from interviews revealed that some older adults who had considerable family support felt that family members would be greatly upset by their deaths and their loss would be difficult to overcome, whereas others felt that their family would miss them but take their passing in stride as an inevitable part of life. Some who had weak or nonexistent family ties felt that family would not care about their deaths or care only about a potential inheritance. Although there were a few individuals in every subgroup, the idea of leaving some kind of legacy for one's children was a response that was found mainly among the men and women of high SES. However, men seemed to view a legacy in terms of money or tangible goods, whereas women viewed it in terms of the transmission of family history and values. The majority of the elders took a philosophical approach to what their death would mean to their families, seeing death as universal and natural and grief as something that would pass as family members adjusted to the death. Most expected to be missed in some way. Among the low SES Whites and African Americans, there were a number of elders who felt that their families really wouldn't care if they died, or that some would miss them and some wouldn't.

CONCLUSIONS

How can one reach some conclusions about the influence of family on older adults' views of death, based on the limited kinds of information we gathered in our interviews? Obviously, full understanding of family influence is impossible at this point in time. However, some conclusions are possible.

The descriptive information about the structural characteristics of these older families revealed that most of the elders still have living family members, although many had lost family members to death, and most felt quite close to these family members. Two aspects of the family, the proportion of deceased family members and feelings of closeness to living family members seemed to be most consistently related to the elders' views of death.

According to Carstensen's (1995) socioemotional selectivity theory, adults tend to limit their social interactions to those relationships that are most rewarding emotionally and the latter occur with people who are familiar and also similar to them. For older adults, these are usually long-term friends and family members. Lang's (2000) recent longitudinal study indicates that such closeness to family is maintained until very late in life, even up through the trajectory of decline prior to death. This reveals how intensely committed older adults are to maintaining these relationships. When members of this close circle die, it represents a great loss to the older adult, particularly because they cannot be replaced. If this is true, then it should follow that older adults who have lost close family members would be more likely to view death as leading to an afterlife rather than extinction because reunion in an afterlife would provide them with an opportunity to renew or maintain the relationships that provide the greatest emotional satisfaction. Loss of a child could be regarded in the same way. The conceptualization of death as involving an afterlife offers the older adult the possibility of regaining the relationships that are most rewarding emotionally. This was partially supported in our study as those older adults with the greatest loss of children were less likely to view death as meaning extinction. The loss of other family members, such as siblings, would also fit such an explanation. Moss and Moss (1989) have noted the great sense of loss felt by many older adults when a sibling has died leading to a sense of existential incompleteness, that is, that the family group is no longer intact. There is a desire to overcome the loss and regain the relationship with siblings. The above hypothesis concerning death as meaning an afterlife in which to renew relationships with either children or siblings certainly needs further testing.

Loss of siblings was related to less fear of the dying process, which we attributed earlier to the pioneering function of siblings. After all, if one's brother or sister has died peacefully (that is, with little or no suffering), there may be little fear for oneself. But in regard to elders' expectations regarding the dying process, both the proportion of dead siblings and the feelings of closeness to living siblings (as well as closeness to living children) were related to fewer rancorous feelings. It would seem that different processes would need to be used to explain such results. If sibling death leads to a less negative view of dying and less fear through a combination of sibling pioneering and greater acceptance of death as afterlife, then one might expect fewer feelings of rancor. From a different perspective, having siblings and adult children to whom one feels close can lead to a general sense of well-being. This kind of emotional support from family could produce expectations of fewer negative feelings during the dying process.

It is surprising that, in the qualitative portion of the study concerned with expected effects of participants' deaths on their families, there was no explicit mention of siblings even though children and grandchildren were mentioned with great frequency. Inasmuch as Moss and Moss (1989) concluded that a substantial portion of elders are greatly affected by a sibling's death, it is puzzling why none of the elders of our study expected that their own death would be mourned by their remaining siblings. The possibility that the older adults may have felt closer to their children than to their siblings does not seem to be an adequate explanation, because the average feeling of closeness to siblings was not greatly lower than the average feeling of closeness to adult children.

Similarly, only a few adults (mainly the low SES African American women) mentioned God and afterlife as a possible reason why they did not expect their loved ones to be upset by their deaths. Given their strong religious faith (see Chapter 6), we might have expected more of these elders to suggest that religious faith could help family members deal with death.

In examining the qualitative interview data on family relationships, one is struck by the way in which dysfunctional family patterns are repeated in certain elders' reports of their relationships with their parents, their siblings, their adult children, and even their grandchildren. These more difficult family relationships were reflected not only in the expectations that family would be little affected by their deaths (or even be glad when they were gone), but also in their meanings, fears of death, and their views of the dying process. At the other end of the spectrum, those elders with the support of close relationships with family are not only able to view death more positively but seem to be motivated to pursue activities during their remaining years for the benefit of their families both before and after their deaths.

9

Death Meanings, Death Fears, and the Dying Process: Some Interrelationships

In earlier chapters, we have examined older adults' death meanings, fears of death, and views of the dying process from both a quantitative and qualitative perspective. We have seen how their views of death varied depending on such demographic background variables as age, gender, marital status, socioeconomic status level, and ethnicity. Also, we have seen how health, religiosity, and family relationships influenced elders' views of death. In these earlier chapters, however, each of these variables was examined separately in order to pay attention to the complexities of the quantitative and qualitative data. In the present chapter, we attempt to bring together the separate threads examined in the preceding chapters to gain a more integrated picture.

One question addressed in the chapter is the extent to which older adults' death meanings, fears of death, and expectations of the dying process are interrelated. Second, inasmuch as cognitive meanings precede emotional reactions, the question is how well older adults' fears of death can be predicted from their death meanings, religious beliefs, family relationships, and health status, along with sociodemographic variables. (Insufficiently established measures of elders' views and expectations about the dying process made it unfeasible to attempt to include them in a multivariate analysis, although some univariate correlations are presented.)

EXISTING STUDIES

Only a few studies thus far have attempted to determine the relationship between various death meanings and fears of death, and those studies that have done so have included only a limited number of variables.

A number of earlier studies reported that those who had the strongest conceptions of death as meaning an afterlife had less fear of death (e.g., Leming, 1979–1980; Pollak, 1979–1980). However, such studies typically considered religiosity to be an indicator of the conceptualization of death as afterlife, thereby confounding this death meaning with religiosity (see Chapter 6). Thus, these studies do not seem to provide an accurate indication of the relationship between the conceptualization of death as afterlife and fear of death. More careful measures of both concepts have enabled more recent researchers to disentangle their effects at least to some degree.

The approach used by Holcomb, Neimeyer, and Moore (1993) to the study of death meanings was to use content coding of respondent's free-response narratives concerning death. By so doing, they identified some 25 death meanings classified into 14 categories (purposefulness of death, negative emotional evaluation, understanding of death, personal involvement, existence, nonexistence, choice, and so on) that were used as a basis for coding death meanings in their further studies. In a study of 504 university students ranging in age from 17 to 64, Holcomb and colleagues correlated students' frequency of use of these categories with their fear of death scores on the MFODS. Among their findings was a relationship between death as meaning continued existence (i.e., some kind of afterlife) and fear of death. That is, the more frequently that death meaning continued existence occurred in their narratives, the less their overall fear of death (total score on the MFODS). More specifically, death as meaning nonexistence, seeing death as purposeless, and seeing death without understanding were related to greater Fear of the Unknown. (Additionally, negative emotional states about death were related to Fear of Being Destroyed and Fear for Significant Others.)

Cicirelli (1998b) constructed an instrument to assess four dimensions of personal death meanings (see Chapter 3). In a sample of 265 university students aged 19–55, these death meanings were related to the eight subscores of the Leming Fear of Death Scale in multiple regression analyses (Leming & Dickinson, 1985). Death as meaning extinction predicted greater fear on seven of the eight subscores on the Leming Measure, with the strongest regression coefficients found in the analyses for fear of isolation, fear of the finality of death, and fear of afterlife concerns. Death as meaning afterlife predicted four subscores, and death as meaning legacy predicted two subscores. Age and gender were also included in these analyses; being younger was associated with greater fear of death on 4 of the 8 subscores (including fear of afterlife concerns, fear of the finality of death, and fear of isolation), whereas being female was associated only with fear of dependency.

A subset of the sample used in the above study was also assessed on the MFODS (Cicirelli, 2001b). In correlational analysis for this group, death as meaning afterlife was related to less Fear of the Unknown and death as meaning extinction was related to greater Fear of the Unknown. Afterlife was also related to less Fear of Being Destroyed and less Fear for Significant Others. Finally, Fear of the Dying Process was greater for those with conceptions of death as meaning extinction and legacy.

The Tomer and Eliason (2000a) structural model of death anxiety has been discussed in an earlier chapters as an example of an attempt to construct a comprehensive theoretical model linking various predictors of death anxiety. These researchers tested their model with samples of young college students and older adults aged 55 and over (Tomer & Eliason, 2000b), using a measure of fear of nonbeing derived from the Revised Death Anxiety Scale (Thorson & Powell, 1994) as the ultimate dependent variable in their hypothesized causal chain. The direct predictors of the fear of nonbeing among older adults included neutral acceptance scale of the Death Attitude Profile—Revised (Wong, Reker, & Gesser,

1994), locus of control (internality, chance, and powerful others, using the multidimensional scale developed by Levenson 1981), meaningfulness of one's life (a feeling that life is worth living), manageability (living the life that one wants), and death salience (the frequency of thinking about circumstances surrounding one's death). Higher scores on neutral acceptance and meaningfulness of one's life were related to less fear of nonbeing, and higher scores on locus of control (regardless of subscale), manageability, and death salience were related to greater fear of nonbeing. Other variables in the causal model had indirect effects on fear of nonbeing, including comprehensibility (a belief that one understands his or her life), religious devotion, and education. Death salience and certain locus of control subscores also had indirect effects. The path model for young adults was quite similar in most respects. (Gender was not included in the path model, although it was correlated with religious devotion and death salience.) It is important to note that Tomer and Eliason did not consider death meanings in their model, but rather beliefs in the meanfulness, manageability, and coherence of one's life.

Cicirelli (1999) also used a path analysis approach to study predictors of Fear of the Dying Process and Fear of the Unknown (as measured by the MFODS) in a sample of 388 older adults aged 60 to 100. Possible predictors included in the model were the externality measure (a combination of the chance and powerful others subscales from Levenson's 1981 locus of control measure), perceived social support, a measure of intrinsic religiosity, ethnicity (White and African American), gender, SES, and age. In the path diagram for Fear of the Dying Process, those with a more external locus of control and women had a greater Fear of the Dying Process, whereas those who had greater religiosity, were older, or were African American, had less Fear of the Dying Process. In indirect effects, those who were older and of lower SES had higher externality, and women and African Americans had greater religiosity. The path diagram for Fear of the Unknown differed in that externality, social support, and religiosity were the only predictors with a direct effect on the fear measure. That is, greater Fear of the Unknown was related to greater externality, less social support, and less religiosity. Age, SES, gender, and ethnicity all had indirect effects. Specifically, those who were older and who had lower SES had a more external locus of control; those who were older, who had lower SES and who were men had less social support; and those who were women and African American had greater religiosity. It is of interest that the factors in the model for Fear of the Unknown were stronger predictors (explaining 28% of the variance) than the variables predicting Fear of the Dying Process (explaining only 14% of the variance). Fear of the Unknown was more influenced by psychosocial factors, whereas Fear of the Dying Process was influenced by both psychosocial and demographic factors.

These existing studies (Cicirelli, 1998b, 2001b; Holcomb et al., 1993; Tomer & Eliason, 2000b) are difficult to compare, because they have not only used different measures of fear of death but have also tended to use different predictor variables. However, some commonalities between the findings are apparent. Death as meaning an afterlife (or some form of continued existence) was related to less fear of death, while death as meaning extinction, nonexistence, or purposelessness was related to a greater number of death fears, especially Fear of the Unknown.

QUANTITATIVE STUDY: INTERRELATIONSHIPS

Interrelationships Between Death Meanings, Fear of Death, and Views of the Dying Process

As a first step in examining the interrelationships between the variables assessed in our empirical study of the death views of older adults, correlations between the three main groups of variables (death meanings, fear of death, and views of the dying process) were computed. These correlations are found in Tables 9.1 and 9.2.

Relation of Death Meanings to Fear of Death

Looking first at how elders' death meanings may have influenced their fears of death (Table 9.1), those who saw death as meaning an afterlife had less Fear of the Unknown, but a greater Fear of Being Destroyed. Those who saw death as meaning extinction had

TABLE 9.1 Correlations of Death Meanings With Fear of Death and Views of the Dying Process

Variable	Death Meanings			
	Afterlife	Motivator	Legacy	Extinction
Fear of Death				
Dying process	–.07	.21*	–.02	.24*
Being destroyed	.22*	.01	.13	–.04
Significant others	–.02	.32**	.17	.25**
The unknown	–.32**	–.05	.13	.33**
Dying Process				
Emotions	–.16	.21*	.05	.21*
Physical survival	–.03	.27**	.11	.31**
Coping with dying	.21*	.30**	.25*	.02
Family	.00	.35**	.08	.12
Rancor	–.50**	–.16	–.11	.21*

* $p < .05$; ** $p < .01$

greater Fear of the Unknown, Fear for Significant Others, and Fear of the Dying Process. These two death meanings are concerned with what may or may not happen after death, with afterlife implying some kind of noncorporeal continuation after death and extinction implying that both physical life and conscious or spiritual life end at death. It is to be expected that those who feel that death means afterlife would feel less fear of death than those who do not share this death meaning. On the other hand, the situation regarding extinction is somewhat puzzling. If one truly feels that death means one's complete end as an individual, why should one fear something unknown that may exist beyond death when death means an absolute end with nothing beyond? This seems illogical. However, some of the items on the MFODS Fear of the Unknown subscales express an uncertainty regarding a possible afterlife; individuals who feel that death means the end of everything may nevertheless feel some degree of uncertainty about their viewpoint.

Those elders who saw death as meaning extinction tended to have a greater Fear of the Dying Process and Fear for Significant Others, whereas those who saw death as meaning afterlife did not manifest these increased fears. It may be the case that belief in an

TABLE 9.2 Correlations of Fear of Death With Views of the Dying Process

Variable	Fear of Death			
	Dying Process	Being Destroyed	Significant Others	The Unknown
Dying Process				
Emotions	.49**	.03	.27**	.21*
Physical survival	.29**	.12	.21*	.12
Coping with dying	.14	.18	.08	.12
Family	.38**	−.16	.39**	.04
Rancor	.11	−.29**	.05	.21*

* $p < .05$; ** $p < .01$

afterlife helps elders to develop an attitude of acceptance of death so that events surrounding the end of life (such as the dying process itself and the loss of loved ones) do not seem as fearful. Belief in an afterlife also promises a reunion with loved ones who have gone before or who will come after. The puzzle still remains why those who see death as afterlife had greater Fear of Being Destroyed. As yet this is unexplained.

Viewing death as meaning an opportunity for legacy was unrelated to any of the four fear of death subscores. Finally, those elders who viewed death as a motivator had greater Fear for Significant Others and Fear of the Dying Process. Both of these death meanings are concerned with activities before death rather than what may take place after death. Establishing some kind of legacy for the time when one is gone is regarded as important from several theoretical perspectives (see Chapter 4) as a form of generativity allowing one to achieve a symbolic immortality by leaving something of oneself for the living and for future generations. One might expect seeing death as an opportunity for legacy to be related to less fear of death. The fact that this was not the case for study participants may be related to the fact that few expressed any concern about a legacy of some sort in the qualitative portion of the study.

Relation of Death Meanings to Views of the Dying Process

As is evident from the correlations displayed in Table 9.1, one's death meanings are indeed related to views of the dying process. Seeing death as afterlife is related to increased concerns about coping with the dying process, but fewer expectations of rancorous feelings. In contrast, seeing death as extinction is related to expectations of greater emotionality in the dying process (both feelings of sadness and depression and feelings of rancor) and to increased concerns about physical survival. Seeing death as meaning an opportunity for legacy is related to concerns about coping with the dying process. Finally, seeing death as a motivator is related to increased expectations of concerns about physical survival, coping with dying, and family, as well as increased expectations of feelings of sadness and depression.

Relation of Views of the Dying Process to Fear of Death

It seems to be a reasonable hypothesis that the way in which one views the dying process would bear a relationship to one's fears of death. If one expects the dying process to be brief and painless, there would seem to be little to fear, whereas if one expects the dying process to be difficult, painful, and protracted, one is naturally fearful of it.

In looking at the correlations of the measures of study participants' views of the dying process with the four fear of death measures from the MFODS (see Table 9.2), one can see that expectations of negative feelings (sorrow, loneliness, uncertainty, depression, etc.), concerns about physical survival, and concerns about family during the dying process are associated with the Fear of the Dying Process measure as well as with Fear for Significant Others. Expectations of emotionality during the dying process, either feelings of sadness and depression or feelings of rancor (anger and bitterness), were associated with Fear of the Unknown. Finally, feelings of rancor were related to less Fear of Being Destroyed.

Predicting Older Adults' Fear of Death

In foregoing chapters, the ways in which older adults' fear of death depends on their demographic background, their religious views, their health, and their family relationships have been explored, and we have just examined the ways in which elders' death meanings and views of the dying process influence their fears of death. The remaining task is to determine how well these factors taken together enable us to predict fear of death. Two general approaches to this task are available: regression analysis and structural equation modeling. Because the number of older adults participating in the empirical study was limited, we opted for the regression approach to avoid the requirements of a larger sample size and more stringent assumptions of structural modeling.

Before proceeding with the analysis, however, some reduction of the number of variables was necessary. Based on factor analysis, a single religiosity score was constructed by combining the nonorganizational religiosity, subjective religiosity, and religious coping subscores, with a high score meaning greater religiosity. Similarly, a single health score was constructed by combining the scores on the health self-rating, the Bradburn affect balance score, number of chronic conditions, number of symptoms experienced, mobility, and independent activities of daily living. A high score on the measure indicated poorer health. With regard to the family variables, only a few selected variables were used in the regression analysis based on correlational findings and the nature of the variables themselves.

A set of hierarchical regression analyses was carried out to explore the prediction of each of the four MFODS fears of death: Fear of the Dying Process, Fear of Being Destroyed, Fear for Significant Others, and Fear of the Unknown. The set of demographic variables (age, gender, ethnicity, SES) was entered first, followed by the health, religiosity, and family variables, and then followed by the death meanings variables (afterlife, extinction, motivator, legacy). (The variables assessing views of the dying process were not included in the regression analyses. One reason was to keep the number of variables from becoming too large in relation to the sample size. A second reason was that, given the constraint on the number of variables, the measures of views of the dying process were considered of secondary importance. Unlike the measures of death meanings and fears of death which are supported by existing research, measures of views of the dying process were exploratory in nature and insufficiently established.)

Fear of the Dying Process

In the analysis for Fear of the Dying Process (see Table 9.3), gender was a significant predictor in the first stage of the analysis (Model 1 in the table), with women having a greater fear of the dying process than men. Age also had a weak effect on fear, with those participants who were older having less fear of the dying process. When adjusted for the effects of religiosity, health, and family variables in the second stage of the analysis (Model 2 in the table), the effect of gender on fear remained significant but age was no longer a significant predictor of fear. Health also had a significant effect on Fear of the Dying Process, with those elders in poorer health having greater fear.

When the death meanings were added in the third stage of the regression analysis (Model 3 in the table), death as motivator and death as extinction were both significant predictors of Fear of the Dying Process, in addition to gender and health, with both death meanings associated with greater fear of the dying process.

Overall, one is able to predict the extent of older adults' fear of the dying process from knowledge of just four variables: gender, health, a conception of death as extinction, and a conception of death as a motivator for accomplishing certain goals during the remaining portion of life. If one is a woman, if one is in poor health, if one sees death as meaning extinction (or the end of everything), and/or if one sees the meaning of death as a motivator for further accomplishment, then one would be predicted to have greater fear of the dying process.

Fear of Being Destroyed

In the analysis for variables predicting Fear of Being Destroyed (see Table 9.4), SES, ethnicity, and age were all significant pre-

TABLE 9.3 Summary of Regression of Fear of the Dying Process on Study Variables

Variable	Standardized ß-Coefficients		
	Model 1	Model 2	Model 3
SES	.04	.13	.16
Gender	.27**	.26**	.25**
Ethnicity	−.19	−.08	−.07
Age	−.19*	−.13	−.05
Religiosity		.01	−.02
Health		.27**	.25**
Proportion of dead children		−.07	.01
Proportion of dead siblings		−.11	−.11
Number of living siblings		.13	.15
Afterlife			.06
Motivator			.30**
Legacy			−.16
Extinction			.28**
Adjusted R^2	.07	.11	.21

R =
* $p < .10$; ** $p < .05$

dictors in the first stage of the analysis (Model 1). Those who were older, who were of lower socioeconomic status, and who were African American were more likely to have a greater fear of bodily destruction after death. However, when religiosity, health, and family variables were added in the second stage of the analysis (Model 2), ethnicity and age were no longer significant predictors after being adjusted for the presence of the stage two variables. Two family variables, the proportion of deceased children and the proportion of deceased siblings, were significant predictors in addition to SES. The addition to the four death meanings to the regression equation in the third stage of the analysis (Model 3) did not appreciably change the prediction.

Thus, Fear of Being Destroyed could be predicted from knowledge of just three variables: the older person's socioeconomic status, and the proportions of deceased siblings in his or her family of origin and deceased children in his or her family of procreation.

TABLE 9.4 Summary of Regression of Fear of Being Destroyed on Study Variables

Variable	Standardized ß-Coefficients		
	Model 1	Model 2	Model 3
SES	−.36**	−.26**	−.30**
Gender	−.06	−.13	−.11
Ethnicity	.27**	.16	.17
Age	.20**	.07	.10
Religiosity		.08	.07
Health		.03	.01
Proportion of dead children		.26**	.24**
Proportion of dead siblings		.31**	.31**
Number of living siblings		.12	.14
Afterlife			.14
Motivator			−.09
Legacy			−.13
Extinction			.08
Adjusted R^2	.23	.29	.29

R =
* $p < .10$; ** $p < .05$

Those elders of higher socioeconomic status seem better able to contemplate the destruction of the body after death without fear than those of lower status levels. Perhaps their additional education helps them to better understand and accept the reasons and processes behind the destruction of the body after death. Regardless of socioeconomic status level, the degree of loss of one's siblings and/or one's children is related to the fear of bodily destruction. The death of two or three siblings from one's family of origin is of course a loss, but the effect of the loss depends on the original family size. For example, losing three siblings from an original group of nine (one-third of the siblings) does not seem to have as great an effect on fear of bodily destruction as losing three siblings from an original group of four (three-fourths of the siblings). The degree of such losses of close family members seems to lead these elders to focus on and become more fearful of the destruction of the body after death.

Fear for Significant Others

In the analysis for variables predicting Fear for Significant Others (see Table 9.5), there were no significant predictors in the first stage of the analysis (Model 1). In the second stage of the analysis (Model 2), once adjusted for the effects of religiosity, health, and family variables, age was a significant predictor along with the proportion of deceased siblings. Those study participants who were older had less fear for significant others, and those who had lost a greater proportion of their siblings had greater fear for their significant others. In the third stage of the analysis (Model 3) when the four death meanings were added to the prediction equation, age and the proportion of deceased siblings were again significant predictors, along with the proportion of deceased children and the two death meanings: death as motivator and death as extinction.

The lower degree of Fear for Significant Others among the older aged participants is perhaps understandable on two counts. For one thing, they are more likely to have lost sizable numbers of family members (spouse, siblings, adult children, and others); thus they have already weathered the deaths of many loved ones and would have fewer family members left to be frightened for. Second, after a long life and many losses, they are more able to deal with loss in a philosophical manner than those who are younger. Many elders have attempted to prepare family members for their own passing and feel that their loved ones will be able to adjust as life goes on.

As was the case for Fear of Being Destroyed, the proportions of deceased siblings and deceased children were related to Fear for Significant Others. It may be the case that having experienced a high degree of loss of close family members, these elders were highly aware of the emotional upheaval that such losses bring and were consequently more fearful of what their own death would mean to others (or what an additional loss of a loved one would mean to them). This argument might seem to be at odds with the

TABLE 9.5 Summary of Regression of Fear for Significant Others on Study Variables

Variable	Standardized ß-Coefficients		
	Model 1	Model 2	Model 3
SES	.01	.05	.14
Gender	.01	−.02	−.03
Ethnicity	.05	−.08	−.04
Age	−.18	−.27**	−.23**
Religiosity		.08	−.06
Health		−.09	−.09
Proportion of dead children		.07	.19*
Proportion of dead siblings		.25*	.23*
Number of living siblings		.10	.10
Afterlife			.16
Motivator			.30**
Legacy			.05
Extinction			.36**
Adjusted R^2	.01	.02	.15

* $p < .10$; ** $p < .05$

explanation in the preceding paragraph that elders seem better able to deal philosophically with deaths of loved ones with increasing age and experience with loss. However, it must be remembered that the effects of the proportions of deceased siblings and deceased children were determined with the effects of age controlled.

The two death meanings related to Fear for Significant Others, death as motivator and death as extinction, are somewhat easier to explain. Those who conceptualize death as motivator feel the need to accomplish certain goals before death, and often these goals involve accomplishing certain tasks for the family. If completion of these tasks were to be cut short by death, it is understandable that the effects of such a premature death on their loved ones would be feared. Similarly, if elders see death as meaning complete extinction without hope of reunion in the afterlife, they may well have greater fear for those loved ones they will leave behind.

Fear of the Unknown

In the analysis of variables predicting Fear of the Unknown (see Table 9.6), none of the demographic variables in the first stage of the analysis (Model 1) was significantly related to Fear of the Unknown, and of the religiosity, health, and family variables entered in the second stage of the analysis (Model 2), only religiosity was a significant predictor. Those elders with greater religiosity had less Fear of the Unknown. When the death meanings variables were added to the prediction equation in the third stage of the analysis (Model 3), two additional predictors were identified: death as afterlife and death as legacy. Having greater religiosity and conceptualizing death as meaning afterlife were both related to less Fear of the Unknown. The death meaning legacy, however, was related to greater Fear of the Unknown. However, this is difficult to interpret, given that no such relationship appeared when the correlations between death meanings and fears of death were examined (Table 9.1).

QUALITATIVE STUDY: INTERPRETATIONS

The strategy used to integrate the findings of the qualitative study with those of the quantitative findings was to examine the interview protocols of those study participants who were in the highest tenth and lowest tenth on each of the four fears of death. The protocols for these two extreme groups were then compared in order to determine whether participants' characteristics and comments made during the interview supported the quantitative results.

Fear of the Dying Process

According to the quantitative findings, the best predictors of Fear of the Dying Process were gender, health, and the meanings of death as extinction and death as a motivator for continued achievement in life. One would expect that those with the greatest fear of the dying process would include a greater proportion of women, those in poor health, and those who saw death as extinction and

TABLE 9.6 Summary of Regression of Fear of the Unknown on Study Variables

Variable	Standardized ß-Coefficients		
	Model 1	Model 2	Model 3
SES	−.16	−.22	−.13
Gender	−.02	.06	.04
Ethnicity	−.03	.06	−.01
Age	−.06	−.01	−.07
Religiosity		−.40**	−.24*
Health		−.10	−.09
Proportion of dead children		.03	.10
Proportion of dead siblings		.10	.09
Number of living children		.21	.20
Afterlife			−.23*
Motivator			−.02
Legacy			.22*
Extinction			.10
Adjusted R^2	.02	.08	.13

* $p < .10$; ** $p < .05$

as a motivator. Conversely, one would expect those with the least fear of the dying process to include a greater proportion of men, those in better health, and those who did not view death as extinction or as a motivator. An examination of the subgroups of study participants who had the greatest and least fears of the dying process revealed some support of these predictions.

Elders with High Fear

Of the subgroup of elders who had the greatest Fear of the Dying Process, all were women. Some mentioned their declining health. Most mentioned some kind of motivation to remain involved in life or to accomplish some goal. Some saw death as the end of everything, and others were skeptical about whether there was anything after death. For example:

Some high SES women in their 80s said:

- As long as I'm productive to somebody and society, I appreciate life. I have to stay well and obey the doctor. I know that as I age, I don't have the stamina . . . anymore. It does limit my physical activity. Death is a big dread.
- I think about death getting closer; I'll take whatever comes. I still want to try to be of value to people. I think they'll bury me and that will be the end of me, I guess.
- I want to complete a piece of writing that I think is pretty good . . . and to spend time with family, a reunion we're planning. Particularly at this age when people are dying off . . . it brings death to your mind. I think a great deal of regret has to come at the end. You might welcome death if you are in a lot of pain. Death is difficult if it is prolonged, but it's inevitable. One uncertainty is . . . that we don't have anything to hold onto, that this [*afterlife*] is going to be.
- I want to see my grandchild grow up. I have this wheelchair problem . . . things are a chore these days. I think dying will be frightening at first, the idea of pain coming with illness. It will depend on the amount of pain I suffer.

A low SES White woman in her 70s said,

- I want to see my granddaughter grow and my other son married. I wonder if I will have more pains [in dying] than I do now. Death is a scary thing. It is difficult when it is prolonged and suffering is involved.

A low SES African American woman said,

- I want to spend more time with family, and try to put my finances in order. Death is difficult when your goals are unfulfilled. I think I will have some feelings of fright [at dying], because it is unknown. My greatest fear is having something like cancer and being in pain for a long time.

Elders with Low Fear

The low fear group contained a few men in addition to several women. Most had little motivation to accomplish any particular goals in their remaining years. Some mentioned their good health, but all spoke of having little fear of dying. For example:

Some high SES White women in their 90s said,

- I have no great desires for anything to be better. I'm satisfied with my present living. Hopefully I will be unconscious [*when dying*]. But I don't dwell on anything like that. I would hope to just lie down and go to sleep. . . . No emotional reaction when it domes to dying. I feel that it is controlled by God.
- I want nothing big [*from life*]. I don't worry about death. I hope things just go on as long as they can and that's it. I think dying will be like putting out the light. . . . I don't think that dying is a terrible thing to experience. No!

A high SES White man in his 90s said,

- I know a lot of people who have gone through a sort of near-death experience and they have a vision. . . . I would expect something of that sort. I think I would feel happiness. I believe the spirit is alive and will continue. The idea that there is no God wouldn't influence my way of thinking.

A high SES White man in his 70s said,

- Right now I've got good health. I see [*dying*] as going to sleep and you wake up in a different place. My soul will go to heaven. [*He wants to continue his present activities.*]

A low SES African American woman in her 80s said,

- I want to keep my health. [*Of dying,*] you just sleep away, I guess. When your time comes, you just go on. Just relax. I think I'd feel happiness. I'm not afraid of dying. I just figure I'm going to heaven.

Some low SES African American women in their 70s said,

- I just take care of business. I see pretty good with my glasses. I get along with my hearing aids. I never think of anything like

death. We've all got to die, so accept what you can't change. I never think about dying. If I wasn't in a lot of pain, I'd just think, well, it's time for me to die. I wish it would be a peaceful place after I die. No, I don't think death is the end of you.
- It [*dying*] is a promise, a promise of glory. We were created for this glory. I don't believe dying is the end, because we have a spirit and a soul.
- I want to continue my life just as it is now. I've got a feeling [*dying*] will be very peaceful, and I'm not going to suffer. I believe that I'll be happy. I hope I'll be going to heaven and not down.

Fear of Being Destroyed

The strongest predictors of a greater fear of bodily destruction after death were a low socioeconomic status level and a high proportion of deceased siblings and children. Conversely, a lower Fear of Being Destroyed was associated with a high socioeconomic status level and a low proportion of deceased siblings and children. This is reflected in the comments of study participants.

Elders with High Fear

In this group of older adults who had a high fear of bodily destruction after death, none mentioned a specific fear about what would happen to the body after death. However, their characteristics fit the prediction equation from the quantitative findings. All were of low socioeconomic status, and all had experienced deaths of a high proportion of their siblings or children or both. For example, note the proportions of deaths in the families of the following participants who had high fear of bodily destruction after death:

- Low SES White woman in her 70s had nine brothers and sisters, all dead. Has three children, but is completely estranged from two of them and has no contact.
- Low SES White woman in her 80s has five of seven brothers and sisters dead, and her only son dead.

- Low SES African American woman in her 70s has two of her three siblings dead, two of her four children dead.
- Low SES African American woman in her 70s has two siblings, both dead, and is childless.
- Low SES African American woman in her 80s has five brothers and sisters, all dead, and one daughter still living.

Elders with Low Fear

In contrast to the elders in the group with a high Fear of Being Destroyed, those with a low fear were all of high socioeconomic status, and they either had all their siblings and children still living or had only a small proportion lost to death. Like the high fear group, some did not speak of what would happen to their body after death. However, others expressed quite definite views. For example:

A high SES White woman in her 80s said,

- I want to be cremated. [*Her only brother is still living, and two of her three children are still living.*]

Another high SES White woman in her 80s also wanted to be cremated, but said,

- I hope they don't cremate me before I'm really dead. That's my only fear about being dead. [*She was an only child, but has two living children.*]

A high SES White woman in her 70s stated,

- Death is just part of the life cycle. [*Her two siblings and four children are all still living.*]

A high SES White man in his 70s was an old child, but has three living children. He was most specific about what would happen to his body after death. He said,

- I have designated that usable parts of my body be harvested . . . I put my machinery to good use for as long as I could. The local mortician . . . is going to render a judgment of whether there is going to be enough left of me to be useful in the laboratory. I don't intend to be put under the ground, I intend to be cremated.

A high SES White woman in her 70s expressed disinterested in what happened to her body after death,

- When I'm dead, I'm dead. I can't do anything about that. I can't have any anxiety over something that has absolutely no solution. [*She has a brother and two children, all of whom are still living.*]

Fear for Significant Others

The strongest predictors of Fear for Significant Others are age (with older adults having less fear), and the death meanings extinction (with high scores associated with greater fear) and motivation (with high scores associated with greater fear). Additionally, higher proportions of deceased siblings and deceased children were associated with greater fear. The prediction regarding age did not appear to be borne out in these comparisons of the subgroups of elders with high and low fear, but differences in the other predictors are easily apparent.

Elders with High Fear

Each of the elders with high Fear for Significant Others exemplifies at least some of the predictors of fear. For example,

One of the elders with high fear was a low SES White woman in her 80s who has no living siblings. The idea of death motivated to get her possessions in order. Of her daughters she said,

- I'm very close to my family and think they will miss me terribly. When I was sick, they all came, and for a long while they called me every night.

- A low SES African American woman in her 70s has no siblings left, and only one son and his family left. She said, "I want to be here for my family. It will be very hard to leave them here." She is unsure about an afterlife, and feels motivated just to "do your duty and so what you have to do."
- Another low SES African American women in her 80s has four of her five siblings dead and one child who died. Of her remaining family she said, "My death would be a loss to them. I've raised them, helped them." She feels motivated to make some changes before death comes, "As death has grown closer, I want to simplify my life."
- A low SES African American man in his 70s has lost two of his four daughters. He was concerned about how his daughters would take his death, "I think they will miss me. Death is difficult when someone is really close to you. No matter how they die, that's bad." He feels motivated to get his house fixed up before he dies.

Elders with Low Fear

Again, those elders with low fear displayed at least some of the predictor characteristics. For example,

- A high SES White woman in her 80s has two siblings and two children, all living. She had little concern about how her family members would be affected by her death, saying merely, "I hope some people will miss me."
- Another high SES White woman in her 80s had all her children and siblings still alive. She felt little motivation to achieve any goal before death, saying, "I can't think of anything new to do [*in life*]. I'm doing well to keep up with things I've already started." She refused to believe that there was no afterlife. She had no fear of how her death would affect her family. She said only, "They'll say she had a good life."
- A low SES African American woman in her 70s had a sister and four children, all living. She has no motivation to achieve anything before death and said, "I'll just go on as I am." She felt

that "people here are going to remember you," and said, "I don't think death is the end of you."

- Another low SES African American woman in her 70s had no siblings but had three living children. She felt that they would not be affected much by her death, "They won't miss me a whole lot. My death won't mean much to any of them." She doesn't feel motivated to do anything more than "continue my life just as I am now."

Fear of the Unknown

In the quantitative analysis, the strongest predictors of Fear of the Unknown were religiosity, death as meaning afterlife, and death as meaning an opportunity for legacy. A stronger meaning of death as legacy, a weaker meaning of death as afterlife, and low religiosity were related to greater fear, whereas a weaker meaning of death as legacy, a stronger meaning of death as afterlife, and high religiosity were related to less fear.

Elders with High Fear

The following comments appear to bear out the quantitative predictions for the group with high Fear of the Unknown.

- A low SES White woman in her 80s said, "I think it would be wonderful if there were a heaven, but I don't really believe it." She had some concerns about a legacy for her family, "I worry how I am going to leave these few assets I have to family, how to distribute those gifts."
- A low SES White woman in her 70s said, "[After I die] I'll just rot. No, I'll be buried. It wouldn't make any difference to me if there was no God." She had some notions of legacy, "I want to do something to help others."
- A high SES White man in his 80s said, "I'm not worried about what will happen after death. . . . Leave me alone in my six-foot grave."
- A low SES African American woman in her 70s felt unconvinced about God and an afterlife, "I'd like to die quick. Beyond that,

I don't know. Even if there was a God, it would be too late. You couldn't change if you wanted to."

- Finally, a high SES White woman in here 80s spoke of a legacy for her family, "I'd like to see that my family's needs are taken care of." She was rather skeptical of the existence of an afterlife, "I would like to find out if there is anything on the other side."

Elders with Low Fear

The quantitative predictions of factors related to low Fear of the Unknown were also reflected in the comments of participants in the low fear group.

- A White man of high SES, in his 90s, felt that "knowing that God exists gives me a great deal of comfort, satisfaction, and anticipation of eternal existence. After all, I look at my body and see 160 pounds of flesh and blood. It's temporal; this is not the real me. This life is a transitory state and I don't fear death. . . . After I die the first thing is to join that wonderful woman who is my wife. Somehow I know that she is waiting for me. That's a tremendous eternity."
- A low SES African American woman in her 80s said, "I want a good Christian life...going to church and service my God . . . when my time comes, I'll be put in the ground until God comes for me."
- A low SES White woman in her 80s said, "I think I will have real peace because absence from the body is presence with the Lord. I couldn't have it any better. And to be in heaven, I'll be happy."
- Finally, a high SES White woman in her 80s said, "I think that after I die, I will go to heaven, my soul will. I want angels to escort me. I have faith that they will."

Despite the fact that many of the questions asked in the qualitative portion of the interview did not pertain specifically to the variables investigated in the quantitative portion of the study, there was a surprising degree of agreement in the findings from the two approaches.

SUMMARY AND CONCLUSIONS

The attempt to reach an integrated picture of the combined effects of the variables investigated in the empirical study on older adults' fears of death was only partially successful. Limitations of sample size also limited the number of variables that could be included in various analyses as well as the investigation of more complex relationships between variables than a linear hypothesis. We elected to eliminate the views and expectations of the dying process altogether from the combined analysis. Despite these limitations, several interesting conclusions emerged. The three groups of variables (demographic variables, religiosity, health, and family variables, and death meanings) will be considered in turn.

The four demographic variables (SES, gender, ethnicity, and age) had limited relationships to fear of death. Ethnicity did not emerge as a predictor of any of the four death fears. Analyses in earlier chapters suggested repeatedly that most differences between African American and White elders were due to differences in socioeconomic status rather than to ethnicity itself. For that matter, SES was a predictor of only Fear of Being Destroyed, with those of higher SES reporting less fear. Gender was related only to Fear of the Dying Process, with women reporting greater fear than men. Finally, age was related only to Fear for Significant Others, with older age associated with less fear.

Religiosity, which was relatively high for the great majority of study participants, was related only to Fear of the Unknown, with higher degrees of religiosity associated with less fear. This relationship was of course expected, in view of the fact that most study participants espoused Christianity, with its promise of a blissful afterlife.

Health was related only to Fear of the Dying Process, with those in poorer health reporting greater fear. Those elders who were already experiencing more severe health problems apparently were quite apprehensive about what they might go through when dying.

Family structure variables were associated with two of the four death fears: Fear of Being Destroyed and Fear for Significant Others. As noted earlier, only a few of the possible family variables could be considered in this analysis; however, the ones selected also appeared in earlier correlations with death fears (Chapter 8). These were the proportion of deceased siblings and the proportion of deceased children in the elder's family. The relationship of these variables to Fear for Significant Others is somewhat easier to understand. The gradual attrition of ascending and many contemporaneous family members through death as the family ages, although an expected part of life, nevertheless leaves the survivor with an incomplete family which can never be restored and which exists only in memory (Cicirelli, 1995a, 1998c). This feeling has been referred to as a sense of "existential incompleteness" (Moss & Moss, 1989), and one which leaves sibling survivors with enduring feelings of loss. Whether they contemplate the way their deaths will affect their remaining loved ones or the way in which they will be affected should another close family member die, those who have already experienced the loss of significant portions of the their family group will have more intense fears of the emotional turmoil that another loss would bring to them. Fears of being the "last leaf on the tree," of being left alone, of abandonment may all enter in.

Explaining the relationship of the proportions of deceased siblings and children to the Fear of Being Destroyed is somewhat more difficult. It is possible that loss of one's siblings and loss of one's children, losses which occur before their naturally expected time, sensitizes the individual to thoughts of bodily destruction to a greater degree than might be the case with other losses.

The relationship of the death meanings to fear of death has been discussed earlier in this chapter. Only those few cases where findings appear to differ need further comment. Death as meaning afterlife was significantly correlated with Fear of Being Destroyed, but was not a significant predictor in the regression analysis. Also, death as meaning extinction was significantly correlated with Fear of the Unknown, but was not a significant predictor in the regression equation. Finally, death as meaning opportunity for legacy was uncorrelated with Fear of the Unknown, but was a significant, albeit weak, predictor in the regression equation. Rather than attempting elaborate explanations of these findings, they can be attributed most simply to the effects of adjusting the relationship of a particular death meaning to a particular fear of death for their overlap with other variables in the regression equation. This can be seen most directly in the case of the positive correlation of death as meaning extinction with Fear of the Unknown. When adjusted for the influence of religiosity (inasmuch as religiosity is negatively correlated with both death meaning extinction and Fear of the Unknown), extinction is no longer a significant predictor of Fear of the Unknown.

Overall, of the four death fears, Fear of Being Destroyed was best predicted by the study variables, with a multiple correlation coefficient, R, of 0.63 and an adjusted R^2 (an indicator of the proportion of variance explained by the predictors) of 0.29. Fear of the Dying process was next with an R of 0.57 and an adjusted R^2 of 0.21, follow by Fear for Significant Others with an R, of 0.56 and an adjusted R^2 of .20. Fear of the Unknown was the most poorly predicted of the four fears of death, with an R, of 0.51 and an adjusted R^2 of only .13. One explanation for the relatively poor prediction of Fear of the Unknown was the fact that these older adults had relatively low Fear of the Unknown and there was not a great deal of variability in their scores. Most of them had strong religious beliefs which included a belief in an joyful afterlife; thus one would not expect to find strong fear of the afterlife in such a population.

The portion of this chapter devoted to the quantitative analyses took the main burden of demonstrating interrelationships among study variables. However, the fact that the quantitative findings were borne out to a large degree by the qualitative results lends support to the conclusions.

10

Conclusions and Implications

If one were to use the conclusions reached in this volume to construct a portrait of the typical views on death held by older adults in the conservative American heartland, it would be something like the following: The central meaning of death is as a transition to a happy afterlife. The dying process will be a simple and painless fading away, perhaps in sleep, accompanied by some sadness and other negative emotions. There is little fear of what lies beyond death, but more fear of the dying process, destruction of the body, and the effects of death on loved ones. Even if one is in good health, it is not desirable to live beyond one's 90s.

Such a portrait can be criticized on at least two counts. First, it doesn't represent the considerable diversity of older adults' views on death and, second, certain aspects of the portrait are internally inconsistent as well as inconsistent with existing research into death and dying.

In this final chapter, we will examine many of the inconsistencies and questions arising from of the conclusions of the previous chapters, attempt to place them in a broader perspective, and identify areas where further research is needed.

INCONSISTENCIES AND QUESTIONS

A Diversity of Personal Meanings of Death in a Multicultural Society

Perhaps the most fundamental idea regarding the relationship between life and death is that death itself is at the core of the renewal of both life and the environment that supports life through its continual development throughout the life span. Without death, evolution and ecology would make no sense.

Within this context, the core functions of society are to nurture the young, protect citizens from premature death, care for the dying, bury the dead, and care for the grieving. The social meanings of death become part of the culture, which in turn regulates the behaviors required to carry out the societal functions related to death.

Personal meanings of death help guide the individual's lifestyle, which includes preparations for death and reactions to it when it occurs. Great variations in personal meanings of death held by members of a society may emerge due to the individual differences of people and the circumstances of their lives. In this sense, diversity is inevitable. However, the degree of diversity of personal meanings of death may go beyond an optimum point, leading to conflict and disruption between subgroups of the society that could eventually disrupt society itself. Some diametrically opposed meanings might be, "death means the elimination of one's competitor in life" compared to "death means sacrifice for the terminally ill," or, "death means that one should always be ready to die for a cause" compared to "death means that one should always be ready to live at any costs." If these differences in personal meanings of death are held by enough individuals, there may be negative consequences for both the individual and society. The question becomes: Can society strive to nurture personal meanings of death that satisfy the needs of the individual in a positive manner and not disrupt the functioning of society? This may become a problem in our increasingly multicultural society where subgroups with widely different values, norms, and beliefs may undercut the common values, norms, and beliefs that once held the society together.

Throughout this volume, the diversity of views on various aspects of death has been evident. Differences in the personal meaning of death as an afterlife is a case in point. Some study participants had no belief in God or the existence of an afterlife and others were frankly skeptical. Although the great majority of older adults participating in the study shared a view that some sort of afterlife exists, their accounts of the nature of that afterlife varied widely. Some were anxious as to whether an afterlife existed or not. Some were exceedingly vague about what an afterlife would be like, even though they were convinced of its existence. Some saw an afterlife as some kind of disembodied floating spirit. Some saw it as a glorious unification with God, whereas others saw it as simply being in the presence of God. Some saw an afterlife as a heaven of eternal peace and beauty. Others saw an afterlife as a time of reunion with loved ones who had gone before, a rejoining with grandparents, parents, siblings, and spouses who have preceded them in death.

This diversity of views about death also characterizes the interviews with individuals in all walks of life included in Studs Terkel's (2001) recent book. The views expressed seem to be a pastiche of ideas gained from personal experiences with the deaths of others, religious teachings, literature, art, the media, interactions with others, and so on.

What is one to make of such a diversity of views? One of the common cultural meanings of death in Western societies is the notion of an afterlife, but the particulars of what an afterlife is like seem to vary. Of course, when attempts to describe the unknowable are made, there is bound to be an abundance of creative ideas of what this unknown afterlife might be like. Each individual is left to sort out images of an afterlife drawn from religion, literature, art, film, and television, reports of near-death experiences and deathbed visions of others, and other manifestations of the culture relative to an afterlife. Finally, that individual seems to reach some distillation of all these images, ideas, and experiences to gain a conception of an afterlife that is personally acceptable. From such a perspective, a diversity of views regarding the meaning of death as afterlife would seem to pose little threat to society as a whole, so long as there is tolerance of the meanings held by others.

Another aspect of the diversity of views concerning an afterlife is that many religious people appeared to feel certain doubts about the existence of God and an afterlife when they were confronted with the prospect of death and dying. Some people who professed a strong belief in God and the afterlife still entertained some degree of doubt that was in the back of their minds.

The existence of such doubts was manifested in inconsistent responses on quantitative fear of death scales and also in various qualitative comments. For example, most participants agreed that religion influences the way they live their life, but on the Death Meaning Scale, many elders agreed that death means personal extinction and/or death means the loss of everything, responses incompatible with a belief that death means afterlife. On the Multidimensional Fear of Death Scale, many elders agreed that no one can say for sure what will happen after death. In the qualitative interviews, various participants indicated that they had doubts at times about an afterlife. For example, some comments already mentioned in the text were, "Supposedly, I will be in heaven, or hope I am." "I wish I could believe like I'm supposed to believe, a Christian afterlife. But I'm not sure anything will happen after I die."

One issue raised by such responses is whether the religious beliefs of some older adults are merely a set of tenets learned in childhood which they have never subjected to adult reflection to reach a mature religious philosophy. If so, lingering doubts about the validity of such ingrained beliefs may surface when questions about their death concerns are raised. This is an area in which further research might be done to more completely explore individual religious beliefs about God and the afterlife and the relationship of such beliefs to death concerns.

What Will Dying Be Like? An Unrealistic Understanding of the Dying Process

When directly asked, the great majority of older adults taking part in the study felt that dying would be a quick and painless event. Some elders described the process of dying but only at the level of metaphor, for example, death is like sleep. Many expected to pass away quietly in their sleep or simply drift off into death. They saw dying as going from being alert to becoming drowsy and finally going into a deep sleep (from which they would awaken in an afterlife). There was no attempt by anyone to provide a literal description of their expected dying process, that is, changes in physical health status, emerging symptoms, increasing physical, emotional, and social needs, possibly increasing pain and mental anguish, and so on. The few who acknowledged the possibility of some kind of pain or distress felt that this would not be a problem because their doctors would keep them "doped up" so that no untoward symptoms would be experienced.

This rosy view of a quick and peaceful dying process as described by study participants is at odds with most existing research studies. Although Fago (2001) noted that many elders have a reduced level of consciousness in the last few days of life, others (e.g., Emanuel & Emanuel, 1998; Field & Cassel, 1997; Gavrin & Chapman, 1995; Hurley, Volicer, and Mahoney, 2001; Lawton, Moss, & Glicksman, 1990; Lynn et al., 1997; Morris, Suissa, Sherwood, Wright, & Greer, 1986; Rees, Hardy, Ling, Broadley, & A'Hern (1998), Turner et al., 1996) have described a wide variety of distressing symptoms during the dying process. Cloud (2000) reported that a third of dying people spent at least 10 days in hospital intensive care units, where they have to deal with pain and suffering; nearly half died in pain. In a survey of the care needs of dying patients (Singer, Martin, & Kelner, 1999), adequate treatment for pain and other symptoms was one of the top five desired domains of care. The overwhelming weight of evidence is that dying is neither quick nor painless for most elders.

In the face of this evidence, how then can one account for study participants' expectations of a benign death? One hypothesis might be that the elderly had no real knowledge or experience as a basis for anticipating their own dying process. However, this seems untenable. Some had come close to dying in previous illnesses of their own, and certainly most older adults in their 70s and beyond have experienced the deaths of many close friends and family members. A goodly proportion of these deaths must have been accompanied by pain and other distressing symptoms during the dying process, if research reports are to be believed.

Another hypothesis might be that they did not have sufficient imagination to contemplate what their own dying process might be like. However, they did show imagination in formulating evaluations of what a good and bad death would be like, as well as in expressing their wishful-thinking about how they would like the dying process to be.

One is then forced to posit that older adults make use of some processes of denial and suppression of evidence that dying may be difficult in order to enable them to cope more readily with the prospect of their own deaths. The anticipation of such a negative event at the end of life evokes coping strategies of denial and distancing themselves from considering or wanting to learn about the dying process. Some study participants commented to the effect that they did not want to think about death because they couldn't do anything and it would be just as well to let it happen when it does and forget it for now. Such processes of denial and suppression may be more successful for some elders than for others. For example, one woman in our study indicated that underneath "we're all a little scared."

A strategy of coping with one's eventual death by suppressing or denying the existence of possible negative events during the dying process precludes any thoughts or planning about improving the quality of life while dying. Such thought processes may be in part responsible for the low participation of older adults in attempts to exert control over their dying process though the use of advance directives (Cicirelli, 2001a). Additionally, older individuals could certainly endeavor to make life more pleasant and meaningful while preparing to die, perhaps even attempting to learn and reflect while dying in order to reach new levels of understanding. For example, it may be emotionally satisfying to feel a sense of gain in wisdom as death approaches.

However, the latter ways of thinking seemed quite alien to most participants in our study. Perhaps such thinking represents the approach of younger generations to dying and death as compared to the approach of most members of an older generation. Nevertheless, preparation for death might include the effort to make life more pleasant and meaningful while dying regardless of one's generation. In any event, most of the older adults we studied seemed to have an unrealistic understanding of the dying process, and consequently would be unable to make any realistic preparation for it. Such a lack of knowledge in itself may make dying more difficult for them.

The Early 80s as a Transition Period

Throughout the study, those older adults in their early 80s not only expressed a greater diversity of views but also differed from those older and younger than themselves on certain quantitative measures. For example, Fear of the Dying Process, Fear of the Unknown, and belief in death as meaning extinction were greater among those aged 80–84 than among older or younger age groups.

Also, those elders in their early 80s anticipated greater concerns about the relationships with their family members, and their own emotional reactions to dying when they are actually going through their own dying process. For those younger and older, the concern for family relationships also had priority but the intensity was less. There was also more concern for physical survival and capacity to cope with dying rather than with emotional reactions to dying.

Although such findings were based on a relatively small sample, they suggest a hypothesis that older adults may be going through a transition period in their early 80s, that is, some kind of a sensitive or critical period. One might speculate that there is a threshold at which elders comes to a recognition of their nearness to death, which in turn triggers a heightened awareness and sensitivity to concerns surrounding death and dying and ultimately leads to some reorganization in thinking in preparation for the final stage in their life.

Large numbers of today's "young-old" seem to go through a postretirement period in which their health is relatively good and they engage in increased social activities with friends and family, travel, and the like. At some point, whether in response to increasing health problems, loss of others in their age group, or subtle signals from their culture that they will soon enter a last stage of life, they appear to enter a transition period as hypothesized above. Clearly, this hypothesis needs to be investigated in further research.

Desire for a Limited Life Span

None of the study participants wanted to live beyond 100 years of age. This is rather surprising in view of the increasing numbers of centenarians in our society (Perls & Silver, 1999). Nevertheless, the elders in our study envisaged a limited life span, both in expected years left to live and desired years left to live. This notion of a limited life span was independent of elders' current age and state of health. Additionally, many elders did not simply accept death as being inevitable; they valued death as something desirable.

Such a finding brings up an interesting question: Why would older adults who are relatively healthy and mobile want to limit their life span and value death? This is especially puzzling since centenarians are treated almost like celebrities at the present time, and many researchers are working on ways to extend life far beyond 100 years. Even though some of our oldest participants were still quite healthy, they felt they were close to the time when they would beginning declining abruptly and they did not want to live longer under those conditions. Perls and Silvers (1999) suggest that a healthy life style may be important to help individuals to reach the early 90s who otherwise would not live that long, but past a certain age genetic factors make it possible for some to reach ages of 100 and beyond regardless of their life style. This may be the case, but elders who are now reaching their 90s do not know whether or not they are the lucky ones genetically endowed for longer life, and hence prefer a limited life rather than gamble on declining abruptly with loss of independence and suffering.

Another point of interest is that older adults in their 80s had a greater belief in death as meaning extinction than other age groups. This is somewhat puzzling when considered in terms of a limited life span. If one is faced with extinction, why not attempt to live longer and become a centenarian or at least promote research concerned with life span extension?

However, a consistent theme represented by the majority of participants in our study leads to another possible interpretation. They did not want to live to age 100 or longer because they might outlive all their friends and family members. The loss of close personal relationships seemed to be essential to the quality of their lives. Even if they could continue living and develop new friendships, it would not be the same for most of them. The advanced technology and knowledge of the new generations would make it increasingly difficult for the very old to understand or communicate with them, and the generation gap in values, norms and beliefs would continue to widen. Thus, new friends could not compensate for the loss of long time close friendships of their own time period. It leads to the idea that close long-term relationships are essential for members of our species if we are to function effectively and efficiently.

Perhaps one could interpret this phenomenon in terms of Antonucci and Akiyama's (1991) convoy theory and Carstensen's (1992, 1995) socioemotional selectivity theory. The convoy theory proposes that individuals go through life with a convoy of close friends and relatives with whom they share social support. Socioemotional selectivity theory hypothesizes that as individuals age, they tend to limit their social interactions to those with whom they have close relationships of long standing. Our earlier findings relating to the influence of the proportions of deceased siblings and children on elders' death views may be interpreted as a recognition of the loss of an important portion of one's convoy, and one that cannot be replaced by new acquaintances. In this context, our finding of elders' desires for a limited life span can be interpreted as a rejection of longer life if they could not continue living that extended life with their convoy of selected close friends and relatives. It also follows that death itself may be actively valued because it provides the possibility of maintaining these close relationships by being able to reunite with them in an afterlife.

Religion and Close Relationships

Regardless of the truth of religion, it serves various psychological needs of older adults. For example, humans have a need to form and maintain attachment relationships to others throughout life to help satisfy their needs for security and comfort. The very old do not seem to be any different in this regard than younger people, and for them (as well as for some younger people), God can become an attachment figure, particularly when they have lost other close relationships. (Attachment to God, of course, seems to vary with personality and ethnicity, for example, it may be more true of African Americans.)

The whole idea of the importance of personal relationships for humans is further reinforced when we look at their religious beliefs.

Many older individuals tend to view God as one who provides security, comfort, and help to them, and as indicated in Chapter 6, God can be viewed as the ultimate attachment figure. Since attachment theory is concerned with relationships, then being with God in an afterlife also represents a close relationship; a special one since it involves the attribute of always being physically or symbolically close to the one that provides such security and comfort. Interestingly, many religious elders indicated that they wanted to be not only with God but also with friends and family members in an afterlife. The relationship with God is important in itself but also becomes a vehicle for the reestablishment of past human relationships.

Thus, the meaning of death seems to encompass notions of the importance of maintaining long-term close relationships and simultaneously avoiding the necessity of compensating for loss of such close relationships by developing new relationships. Both cases suggest that death has a deeper meaning for the elderly, representing the importance of close personal relationships.

Fear of Dying: Inconsistencies Between the Literature and Present Study

Various studies in the literature (e.g., Johnson & Barer, 1997; Tobin, 1991, 1996) report that elderly do not fear death but they do fear the dying process. In our present study, we did not find this to be the case, as the majority of participants claimed that they did not fear dying. For example, in regard to pain, they felt that powerful medications would alleviate any concern for pain, or God would protect them from such pain.

The literature (e.g., Bradley, Fried, Kasl, & Idler, 2001; Cicirelli, 2001a) indicates how important it is for the elderly to feel a greater sense of control over when, how, and where they will die. This certainly sounds logical as we all know how important it is to have control over our lives. Yet many older adults in the present study did not seem to feel that control of the dying process itself was important. A common position was that since one is so close to death, what difference does it make whether or not one attempts to control one's dying. It seems almost foolish since there is no future to be concerned about.

Finally, the evidence in the research literature (e.g., DeVries & Blando, 2001) seems to indicate that the majority of elders prefer to have someone to whom they are close (e.g. family members) with them when they are dying. However, we found this to be only partially true. Many elders did prefer to have someone with them when dying, but at least half did not want others with them or were indifferent about it. This phenomenon increased with age, in that most of the 90-year-olds did not seem to need or care about having others with them when dying. Perhaps they felt that they had lived their life fully and completely accepted death without the need for goodbyes. Or perhaps, at their age, there weren't any close family or friends left to be with. Other older adults did not want to burden family members or friends with their dying. Such comments were typically made by those elders who did not want to have others present. Those who were indifferent did not seem that closely attached to other people. Obviously, various reasons might exist for elders' preferences, but the results from this study indicate that a more complete explanation than now exists is needed as to why many have a fear of death and others do not, why some need to control the dying process and others do not, and why some prefer to have others with them when dying while others do not.

Fear of the Unknown vs. Fear of Annihilation/Extinction

A number of dimensions of the fear of death exist, depending on the particular measuring instrument used. The content of these dimensions varies considerably from instrument to instrument, but one which is common to many instruments is the fear of extinction or annihilation (a total end to existence) and the allied fear of the unknown (what may or may not happen after death). Although these fears are often considered to be synonymous, it is not clear from a methodological viewpoint whether this is really the case. Previous research has often assumed that these fears were synonymous. It was felt that, at the least, sufficient overlap existed that one term could substitute for the other. For example if one had a fear of annihilation or extinction, then one would fear the end of one's existence, with nothing but an unknown remaining.

However, one can apply an analogy to the positions of an atheist and an agnostic here. An atheist would state there is definitely no God and attempt to provide evidence for this position, whereas an agnostic would question whether a God exists but recognize that there is insufficient evidence to decide this question. By analogy, those referring to fear of annihilation would argue that total annihilation takes place with an extinction of earthly life and no afterlife, whereas those referring to fear of the unknown might argue that they are skeptical of what might happen after death because there is insufficient evidence to know whether there is a continuation of existence as some kind of noncorporeal being and what kind of existence this might be. What is needed is to attempt to construct separate measures of each of these concepts. One could then better determine whether the fears are independent of one another, synonymous, or correlated to some degree. As far as I know, this has not been done. There may be distinctions here that should be considered in further studies in this domain.

Significance of Socioeconomic Status, Ethnicity, Gender, and Age

Findings of the present study indicate that older adults' socioeconomic status level is an important factor influencing their views on death and dying. In most comparisons, SES was more influential than gender or ethnic differences.

Admittedly, our study was limited not only in terms of sample size and representativeness but in terms of measures of contextual factors and changes over time. There was little or no opportunity to determine how sociodemographic factors might interact in different situations or at different time periods. Under the latter conditions, the sociodemographic factors might be a more powerful influence than when considered only under a single situation at one time period. Nevertheless, even under a single condition, the present study provides clues as to their potential importance.

Our study indicated that, in comparison to lower SES Whites and African Americans, higher SES White men and women were limited in their personal death meanings to broad and widely shared conceptions. Men tended to be more philosophical and women were more concerned with relationships. The lower SES Whites and African Americans displayed not only greater individual differences in death meanings, but these differences included a much wider variety of death meanings. For elders at the higher socioeconomic status levels, death meanings seemed abstract and concerned with definitions whereas for elders at the lower socioeconomic status levels, death meanings included metaphors and were associated with emotions. In short, not only did the death meanings of the two socioeconomic status levels differ, but these differences seemed to be related to different ways of cognitive thinking. The implication is that strategies of cognitive functioning may be important to investigate as mediators of death meanings.

The reader will recall that, for certain measures of death views, ethnicity and gender took on greater importance, sometimes overriding socioeconomic status level. For example, in expectations of the dying process, Whites anticipated more emotional reactions and more family concerns than African Americans. The latter were more concerned in coping with dying. In regard to fears of death, women had more Fear of the Dying Process than did men. These examples not only illustrate the importance of the sociodemographic variables but their interaction at a given moment in time. Again, additional assessments under different conditions and at different time periods would be of great interest in future research inasmuch as sociodemographic variables are a reflection of basic sociocultural conditions that are continually evolving.

Significance of the Family in Relation to Death Concerns

The present study indicated that family is a far more important influence on the death views of older adults than previously expected, especially such family members as siblings, adult children, and grandchildren. However, there are few if any studies relating the influence of family members to elders' personal meanings of death, death fears, and views of the dying process. In recent years, changes in the structure and nature of the family are accelerating, with large increases over earlier times in the numbers of half-siblings, stepsiblings, and adoptive siblings, along with stepchildren, adopted children, fictive children, and so on. These changes

affect not only the structural characteristics of the family, but relationships between family members as well (e.g., White, 1998, 2001).
Thus, studies aimed at understanding the influence of family on
elders' death views will produce biased results if only biological
relatives are studied. (Particularly for older adults, relationships
with "in-laws" may also be important.) In addition to a more careful assessment of the structural characteristics of older adults' families, future studies also need to assess the quality of family
relationships, including such factors as frequency of contact, closeness of feelings, helping patterns, and mutual influences. Each of
these attributes of family may vary independently and have its effect.
This is important because theories of personal relationships indicate the importance of closeness of feeling, but influence or help
do not automatically follow closeness. For example, an elderly
mother may feel close to her daughter, but one cannot assume that
she was influenced or helped by the daughter, and each variable
may be related to her death concerns in a different manner.

God as the Ultimate Attachment Figure

From a theoretical viewpoint, one may ask why a belief in God
seems to be so important in the lives of the elderly. The data from
our study indicate that older adults' belief in God is not based on
any reasoning that such a God would be necessary to account for
their own existence and the existence of the world. Nor did the
data indicate a conception of a God who expects people to follow
certain rules of behavior, with punishment if these rules are not
followed. In short, there is little mention of an ethical component
by the older adults we studied. Nor was there much concern for a
spiritual component (with only a few elders mentioning it). There
was little reflection on such questions as how the existence of God
might account for the evils in the world or the catastrophic events
that harm many good and innocent people. Nor was there any
reflection on the fact that people of different religious backgrounds
involved in conflict all feel that God is on their side, that is, that
God endorses their viewpoint above that of others. In short, the
great majority of the elders we studied did not seem to conceptualize God or their relationship to God in broad ways.

Their belief in God seems focused on the conception of a personal, caring God who is more powerful than themselves and who can not only satisfy their physical and emotional needs but who can help give them a vicarious sense of control over an unpredictable world now and in a future life. When we asked elders to describe God or to indicate the things that they pray for, they were concerned primarily with seeking things for themselves. They asked for God to always be there to help them, to satisfy their needs, to love them, and to forgive any transgressions. Obviously, it is important for these older adults to be with such a God, and to experience the resulting security and comfort. These are the same criteria used to establish a relationship with an attachment figure. From a psychological viewpoint, God can be conceptualized as the ultimate attachment figure for religious people.

Other researchers (e.g., Kirkpatrick, 1998, 1999; Pargament, 1997) have already suggested that God is an attachment figure for religious people. Up to a point, our data confirms this viewpoint. However, there were also many individuals who did not seem to fit the characteristics of a religious attachment. The issue then is whether the acceptance of God as an attachment figure depends upon the personality of the individuals involved. Further research is needed to investigate this question in relation to older adults.

Perceived vs. Objective Health Status

Many individuals in our study had health problems and yet they rated themselves as being in good, very good, or excellent health. Most rated their own health positively even in comparison to younger adults. Certainly, self-ratings of health have demonstrated validity and have been found to be excellent predictors of mortality (e.g., Ferraro & Kelley-Moore, 2001). One possibility is that the high self-ratings of health of the older adults we studied were derived from a functional adequacy conception of health. According to a functional adequacy criterion, health is defined in terms of what a person can do regardless of any diseases or symptoms he or she manifests. For example, a person may experience pain and certain other symptoms, but still be able to carry out the everyday activities of living. In this sense, that person would still be defined as healthy. Another possibility is that study participants were being defensive and attempting to maintain self-esteem by evaluating their health as good. There is certainly evidence in the literature for this viewpoint. In the face of adversity, older people make use of many strategies in an attempt to maintain their self concept and self-esteem for as long as possible (e.g., Brandstaedter & Greve, 1994; McCoy, Pyszczynski, Solomon, & Greenberg, 2000). Perhaps more research is needed as to how perceived and objective health may differentially influence older adults' views of death.

Fear of Bodily Destruction

Among the topics discussed in Chapter 9, the paradoxical nature of the fear of bodily destruction found in highly religious older adults who saw death as meaning afterlife was mentioned. If one truly believes that death means the beginning of a joyful afterlife as a noncorporeal spirit, why should one be afraid of the destruction of the body after death. Those who were older, who were of lower socioeconomic status, and who were African American were more likely to have a greater fear of bodily destruction after death. All these subgroups of elders were more likely to be religious and to see death as meaning afterlife. Also, those who had greater proportions of deceased siblings and children were also more likely to have a greater Fear of Being Destroyed. When effects of predictor variables were adjusted in the regression analysis, death as meaning afterlife dropped out of the prediction equation, as did age and ethnicity. If Fear of Being Destroyed is no longer predicted by the death meaning afterlife, but by such life events as the deaths of siblings and children, this suggests that fear of bodily destruction may be related to a more general fear of bodily mutilation (e.g., loss of blood, loss of limbs, etc.) that is rather universal throughout life rather than a specific death-related fear. Those elders of higher socioeconomic status levels seemed better able to separate what happens to the body after death (e.g., autopsy, burial, putrefaction, cremation, etc.) from the more elemental fear of bodily mutilation in life. This is a topic to be explored further in research.

Never Thinking of Death: Defense or Mature Philosophy

During the qualitative interviews, a considerable number of study participants insisted that they simply never thought of death and consequently were not worried or afraid of it. This is particularly puzzling when taken in conjunction with their expectations of having only a limited number of years left to live. We are left with the task of attempting to interpret such a view.

On the one hand, the lack of thoughts of death could be the result of strong defense mechanisms, in which any emerging thoughts of death are denied or repressed, to be dealt with outside of conscious awareness as earlier forms of terror management theory (e. g., Solomon, Greenberg, & Pyszczynski, 1991a) would predict. This is a possible explanation, although it leaves one with the further task of explaining why older adults who don't want to think about death would voluntarily take part in a study in which they were to be interviewed extensively about death.

Another possible explanation is that suggested by various authors (e.g., Johnson & Barer, 1997; McCoy et al., 2000; Neimeyer, Fontana, & Gold, 1984; Wong, 2000) that those who have less fear of death have developed a mature philosophical approach to it. Wong suggests that to overcome the fear of death, individuals need to come to terms with the inevitable reality of death as part of the natural cycle of life, first cognitively and then affectively. He advocates making good use of one's time in life through self-actualization in the accomplishment of meaningful goals. McCoy and colleagues (2000) have outlined a number of strategies that older adults use to deal with the realities of their impending death. Included among these are ways to maintain self-esteem (e.g., downward social comparisons, optimism, redefining standards, minimizing exposure to dissenting opinions, readjusting goals, and reinterpreting events), attaining independence from social validation, creating a more individualized conception of self and the world, increasing self-understanding through life review, and attaining a sense of transcendence through generativity (creating legacies for future generations). The last of these strategies, generativity, had little support from our empirical data. Elders' conception of death as an opportunity for legacy was unrelated to Fear of the Dying

Process, Fear of Being Destroyed, and Fear for Significant Others, and was weakly related to greater Fear of the Unknown. Also, in the qualitative interviews, relatively few elders spoke of any kind of legacy for their heirs or for society at large. Thus one can assume that generativity is not an avenue by which most of the elders we studied attained reduced fear of death. Whether other strategies outlined by McCoy et al. are responsible for the elders' lack of concern with death should be determined in further research.

LIMITATIONS OF THE STUDY: A FURTHER WORD

Many limitations of our empirical study were noted early in this volume, among them the relatively small size and representativeness of the sample. Also, with the possible exception of the fear of death measure (MFODS), the measures of death meanings and the dying process were either relatively new or were devised for the present study.

In addition to the above limitations, the study did not take account of the varying contexts in which study participants lived. Also, even though the study was an exploratory venture into a relatively new field, a better integration of the quantitative and qualitative approaches was needed. In many cases, we were unable to compare findings of the two approaches because relevant questions were not asked in the qualitative interviews. A final limitation of the study was that it was not guided by theory. In one sense, this was an asset because we were free to investigate certain topics that might not have been included in a theory-based study, but use of a theory to guide the study might have led to findings that could confirm or disconfirm predictions from theory.

Despite its limitations and exploratory nature, we were able to summarize some trends in the empirical data and attempt some explanations of study findings. In many cases there was a convergence of findings from the quantitative study, the qualitative study, and the existing literature that increased confidence in the conclusions. Finally, the study enabled us to identify some issues that need to be explored in further study, and to formulate some tentative hypotheses for future research.

ISSUES AND HYPOTHESES FOR FUTURE STUDIES

One aim of the present study was to gain new insights into older adults views of death and factors influencing these views that could be followed up in a more comprehensive study. Although some specific areas for further research were identified in the first portion of this chapter, some more general issues and hypotheses for further study are discussed below.

Age differences and age changes need to be taken more seriously in any future studies of elders' views of death. This study made it clear that one cannot generalize research findings on views of death to all older adults, but must qualify one's conclusions in relation to the age of the individuals in question. Some views varied with age, and a simple young-old and old-old classification was insufficient to demonstrate these age differences when U-shaped age curves were involved. Cross-sectional samples using smaller age categories may better reflect important life changes with age. Of course, studying hypotheses about older adults' changing views of death in longitudinal studies is essential if one is to gain evidence that the early 80s do constitute some kind of transition period when older adults' views change in regard to death. Even short-term longitudinal studies, perhaps over a five-year period, could be of value in determining how death views change over time. They may also be of value in learning how older adults' views of death change in response to contemporary events, such as the terrorist attack on the World Trade Center in New York with its catastrophic loss of life. These are turbulent times, and longitudinal studies may give us insights into how elders' views of death change in response to large numbers of deaths of societal members and to a continuing threat to members of the society.

Second, we were hoping to find some relationships between elders' personal meanings of death, death fears, and views of the dying process, and their reports of personal health, religious beliefs, and relationships with family members. These latter three factors are core areas that pervade and influence many aspects of elders' thoughts and lives. Their hypothesized impact on older adults' personal meanings of death, death fears, and views of the dying process was supported by our empirical study, but needs to be confirmed in larger and more carefully designed studies. The ways in which these variables depend on sociodemographic variables such as gender, ethnicity, socioeconomic status, and age also needs more careful investigation. Future research needs to look for patterns in the relationships of family, health, and religiosity to death views as they vary among subgroups differing on combinations of the sociodemographic variables.

However, any future study needs more refined measures to capture the full impact of these three key factors. This is particularly true in the area of family relationships, where the quality of relationships needs to be taken into account in addition to the family structural characteristics. Families are extremely important to elderly people, but careful distinctions need to be made between closeness of feelings, helping behaviors, and influence of family members on elders' views.

In the case of religion, the relationship between religious beliefs and attachment to God should be clarified. The emotional turmoil revealed by some study participants when a core tenet of religious belief, the existence of God, was challenged as well as the doubts voiced by some participants as to the existence of an afterlife suggests that some measure of strength of beliefs or degree of confidence in beliefs would be useful. Also, further research is needed into the ways in which religious beliefs and behaviors change with increasing age and perceived closeness to death.

Our empirical study did not consider contextual and personality factors, and the influence of these factors has not been studied in previous research, at least insofar as we were able to find in the existing research literature. Future research in this area needs to include basic personality variables. Aspects of personality (both stable and changing aspects) that are related to the way older adults live are also likely to be related to their views about death and may account for some of the differences between subgroups that we observed. Certainly contextual factors should be also given more consideration. The kinds of housing that elder adults live in, different types of neighborhoods, availability of transportation and services, and availability of useful roles for elders are all contextual factors that may influence older adults' feelings of efficacy and participation in ongoing community life and in turn influence their views of death.

Future studies need to investigate further the factors influencing elders' desired time left to live in view of the fact that no one wished to become a centenarian. Although poor health and lack of close relationships may be understandable reasons for desiring a shorter life span, the effect of religious beliefs, lack of meaningful roles in later life, and various cultural signals on older adults' desired life span needs to be investigated.

Finally, earlier studies established some connections between older adults' fear of death and their end-of-life decision preferences. Including knowledge of elders' personal meanings of death and their expectations about the dying process in such studies should lead to a better understanding of their end-of-life decisions and suggestions for improved care during the dying process.

A FUTURE PERSPECTIVE

We have pointed out a number of questions and issues in connection with older adults' views on death, as well as suggestions for further research. However, approaching research questions item by item will not yield a full understanding of a complex area such as older adults' views on death. One needs to look at the data provided in this and other studies as a basis for formulating a broad perspective on how individuals cope with perceptions of death, that is, the meanings they give to death, their understanding and expectations about the dying process, and their fears of death and the dying process. For some individuals, death and dying will be very stressful events. The extent to which this is true may depend on various sociocultural influences as well as on specific cognitions, feelings, and experiences of the individual. Gaining an understanding of all the factors influencing the older individual's views of death may enable gerontologists to suggests appropriate kinds of emotional support and coping strategies to help that person deal with fears of approaching death. Interventions based on family relationships, religious beliefs, age related health changes, and so on, can aim to instill more positive meanings of death, reduce fears of death, and provide a more realistic understanding of the dying process.

Existing theoretical approaches such as terror management theory (e.g., Solomon et al., 1991a; McCoy et al., 2000) or the Tomer and Eliason (2000a) comprehensive model of death anxiety offer possible starting points for a broad perspective for future research. Another possibility is to start with an empirically based path modeling scheme, fitting known variables influencing elders' death views into a more comprehensive causal model. However, any such attempts need to include a broader cultural framework that explains the effects of the larger culture on the individual's views of death.

The fact of death itself is the core idea that generates and integrates the social and personal meanings of death and fears about death and/or dying. Becoming aware of the fact that death ends man's earthly existence produces a basic fear of death. The fact of death and the fear of death have led to the development of social and cultural institutions to prevent premature death and provide care during the dying process. The societal meanings of death that are generated become part of the culture that helps to regulate the societal functions necessary to carry out the protective and caring functions (as well as the utilitarian functions of dealing with the dead). How we as individuals cope with the phenomena of death is related to the functions of these societal institutions. They provide emotional support as well as opportunities to learn and develop the knowledge, skills, and maturity of personality to deal with death.

We started this book based on the idea of many other researchers and scholars that death itself is the driving force that generates societies to help protect individuals from premature death and to care for them during the dying process, and that one task of the culture is to establish social meanings of death which regulate group behavior to carry out the tasks necessarily to accomplish these goals. Eventually, the personal meanings and fears of death on the individual level not only influence the daily living of people but also may feed back to modify the social meanings of death and the functioning of society. In effect, such thinking is a modification of Kastenbaum's (1995, 2000b) conception of the death system.

The death system itself can be looked upon as only a subsystem of a broader societal system. Thus, the death subsystem should have the properties of any system, with all the components inter-dependent and mutually influencing each other. Also, it fits the category of a dynamic nonlinear system, in that change over time is inevitable as society evolves and that relatively small changes in one part of the system may have large repercussions in changing the system itself.

For example, the death of more than 3,000 people as the result of the recent terrorist attacks may be a small number relative to the total society, but its effect has led to many subsequent changes in society to protect other citizens from such premature death. As these changes take place, those members of society assuming responsibility for regulating the death system need to develop a more efficient procedure for dealing with catastrophic events that are quite disruptive of society's functions.

We live in a society that is a highly technical and complex system, such that catastrophic current events have rapid effects and can influence many kinds of future events that could threaten the society as a whole. To avoid these possibilities, an interventionist perspective should be a strong component of the death system in order to anticipate and deal with negative changes in social and personal meanings of death that may be disruptive of the death system and society itself. One general strategy would be to determine where small interventions in the death system could produce large positive effects, that is, nonlinear change. For example, one might support and promote the religious beliefs of societal members to a greater extent if they lead to changes in personal meanings of death that reduce the stress on individuals caused by fear of death. Many other ideas could be considered at multiple levels of the system, e.g., intervening at the level of personal meanings, social meanings, the functioning of society itself, or developing a system to anticipate and lessen the impact of negative events. Whatever improvements that interventions can bring about in the larger system should eventually lead to positive changes in older adults' views of death and enable them to proceed through the dying process more easily.

References

"A nation challenged: dead and missing." (2002, February 24). *New York Times*, p. A12.

Addison, R. B. (1992). Grounded hermeneutic research. In B. F. Crabtree & W. L. Miller (Eds.), *Doing qualitative research* (pp. 110–124). Newbury Park, CA: Sage.

Aiken, L. R. (2001) (4th Ed.). *Dying, death, and bereavement.* Mahwah, NJ: Lawrence Erlbaum Associates.

Ainlay, S. C., & Smith, R. (1984). Aging and religious participation. *Journal of Gerontology, 39,* 357–63.

Ainsworth, M. D. S. (1989). Attachments beyond infancy. *American Psychologist, 44,* 709–716.

Angier, N. (2001, May 6). Together, in sickness and in health. *New York Times Magazine,* pp. 67–69.

Antonucci, T. C., & Akiyama, H. (1991). Convoys of social support: Generational issues. *Marriage and Family Review, 16,* 103–123.

Baltes, P. B. (1997). On the incomplete architecture of human ontogeny: Selection, optimization, and compensation as foundation of developmental theory. *American Psychologist, 52,* 366–380.

Baumeister, R. F. (1991). *Meanings of life.* New York: The Guilford Press.

Becker, E. (1973). *The denial of death.* New York: Free Press.

Bengtson, V. I., Cuellar, J. B., & Ragan, P. K. (1977). Stratum contrasts and similarities in attitudes toward death. *Journal of Gerontology, 32,* 76–88.

Bengtson, V. L., Reedy, M. N., & Gordon, C. (1985). Aging and self-conceptions: Personality processes and social contexts. In J. E. Birren & K. W. Schaie (Eds.), *Handbook of the psychology of aging* (2nd ed., pp. 544–594). New York: Van Nostrand Reinhold.

Benyamini, Y., & Idler, E. I. (1999). Community studies reporting association between self-rated health and mortality. *Research on Aging, 21,* 392–401.

Birren, J. E., & Zarit, J. M. (1985). Concepts of health, behavior, and aging. In J. E. Birren & J. Livingston (Eds.), *Cognition, stress, and aging* (pp. 1–20). Englewood Cliffs, NJ: Prentice-Hall.

Blendon, R. J., Szalay, U. S., & Knox, R. A. (1992). Should physicians aid their patients in dying? The patient's perspective. *Journal of the American Medical Association, 267,* 2658–2662.

Bowlby, J. (1979). *The making and breaking of affectional bonds.* London: Tavistock.

Bowlby, J. (1980). *Attachment and loss. Vol. 3. Loss, stress, and depression.* New York: Basic books.

Bradburn, N. M. (1969). *The structure of psychological well being.* Chicago: Aldine.

Bradley, E. H., Fried, T. R., Kasl, S. V., & Idler, E. (2001). Quality-of-life-trajectories of elders in the end of life. In M. P. Lawton (Series & Vol. Ed.), *Annual Review of Gerontology and Geriatrics: Vol. 20, 2000. Focus on the end of life: Scientific and social issues* (pp. 64–96). New York: Springer Publishing Company.

Brandstaedter, J., & Greve, W. (1994). The aging self: Stabilizing and protective processes. *Developmental Review, 14,* 52–80.

Brent, S. R., & Speece, M. W. (1993). "Adult" conceptions of irreversibility: Implications for the development of a concept of death. *Death Studies, 17,* 203–224.

Brubaker, T. H. (1983). Introduction. In T. H. Brubaker (Ed.), *Family relationships in later life* (pp. 9–18). Beverly Hills, CA: Sage.

Brunner, B. (Ed.). (1999). *The Time Almanac 1999.* Boston: Information Please, LLC.

Butler, R. N. (1963). The life review: An interpretation of reminiscence in the aged. *Psychiatry, 26,* 65–76.

Callahan, D. (1995). No one has the right to make decisions in support of euthanasia. In C. Wekesser (Ed.), *Euthanasia: Opposing viewpoints* (pp. 115–119). San Diego, CA: Greenhaven Press.

Capital punishment and homicide rates. (2001, July 22). *New York Times,* p. 21.

Capuzzo, M. (2001). *Close to shore: A true story of terror in an age of innocence.* New York: Broadway Books.

Carney, S. S., Rich, C. L., Burke, P. A., & Fowler, R. C. (1994). Suicide over 60: The San Diego study. *Journal of the American Geriatrics Society, 42,* 174–180.

Carstensen, L. L. (1992). Motivation for social contact across the lifespan: A theory of socioemotional selectivity. In J. E. Jacobs (Ed.), *Nebraska Symposium on Motivation, 1992. Developmental perspectives on motivation* (pp. 209–254). Lincoln, NE: University of Nebraska Press.

Carstensen, L. L. (1995). Evidence for a life-span theory of socioemotional selectivity. *Current Directions in Psychological Science, 4,* 151–156.

Chatters, L. M., Levin, J. S., & Taylor, R. J. (1992). Antecedents and dimension of religious involvement among older Black adults. *Journal of Gerontology, 47,* S269–S278.

Chochinov, H. M., Tataryn, D., Clinch, J. J., & Dudgeon, D. (1999). Will to live in the terminally ill. *The Lancet, 354,* 816–819.

Choice in Dying, Inc. (1993). *State statutes governing living wills and appointment of health care agents.* New York: Author.

Cicirelli, V. G. (1982, December). *Influence of adult children on health and health problems of advanced elderly parents.* Report to the AARP Andrus Foundation. West Lafayette, IN: Author.

Cicirelli, V. G. (1989, July). *Influence of siblings' death on subjective well-being in old age.* Paper presented at the Xth Biennial Meetings of the International Society for the Study of Behavioural Development, Jyvaskyla, Finland.

Cicirelli, V. G. (1991). Attachment theory in old age: Protection of the attached figure. In K. Pillemer & K. McCartney (Eds.), *Parent-child relations across the life span* (pp. 25–42). Hillsdale, NJ: Erlbaum.

Cicirelli, V. G. (1995a). A measure of caregiving daughters' attachment to elderly mothers. *Journal of Family Psychology, 9,* 89–94.

Cicirelli, V. G. (1995b, December). *Personality factors related to elders' end-of-life decisions. Study I.* Report to the AARP Andrus Foundation. West Lafayette, IN: Author.

Cicirelli, V. G. (1995c). *Sibling relationships across the life span.* New York: Plenum.

Cicirelli, V. G. (1997). Relationship of psychosocial and background variables to older adults' end-of-life decisions. *Psychology and Aging, 12,* 72–83.

Cicirelli, V. G. (1998a). Intergenerational relationships in modern families. In L. L'Abate (Ed.), *Handbook of family psychopathology* (pp. 185–206). New York: Guilford Press.

Cicirelli, V. G. (1998b). Personal meanings of death in relation to fear of death. *Death Studies, 22,* 713–733.

Cicirelli, V. G. (1998c). Views of elderly people concerning end-of-life decisions. *Journal of Applied Gerontology, 17,* 186–203.

Cicirelli, V. G. (1999). Personality and demographic factors in older adults' fear of death. *The Gerontologist, 39,* 569–579.

Cicirelli, V. G. (2000). Older adults' ethnicity, fear of death, and end-of-life decisions. In A. Tomer (Ed.), *Death attitudes and the older adult: Theories, concepts, and applications* (pp. 175–191). Philadelphia, PA: Taylor & Francis.

Cicirelli, V. G. (2001a). Healthy elders' early decisions for end-of-life living and dying. In M. P. Lawton (Vol. & Series Ed.), *Focus on the end* of life: Scientific and social issues. Vol. 20. Annual Review of Gerontology and Geriatrics (pp. 163–192). New York: Springer Publishing.

Cicirelli, V. G. (2001b). Personal meanings of death in older adults and young adults in relation to their fears of death. *Death Studies, 25,* 663–683.

Clement, R. (1998). Intrinsic religious motivation and attitudes toward death among the elderly. *Current Psychology: Developmental, Learning, Personality, Social, 17,* 237–248.

Cloud, J. A. (2000, September 18). A kinder, gentler death. *Time, 156*(12), 60–67.

Cohen-Mansfield, J., Droge, J. A., & Billig, N. (1992). Factors influencing hospital patients preferences in the utilization of life-sustaining treatments. *Gerontologist, 32,* 89–95.

Connidis, I. A. (2001). *Family ties and aging.* Thousand Oaks, CA: Sage.

Conte, H. R., Weiner, M. B., & Plutchik, R. (1982). Measuring death anxiety: Conceptual, psychometric, and factor analytic aspects. *Journal of Personality and Social Psychology, 43,* 775–785.

Cook, A. S., & Oltjenbruns, K. A. (1998). *Dying and grieving: Life span and family perspective* (2nd ed.). Fort Worth, TX: Harcourt Brace.

Corr, C. A., Nabe, M. C., & Corr, D. M. (2000). *Death and dying, life and living* (3rd ed.). Belmont, CA: Wadsworth.

Crimmins, E. M., Saito, Y., & Reynolds, S. L. (1997). Further evidence on recent trends in the prevalence and incidence of disability among older Americans from two sources: the LSOA and the NHIS. *Journal of Gerontology: Social Sciences, 52B,* S59–S71.

Danis, M., Garrett, J., Harris, R., & Patrick, D. L. (1994). Stability of choices about life-sustaining treatments. *Annals of Internal Medicine, 120,* 567–573.

Danis, M., Patrick, D. L., Southerland, L. I., & Green, M. (1988). Patients' and families' preferences for medical intensive care. *Journal of the American Medical Association, 260,* 797–802.

Dattel, A. R., & Neimeyer, R. A. (1990). Sex differences in death anxiety: Testing the emotional expressiveness hypothesis. *Death Studies, 14,* 1–11.

Davies, N. (1996). *Europe: A history.* New York: Oxford University Press.

Davis, S. F., Bremer, S. A., Anderson, B. J., & Tramill, J. L. (1983). The interrelationships of ego strength, self-esteem, death anxiety and gender in undergraduate college students. *Journal of General Psychology, 108,* 419–422.

Davis, S. F., Martin, D. A., Wilee, C. T., & Voorhees, J. W. (1980). Relationship of fear of death and level of self-esteem in college students. *Psychological Reports, 42,* 419–422.

Deeg, D. J. H., Kardaun, J. W. P. F., & Fozard, J. L. (1996). Health, behavior, and aging. In K. W. Schaie & J. E. Birren (Eds.), *Handbook of the psychology of aging* (4th ed., pp. 129–149). San Diego: Academic Press.

DeSpelder, L. A., & Strickland, A. L. (2002). *The last dance* (6th ed.). Boston: McGraw-Hill.

deVries, B., & Blando, J. A. (2001). Friendship at the end of life. In M. P. Lawton (Vol. & Series Ed.), *Focus on the end of life: Scientific and social issues. Vol. 20. Annual Review of Gerontology and Geriatrics* (pp. 144–162). New York: Springer Publishing.

Diamond, E. L., Jernigan, J. A., Moseley, R. A., Messina, V., & McKeown, R. A. (1989). Decision-making abilities and advance directive preferences in nursing home patients and proxies. *Gerontologist, 29,* 622–626.

Dietz, B. E. (1996). The relationship of aging to self-esteem: The relative effects of maturation and role accumulation. *International Journal of Aging and Human Development, 43,* 249–266.

Ditto, P. H., Druley, J. A., Moore, K. A., Danks, J. H., & Smucker, W. D. (1996). Fates worse than death: The role of valued life activities in health-state evaluation. *Health Psychology, 15,* 332–343.

Dixon, N. (1998). On the difference between physician-assisted suicide and active euthanasia. *Hastings Center Report, 28,* 25–29.

Dodd, D. K., & Mills, L. L. (1985). FADIS: A measure of the fear of accidental death and injury. *Psychological Record, 35,* 269–275.

Downey, A. M. (1984). Relationship of religiosity to death anxiety in middle-aged males. *Psychological Reports, 54,* 811–822.

Dugger, C. W. (2001, May 6). Why abortions of female fetuses are rising in China and India. *New York Times,* p. 4.

Dunkle, R., Roberts, B., & Haug, M. (2001). *The oldest old in everyday life.* New York: Springer Publishing.

Durlak, J. A., Horn, W., & Kass, R.A. (1990). A self-administering assessment of personal meanings of death. *Omega, 21,* 301–309.

Ehrlich, P. R., (1968). *The population bomb.* New York: Ballantine Books.

Ehrlich, P. R., &, Ehrlich, A. (1990). *The population explosion.* New York: Simon & Shuster.

Eleazar, G. P., Hornung, C. A., Egbert, C. B., Egbert, J. R., Eng, C., Hedgepeth, J., McCann, R., Strothers, J., III, Sapir, M., Wei, M., & Wilson, M. (1996). The relationship between ethnicity and advance directives in a frail older population. *Journal of the American Geriatrics Society, 44,* 938–943.

Emanuel, E. J., & Emanuel, L. L.(1998). The promise of a good death. *The Lancet, 351 (Suppl II),* 21–29.

Erikson, E. (1959). Identity and the life cycle: Selected papers. *Psychological Issues, 1*, 1–171.

Erikson, E. H. (1963). *Childhood and society* (Rev. ed.). New York: Norton.

Erikson, E. H. (1982). *The life cycle completed.* New York: Norton.

Everhart, B. S., & Pearlman, R. A. (1990). Stability of patient preferences regarding life-sustaining treatments. *Chest, 97*, 159–164.

Fago, J. A. P. (2001). Physical aspects of dying. In K. L. Braun, J. H. Pietsch, & P. L. Blanchette (Eds.), *Cultural issues in end-of-life decision making* (pp. 13–22). Thousand Oaks, CA: Sage.

Feifel, H. (1990). Psychology and death: Meaningful rediscovery. *American Psychologist, 45*, 537–543.

Ferraro, K. (1985). The effect of widowhood on the health status of older persons. *International Journal of Aging and Human Development, 21*, 9–25.

Ferraro, K., & Kelley-Moore, J. A. (2001). Self-rated health and mortality among Black and White adults: Examining the dynamic evaluation thesis. *Journal of Gerontology: Social Sciences, 56B*, S195–S205.

Field, M. J., & Cassel, C. K. (Eds.).(1997). *Approaching death: Improving care at the end of life.* Washington, DC: National Academy Press.

Florian, V., & Kravitz, S. (1983). Fear of personal death: Attribution, structure, and relation to religious belief. *Journal of Personality and Social Psychology, 44*, 600–607.

Fortner, B. V., Neimeyer, R. A., & Rybarczyk, B. (2000). Correlates of death anxiety in older adults: A comprehensive review. In A. Tomer (Ed.), *Death attitudes and the older adult: Theories, concepts, and applications* (pp. 95–108). Philadelphia, PA: Taylor & Francis.

Frankl, V. E. (1963). *Man's search for meaning.* Boston: Beacon Press. (Original work published in 1959).

Fry, P. S. (1990). A factor analytic investigation of home-bound elderly individuals' concerns about death and dying, and their coping responses. *Journal of Clinical Psychologicy, 46*, 737–748.

Galt, C. P., & Hayslip, B., Jr. (1998). Age differences in the level of overt and covert death anxiety. *Omega, 37*, 187–202.

Gavrin, J. K., & Chapman, C. R. (1995). Clinical management of dying patients, *Western Journal of Medicine, 163*, 268–277.

Gelles, R., & Levine, A. (1999). *Sociology* (6th ed.). Boston: McGraw-Hill.

Gesser, G., Wong, P. T. P., & Reker, G. T. (1987–1988). Death attitudes across the life span: The development and validation of the death attitude profile (DAP). *Omega, 18*, 113–128.

Glaser, B. G., & Strauss, A. L. (1968). *Time for dying.* Chicago. Aldine Publishing Company.

Greenberg, J., Pyszczynski, T., Solomon, S., Simon, L., & Breus, M. (1994). Role of consciousness and accessibility of death-related thoughts in mortality salience effects. *Journal of Personality and Social Psychology*, *67*, 627–637.

Greenberg, J., Solomon, S, & Pyszczynski, T. (1997). Terror management theory of self-esteem and cultural worldviews: Empirical assessments and conceptual refinements. In M. P. Zanna (Ed.), *Advances in Experimental Social Psychology. Vol. 29* (pp. 61–139). San Diego: Academic Press.

Greyson, B. (1994). Reduced death threat in near-death experiencers. In R. A. Neimeyer (Ed.), *Death anxiety handbook: Research, instrumentation, and application* (pp. 169–179). Washington, DC: Taylor & Francis.

Guralnik, J. M., & Kaplan, G. A. (1989). Predictors of healthy aging: Prospective evidence from the Alameda County study. *American Journal of Public Health, 79*, 703–708.

Heckler, R. A. (1994). *Waking up, alive.* New York: Ballantine Books.

Heidegger, M. (1962). *Being and time* (J. Macquarrie & E. Robinson, Trans.). London: SCM Press, Ltd. (Original work published 1927).

Henderson, M. (1990). Beyond the living will. *Gerontologist, 30*, 480–485.

Hendin, D. (1973). *Death as a fact of life.* New York: Warner Paperback Library.

Hendon, M. K., & Epting, F. R. (1989). A comparison of hospice patients with recovering and ill patients. *Death Studies, 13*, 567–578.

Hendricks, J. (1996). Qualitative research: Contributions and advances. In R. H. Binstock & L. K. George (Eds.), *Handbook of aging and the social sciences* (4th ed., pp. 52–72). San Diego: Academic Press.

High, D. M. (1993a). Advance directives and the elderly: A study of intervention strategies to increase use. *Gerontologist, 33*, 342–350.

High, D. M. (1993b). Why are elderly people not using advance directives? *Journal of Aging and Health, 5*, 497–515.

Hintze, J., Templer, D. I., Capelletty, G. G., & Frederick, W. (1994). Death depression and death anxiety in HIV-infected males. In R. A. Neimeyer (Ed.), *Death anxiety handbook: Research, instrumentation, and application* (pp. 193–200). Washington, DC: Taylor & Francis.

Hoelter, J. W. (1979). Multidimensional treatment of death. *Journal of Consulting and Clinical Psychology, 47*, 996–999.

Holcomb, L. E., Neimeyer, R. A., & Moore, M. K. (1993). Personal meanings of death: A content analysis of free-response narratives. *Death Studies, 17*, 299–318.

Hollingshead, A. B. (1957). *Two-factor index of social position.* New Haven, CT: Author.

Hood, R. W., Jr., Spilka, B., Hunsberger, B., & Gorsuch, R. (1996). *The psychology of religion: An empirical approach* (2nd ed.). New York: Guilford Press.

Hurley, A. C., Volicer, L., & Mahoney, E. K. (2001). Comfort in older adults at the end of life. In M. P. Lawton (Series & Vol. Ed.), *Annual Review of Gerontology and Geriatrics. Vol. 20, 2000. Focus on the end of life: Scientific and social issues* (pp. 120–143). New York: Springer Publishing.

Institute of Medicine. (1997). *Approaching death: Improving care at the end of life.* Washington, DC.: National Academy Press.

Johnson, C. L., & Barer, B. M. (1997). *Life beyond 85 years: The aura of survivorship.* New York: Springer Publishing.

Kalish, R. A. (1981). *Death, grief, and caring relationships.* Monterey, CA: Brooks-Cole.

Kalish, R. A. (1985). The social context of death and dying. In R. H. Binstock & E. Shanas (Eds.), *Handbook of aging and the social sciences* (2nd ed., pp. 149–170). New York: Van Nostrand Reinhold.

Kart, C. S., & Kinney, J. M. (2001). *The realities of aging.* Boston: Allyn & Bacon.

Kastenbaum, R. J. (1992). *The psychology of death* (2nd ed.). New York: Springer Publishing.

Kastenbaum, R. (1995). *Death, society, and human experience* (5th ed.). Boston: Allyn & Bacon.

Kastenbaum, R. (1996). A world without death? First and second thoughts. *Mortality, 1,* 141–153.

Kastenbaum, R. (2000a). Death attitudes and aging in the 21st century. In A. Tomer (Ed.), *Death attitudes and the older adult: Theories, concepts, and applications* (pp. 257–280). Philadelphia, PA: Taylor & Francis.

Kastenbaum, R. (2000b). *The psychology of death* (3rd ed.). New York: Springer Publishing.

Kastenbaum, R., & Herman, C. (1997). Death personifications in the Kevorkian era. *Death Studies, 21,* 115–130.

Kearl, M. C. (1989). *Endings: A sociology of death and dying.* New York: Oxford University Press.

Kelly, G. (1955). *The psychology of personal constructs.* New York: Norton.

Kight, M. (1998). *Forever changed: Remembering Oklahoma City, April 19, 1995.* Amherst, NY: Prometheus Books.

Kirkpatrick, L. A. (1998). God as a substitute attachment figure: A longitudinal study of adult attachment style and religious change in college students. *Personality and Social Psychology Bulletin, 24,* 961–973.

Kirkpatrick, L. A. (1999). Attachment and religious representations and behavior. In J. Cassidy & P. Shaver (Eds.), *Handbook of attachment: Theory, research, and clinical applications* (pp. 803–822). New York: Guilford Press.

Koenig, H. G., Smiley, M., & Gonzales, J. A. P. (1988). *Religion, health, and aging.* New York: Greenwood.

Krause, N. (1993). Measuring religiosity in late life. *Research on Aging, 15,* 170–197.

Krause, N., Chatters, L. M., Meltzer, T., & Morgan, D. L. (2000). Using focus groups to explore the nature of prayer in late life. *Journal of Aging Studies, 14,* 191–212.

Krause, N., & Tran, T. V. (1989). Stress and religious involvement among older Blacks. *Journal of Gerontology: Social Sciences, 44,* S4–S13.

Kubler-Ross, E. (1969). *On death and dying.* New York: Macmillan.

Kubler-Ross, E. (1997). *The wheel of life: A memoir of living and dying.* New York: Simon & Schuster.

Kunkel, S. R., & Applebaum, R. A. (1992). Estimating the prevalence of long-term disability for an aging society. *Journal of Gerontology: Social Sciences, 47B,* S253–S260.

Kureshi, A., & Husain, A. (1981). Death anxiety in intrapunitiveness among smokers and nonsmokers: A comparative study. *Journal of Psychological Research, 25,* 42–45.

Labouvie-Vief, G. (1982). Dynamic development and mature autonomy: A theoretical prologue. *Human Development, 25,* 161–191.

Lang, F. R. (2000). Endings and continuities of social relationships: Maximizing intrinsic benefits within personal networks when feeling near to death. *Journal of Social and Personal Relationships, 17,* 155–182.

LaRue, A., Bank, I., Jarvik, L., & Hetland, M. (1979). Health in old age: How do physicians' ratings and self-ratings compare? *Journal of Gerontology, 8,* 108–115.

Lawton, M. P. (1972). Assessing the competence of older people. In D. Kent, R. Kastenbaum, & R. Sherwood (Eds.), *Research planning and action for the elderly* (pp. 122–143). New York: Behavioral Publications.

Lawton, M. P. (2000). Quality of life, depression, and end-of-life attitudes and behaviors. In G. M. Williamson, D. R. Shaffer, & P. A. Parmelee (Eds.), *Physical illness and depression in older adults: A handbook of theory, research, and practice* (pp. 229–258). New York: Plenum.

Lawton, M. P., Moss, M., Fulcomer, M., & Kleban, M. H. (1982). A research and service-oriented multilevel assessment instrument. *Journal of Gerontology, 37,* 91–99.

Lawton, M. P., Moss, M., & Glicksman, A. (1990). The quality of the last year of life of older persons. *Milbank Quarterly, 68,* 1–28.

Leinbach, R. M. (1993). Euthanasia attitudes of older persons: A cohort analysis. *Research on Aging, 15,* 433–445.

Leming, M. R. (1979–1980). Religion and death: A test of Homan's thesis. *Omega, 10,* 347–364.

Leming, M. R., & Dickinson, G. E. (1985). *Understanding death, dying, and bereavement.* New York: Holt, Rinehart, & Winston.

Lester, D. (1994). The Collett-Lester Fear of Death Scale. In R. A. Neimeyer (Ed.), *The death anxiety handbook: Research, instrumentation, and application* (pp. 45–60). Washington, DC: Taylor & Francis.

Levin, J. S. (1997). Religious research in gerontology 1980–1994: A systematic review. *Journal of Religious Gerontology, 10,* 3–31.

Levenson, H. (1981). Differentiating among internality, powerful others, and change. In H. M. Lefcourt (Ed.), *Research with the locus of control concept* (Vol. 1, pp. 15–63). New York: Academic Press.

Levenson, J. W., McCarthy, E. P., Lynn, J., Davis, R. B., & Phillips, R. S. (2000). The last six months of life for patients with congestive heart failure. *Journal of the American Geriatrics Society, 48,* S101–S109.

Lifton, R. J. (1983). *The broken connection: On death and continuity of life.* New York: Basic Books.

Lonetto, R., & Templer, D. I. (1986). *Death anxiety.* Washington, DC: Hemisphere Publishing.

Lynn, J., Teno, J. M., Phillips, R. S., Wu, A. W., Desbiens, N., Harrold, J., Claessens, M. T., Wenger, N., Kreling, B., & Connors., A. F. Jr. (1997). Perceptions by faculty members of the dying experience of older and seriously ill patients: SUPPORT investigators—Study to understand prognoses and preferences for outcomes and risks of treatments. *Annals of Internal Medicine, 126,* 97–106.

MacDonald, W. L. (1998). Situational factors and attitudes toward voluntary euthanasia. *Social Science and Medicine, 46,* 73–81.

Maddi, S. (1970). The search for meaning. In W. J. Arnold, & M. Page (Eds.), *Nebraska symposium on motivation* (pp. 137–186). Lincoln: University of Nebraska Press.

Malloy, T. R., Wigton, R. S., Meeske, J., & Tape, T. G. (1992). The influence of treatment descriptions on advance medical directive decisions. *Journal of the American Geriatrics Society, 40,* 1255–1260.

Manton, K. G. (1992). Mortality and life expectancy changes among the oldest old. In R. M. Suzman, D. P. Willis, & K. G. Manton (Eds.), *The oldest old* (pp. 157–182), New York: Oxford University Press.

Marshall, V. W. (1980). *Last chapters: A sociology of aging and dying.* Monterey, CA: Brooks/Cole Publishing.

Maslow, A. H. (1968). *Toward a psychology of being* (2nd ed.). New York: Van Nostrand Reinhold.

Maslow, A. H. (1970). *Motivation and personality* (2nd ed.). New York: Harper and Row.

Mazur, D. J., & Merz, J. F. (1996). Patients' willingness to accept life-sustaining treatment which the expected outcome is a diminished mental health state: An exploratory study. *Journal of the American Geriatrics Society, 44,* 565–568.

McCoy, S. K., Pyszczynski,, T., Solomon, S., & Greenberg, J. (2000). Transcending the self: A terror management perspective on successful aging. In A. Tomer (Ed.), *Death attitudes and the older adult: Theories, concepts, and applications* (pp. 37–63). Philadelphia, PA: Taylor & Francis.

McFadden, S. H., & Levin, J. S. (1996). Religion, emotions, and health. In C. Magai & S. H. McFadden (Eds.), *Handbook of emotion, adult development, and aging* (pp. 349–362). San Diego, CA: Academic Press.

McGuire, F. L. (1976). Personality factors in highway accidents. *Human Factors, 18,* 433–442.

Moller, D. W. (1996). *Confronting death.* New York: Oxford University Press.

Moody, R. A. (1975). *Life after life.* Covington, GA: Mockingbird Books.

Moore, C. D., & Sherman, S. R. (1999). Factors that influence elders' decisions to formulate advance directives. *Journal of Gerontological Social Work, 34,* 21–37.

Moore, D. W. (1997, January). Willingness to support doctor-assisted suicide—only slightly affected by whether pain is mentioned in the question. *Gallup Poll Monthly, 376,* 28–30.

Morris, J. N., Suissa, S., Sherwood, S., Wright, S. M., & Greer, D. (1986). Last days: A study of the quality of life of terminally ill cancer patients. *Journal of Chronic Disease, 39,* 47–62.

Moss, M., Lawton, M. P., & Glicksman, A. (1991). The role of pain in the last year of life of older persons. *Journal of Gerontology: Psychological Sciences, 46,* P51–P57.

Moss, S. Z., & Moss, M. S. (1989). Death of an elderly sibling. *American Behavioral Scientist, 33,* 94–108.

Mullins, L. C., & Lopez, M. A. (1982). Death anxiety among nursing home residents: A comparison of the young-old and the old-old. *Death Education, 6,* 75–86.

Mutran, E. J., Danis, M., Bratton, K. A., Sudha, S., & Hanson, L. (1997). Attitudes of the critically ill toward prolonging life: The role of social support. *Gerontologist, 37,* 192–199.

Nadeau, J. W. (1998). *Families making sense of death.* Thousand Oaks: CA. Sage Publications.

Nagy, M. (1948). The child's theories concerning death. *Journal of Genetic Psychology, 73,* 3–27.

National Safety Council (1999). *Injury facts, 1999 edition.* Chicago: Author.

Neimeyer, R. A. (1988). Death anxiety. In H. Wass, R. Berardo, & R. A. Neimeyer (Eds.), *Dying: Facing the facts* (2nd ed., pp. 97–136). Washington, DC: Hemisphere Publishing.

Neimeyer, R. A. (Ed.).(1994a). *Death anxiety handbook: Research, instrumentation, and application.* Washington, DC: Taylor & Francis.

Neimeyer, R. A. (1994b). The Threat Index and related methods. In R. A. Neimeyer (Ed.), *Death anxiety handbook: Research, instrumentation, and application* (pp. 61–101). Washington, DC: Taylor & Francis.

Neimeyer, R. A., & Dingemans, P. (1980). Death orientation in the suicide intervention worker. *Omega, 11,* 15–23.

Neimeyer, R. A., Dingemans, P., & Epting, F. R. (1977). Convergent validity, situational stability, and meaningfulness of the Threat Index. *Omega, 8,* 251–265.

Neimeyer, R. A., Fontana, D. J., & Gold, K. (1984). A manual for content analysis of death constructs. In F. R. Epting & R. A. Neimeyer (Eds.), *Personal meanings of death* (pp. 213–234). Washington, DC: Hemisphere Publishing.

Neimeyer, R. A., & Moore, M. K. (1994). Validation and reliability of the Multidimensional Fear of Death Scale. In R. A. Neimeyer (Ed.), *Death anxiety handbook: Research, instrumentation, and application* (pp. 103–119). Washington, DC: Taylor & Francis.

Neimeyer, R. A., & Van Brunt, D. (1995). Death anxiety. In H. Wass & R. A. Neimeyer (Eds.), *Dying: Facing the facts* (3rd ed.) (pp. 49–88). Washington, DC: Taylor & Francis.

Noppe, I. C., & Noppe, L. D. (1997). Evolving meanings of death during early, middle, and later adolescence. *Death Studies, 21,* 253–275.

Pargament, K. I. (1997). *The psychology of religion and coping: Theory, research, and practice.* New York: Guilford Press.

Pargament, K. I., Koenig, H. G., Tarakeshwar, N., & Hahn, J. (2001). Religious struggle as a predictor of mortality among medically ill elderly patients: A 2-year longitudinal study. *Archives of Internal Medicine, 161,* 1881–1885.

Parkes, C. M. (1996). Genocide in Rwanda: Personal reflections. *Mortality, 1,* 95–110.

Pattison, E. M. (1977). *The experience of dying.* Englewood Cliffs, NJ: Prentice Hall.

Perls, T. T. (1998). The oldest old. *Scientific American, 272*(1), 70–75.

Perls, T. T., & Silver, M. H. (1999). *Living to 100: Lessons in living to your maximum potential at any age.* New York: Basic Books.

Petrisek, A. C., & Mor, V. (1999). Hospice in nursing homes: A facility-level analysis of the distribution of hospice beneficiaries. *Gerontologist, 39,* 279–290.

Pollak, J. M. (1979–1980). Correlates of death anxiety: A review of empirical studies. *Omega, 10,* 97–121.

Potter, J. M., Stewart, D., & Duncan, G. (1994). Living wills: Would sick people change their minds? *Postgraduate Medicine, 70,* 818–820.

Prado, C. G. (1998). *The last choice: Preemptive suicide in advanced old age* (2nd ed.). Westport, CT: Praeger.

Pyszczynski, T., Greenberg, J., & Solomon, S. (1999). A dual-process model of defense against conscious and unconscious death-related thoughts: An extension of terror management theory. *Psychological Review, 106,* 835–845.

Rees, E., Hardy, J., Ling, J., Broadley, K., & A'Hern, R. (1998). The use of the Edmonton Symptom Assessment Scale (ESAS) within a palliative care unit in the UK. *Palliative Medicine, 12,* 75–82.

Richards, L. (1999). *Using NVivo in qualitative research.* Melbourne, Australia: Qualitative Solutions and Research.

Rigdon, M. A., & Epting, F. R. (1985). Reduction in death threat as a basis for optimal functioning. *Death Studies, 9,* 427–448.

Rimer, S. (1998, June 22). As centenarians thrive, "old" is redefined. *The New York Times,* pp. A1, A14.

Robinson, P. J., & Wood, K. (1983). Fear of death and physical illness. *Death Education, 7,* 139–144.

Rogers, C. R. (1959). A theory of therapy, personality, and interpersonal relationships, as developed in the client-centered framework. In S. Koch (Ed.), *Psychology: A study of a science* (Vol. 3, pp. 184–256). New York: McGraw-Hill.

Roof, W. C., & McKinney, W. (1987). *American mainline religion: Its changing shape and future.* New Brunswick, NJ: Rutgers University Press.

Ross, L. M., & Pollio, H. R. (1991). Metaphors of death: A thematic analysis of personal measures. *Omega, 23,* 291–307.

Rothbard, J. C., & Shaver, P. R. (1994). Continuity of attachment across the life span. In M. B. Sperling & W. H. Berman (Eds.), *Attachment in adults: Clinical and developmental perspectives* (pp. 31–71). New York: Guilford Press.

Rowe, J. W., & Kahn, R. L. (1998). *Successful aging.* New York: Pantheon Books.

Rubin, S. B. (1998). *When doctors say no: The battleground of medical futility.* Bloomington, IN: Indiana University Press.

Rummel, R. J. (1995). Megamurders. In J. B. Williamson, & E. S. Shneidman (Eds.), *Death: Current perspectives* (4th ed., pp. 425–433). Mountain View, CA: Mayfield Publishing.

Ryff, C. D. (1991). Possible selves in adulthood and old age: A tale of shifting horizons. *Psychology and Aging, 6,* 286–295.

Sabom, M. B. (1982). *Recollections of death: A medical investigation.* New York: Harper & Row.

Salovey, P., Rothman, A. J., & Rodin, J. (1998). Health behavior. In D. T. Gilbert, S. T. Fiske, & G. Lindzey (Eds.), *The handbook of social psychology. Vol. II* (4th ed.; pp. 633–683). Boston: McGraw-Hill.

Sankar, A., & Gubrium, J. F. (1994). *Qualitative methods in aging research.* Thousand Oaks, CA: Sage.

Sartre, J. P. (1966). *Being and nothingness: An essay on phenomenological ontology* (H. Barnes, trans.) New York: Citadel Press. (Original work published 1943.)

Schoenfeld, D. E., Malmrose, L. C., Blazer, D. G., Gold, D. T., & Seeman, T. E. (1994). Self-rated health and mortality in the high-functioning elderly—a closer look at healthy individuals. MacArthur field study of successful aging. *Journal of Gerontology: Medical Sciences, 49A,* M109–M115.

Schoeni, R. F., Freedman, V. A., & Wallace, R. B. (2001). Persistent, consistent, widespread, and robust? Another look at recent trends in old age disability. *Journal of Gerontology: Social Sciences, 56B,* S206–S218.

Schonwetter, R. S., Teasdale, T. A., Taffet, G., Robinson, B. E., & Luchi, R. J. (1991). Educating the elderly: Cardiopulmonary resuscitation decisions before and after intervention. *Journal of the American Geriatrics Society, 39,* 372–377.

Schonwetter, R. S., Walker, R. M., Kramer, D. R., & Robinson, B. E. (1994). Socioeconomic status and resuscitation preferences in the elderly. *Journal of Applied Gerontology, 13,* 157–171.

Schonwetter, R. S., Walker, R. M., Solomon, M., Indurkhya, A., & Robinson, B. E. (1996). Life values, resuscitation prefereences, and the applicability of living wills in an older population. *Journal of the American Geriatrics Society, 44,* 954–958.

Schroepfer, T. (1999). Facilitating perceived control in the dying process. In B. de Vries, (Ed.), *End of life issues: Interdisciplinary and multidimensional perspectives* (pp. 57–76). New York: Springer Publishing.

Schulz, R., Martire, L. M., Beach, S. R., & Scheier, M. F. (2000). Depression and mortality in the elderly. *Current Directions in Psychological Science, 9,* 204–208.

Schulz, R., & Schlarb, J. (1987–1988) Two decades of research on dying: What do we know about the patient? *Omega, 18,* 299–317.

Seale, C., Addington-Hall, J., & McCarthy, M. (1997). Awareness of dying: Prevalence, causes and consequences. *Social Science & Medicine, 45,* 477–484.

Seckler, A. B., Meier, D. E., Mulvihill, M., & Paris, B. E. C. (1991). Substituted judgment: How accurate are proxy predictions? *Annals of Internal Medicine, 115,* 90–92.

Seidlitz, L., Duberstein, P. R., Cox, C., & Conwell, Y. (1995). Attitudes of older people toward suicide and assisted suicide: An analysis of Gallup poll findings. *Journal of the American Geriatrics Association, 43,* 993–998.

Shaw, L., & Sichel, H. S. (1971). *Accident proneness: Research on the occurrence, causation, and prevention of road accidents.* New York: Pergamon.

Singer, M. (1999, August). The population surprise. *Atlantic Monthly*, pp. 22–25.

Singer, P. A., Martin, D. K., & Kelner, M. (1999). Quality end-of-life care: Patients' perspectives. *JAMA, 281*, 163–168.

Solomon, S., Greenberg, J., & Pyszczynski, T. (1991a). A terror management theory of social behavior: The psychological functions of self-esteem and cultural worldviews. In M. P. Zanna (Ed.), *Advances in experimental social psychology* (Vol. 24, pp. 93–159). San Diego: Academic Press.

Solomon, S., Greenberg, J., & Pyszczynski, T. (1991b). Terror management theory of self esteem. In C. R. Snyder & R. D. Forsyth (Eds.), *Handbook of social and clinical psycology: The health perspective* (pp. 21–40). New York: Pergamon Press.

Sonnenblick, M., Friedlander, Y., & Steinberg, A. (1993). Dissociation between the wishes of terminally ill parents and decisions by their offspring. *Journal of the American Geriatrics Society, 41*, 599–604.

Speece, M. W., & Brent, S. B. (1996). The development of children's understanding of death. In C. A. Corr & N. B. Corr (Eds.), *Handbook of childhood death and bereavement* (pp. 29–50). New York: Springer Publishing.

Staton, J., Shuy, R., & Byock, R. (2001). *A few months to live: Different paths to life's end.* Washington, DC: Georgetown University Press.

Steinhauser, K. E., Christakis, N. A., Clipp, E. C., McNeilly, M., McIntyre, L., & Tulsky, J. A. (2000). Factors considered important at the end of life by patients, family, physicians, and other care providers. *JAMA, 284*, 2476–2482.

Strauss, A., & Corbin, J. (1990). *Basics of qualitative research: Grounded theory procedures and techniques.* Newbury Park, CA: Sage.

Suicide rate among elderly climbs by 9% over 12 years. (1996, January 12). *The New York Times*, p. A11.

Suzman, R. M., Manton, K. G., & Willis, D. P. (1992). Introducing the oldest old. In R. M. Suzman, D. P. Willis, & K. G. Manton (Eds.), *The oldest old* (pp. 3–14). New York: Oxford University Press.

Tamm, M.E. (1996). Personification of life and death among Swedish health care professionals. *Death Studies, 20*, 1–22.

Templer, D. E. (1972). The construction and validation of a death anxiety scale. *Journal of General Psychology, 82*, 165–167.

Terkel, S. (2001). *Will the circle be unbroken? Reflections on death, rebirth, and hunger for a faith.* New York: The New Press.

Thorson, J. A., & Powell, F. C. (1990). Meanings of death and intrinsic religiosity. *Journal of Clinical Psychology, 46*, 379–391.

Thorson, J. A., & Powell, F. C. (1994). A Revised Death Anxiety Scale. In R. A. Neimeyer (Ed.), *Death anxiety handbook: Research, instrumenta-*

tion, and application (pp. 31–43). Washington, DC: Taylor & Francis.

Thorson, J. A., & Powell, F. C. (2000). Death anxiety in younger and older adults. In A. Tomer (Ed.), *Death attitudes and the older adult: Theories, concepts, and applications* (pp. 123–136). Philadelphia, PA: Taylor & Francis.

Tobin, S. S. (1991). *Personhood in advanced old age: Implications for practice.* New York: Springer Publishing.

Tobin, S. S. (1996). A non-normative old age contrast: Elderly parents caring for offspring with mental retardation. In V. L. Bengtson (Ed.), *Adulthood and aging: Research on continuities and discontinuities* (pp. 124–142). New York: Springer Publishing.

Tomer, A. (1994). Death anxiety in adult life: Theoretical perspectives. In R. A. Neimeyer (Ed.), *Death anxiety handbook: Research, instrumentation, and application* (pp. 3–28). Washington, DC: Taylor & Francis.

Tomer, A. (2000a). Death attitudes and the older adult: Closing thoughts and open questions. In A. Tomer (Ed.), *Death attitudes and the older adult: Theories, concepts, and applications* (pp. 281–288). Philadelphia, PA: Taylor & Francis.

Tomer, A. (2000b). Death-related attitudes: Conceptual distinctions. In A. Tomer (Ed.), *Death attitudes and the older adult: Theories, concepts, and applications* (pp. 87–94). Philadelphia, PA: Taylor & Francis.

Tomer, A., & Eliason, G. (1996). Toward a comprehensive model of death anxiety. *Death Studies, 20,* 343–365.

Tomer, A., & Eliason, G. (2000a). Attitudes about life and death: Toward a comprehensive model of death anxiety. In A. Tomer (Ed.), *Death attitudes and the older adult: Theories, concepts, and applications* (pp. 3–22). Philadelphia, PA: Taylor & Francis.

Tomer, A., & Eliason, G. (2000b). Beliefs about self, life, and death: Testing aspects of a comprehensive model of death anxiety and death attitudes. In A. Tomer (Ed.), *Death attitudes and the older adult: Theories, concepts, and applications* (pp. 137–153). Philadelphia, PA: Taylor & Francis.

Tomer, A., Eliason, G., & Smith, J. (2000). The structure of the Revised Death Anxiety Scale in young and old adults. In A. Tomer (Ed.), *Death attitudes and older adults: Theories, concepts, and applications* (pp. 109–122). Philadelphia: Taylor & Francis.

Tomlinson, R., Howe, K., Notman, M., & Rossmiller, D. (1990). An empirical study of proxy consent for elderly persons. *Gerontologist, 30,* 54–64.

Tsevat, J., Cook, E. F., Green, M. L., Matchar, D. B., Dawson, N. V., Broste, N. K., Wu, A. W., Phillips, R. S., Oye, R. K., & Goldman, L. (1994). Health values of the seriously ill. *Annals of Internal Medicine, 122,* 514–520.

Tsevat, J., Dawson, N. V., Wu, A. W., Lunn, J., Soukup, J. R., Cook, E. F., Vidaillet, H., & Phillips, R. S. (1998). Health values of hospitalized patients 80 years or older. *Journal of the American Medical Association, 279,* 371–375.

Turner, K., Chye, R., Aggarwal, K.G., Philip, J., Skeels, A., & Lickiss, J. N. (1996). Dignity in dying. A preliminary study of patients in the last three days of life. *Journal of Palliative Care, 12,* 7–13.

U. S. attacked (2001, September 12). *New York Times,* pp. A1–A25.

U. S. Bureau of the Census (1991). *Household and family characteristics. March, 1991.* (Publication No. AP-20–458). Washington, DC: U. S. Government Printing Office.

U. S. Bureau of the Census (1994). *Statistical Abstracts of the United States. 1994* (114th ed.). Washington, DC: U. S. Government Printing Office.

U. S. Bureau of the Census (1997). *Statistical Abstracts of the United States. 1997* (117th ed.). Washington, DC: U. S. Government Printing Office.

U. S. Bureau of the Census (1998). *Statistical Abstracts of the United States. 1998* (118th ed.). Washington, DC: U. S. Government Printing Office.

van Doorn, C., Bradley, E. H., Curry, L. A., Fried, T. R., Williams, C. R., Fortinsky, R., Glass, T., & Kasl, S. V. (1999). Social support and social ties in the last year of life. *Gerontologist, 39* (Suppl.), 126.

Verbrugge, L. M. (1989). Gender, aging, and health. In K. S. Markides (Ed.), *Aging and health* (pp. 22–78). Newbury Park, CA: Sage.

Verbrugge, L. M. (1994). Disability in late life. In R. P. Abeles, H. C. Gift, and M. G. Ory (Eds.), *Aging and quality of life* (pp 79–98). New York: Springer Publishing.

Villaverde, M. M., & MacMillan, C. W. (1980). *Ailments of aging: From symptom to treatment.* New York: Van Nostrand Reinhold.

Viney, L. L. (1984). Concerns about death among severely ill people. In F. R. Epting & R. A. Neimeyer (Eds.), *Personal meanings of death* (pp. 143–158). Washington, DC: Hemisphere.

Webster, J. T. (1997). Attachment style and well-being in elderly adults: A preliminary investigation. *Canadian Journal on Aging, 16,* 101–111.

Wenestam, C. G., & Wass, H. (1987). Swedish and U.S. children's thinking about death: A qualitative study and cross-cultural comparison. *Death Studies, 11,* 99–121.

Whitbourne, S. K. (2001). *Adult development and aging: A biopsychosocial perspective.* New York: Wiley & Sons.

White, L. (1998). Who's counting? Quasi-facts and stepfamilies in reports of number of siblings. *Journal of Marriage and the Family, 60,* 725–733.

White, L. (2001). Sibling relationships over the life course: A panel analysis. *Journal of Marriage and the Family, 63,* 555–568.

Williams, C. J. (2001, March 11). Dutch make euthanasia legal. *Lafayette Journal & Courier*, p. 3.

Wolk, R. L., & Wolk, R. B. (1971). *Manual: The Gerontological Apperception Test*. New York: Behavioral Publications.

Wong, P. T. P. (2000). Meaning of life and meaning of death in successful aging. In A. Tomer (Ed.), *Death attitudes and the older adult* (pp. 23–35). Philadelphia: Taylor & Francis.

Wong, P. T. P, Reker, G. T., & Gesser, G. (1994). Death Attitude Profile— Revised: A multidimensional measure of attitudes toward death. In R. A. Neimeyer (Ed.), *Death anxiety handbook: Research, instrumentation, and application* (pp. 121–148). Washington, DC: Taylor and Francis.

Wood, J. V., Taylor, S. E., & Lichtman, R. R. (1985). Social comparison in adjustment to breast cancer. *Journal of Personality and Social Psychology, 49*, 1169–1183.

Young, M., & Daniels, S. (1980). Born again status as a factor in death anxiety. *Psychological Reports, 47*, 367–370.

Zweibel, N. R., & Cassel, C. K. (1989). Treatment choices at the end-of-life: A comparison of decisions by older patients and their physician-selected proxies. *The Gerontologist, 29*, 615–621.

Index